Dietary Fiber Functionality in Food and Nutraceuticals

Functional Foods Science and Technology Series

Functional foods resemble traditional foods but are designed to confer physiological benefits beyond their nutritional function. Sources, ingredients, product development, processing, and international regulatory issues are among the topics addressed in Wiley's Functional Food Science and Technology book series. Coverage extends to the improvement of traditional foods by cultivation, biotechnological, and other means, including novel physical fortification techniques and delivery systems such as nanotechnology. Extraction, isolation, identification, and application of bioactives from food and food processing by-products are among other subjects considered for inclusion in the series.

Series Editor: Professor Fereidoon Shahidi, PhD, Department of Biochemistry, Memorial University of Newfoundland, St. John's, Newfoundland, Canada.

The books under the series are as follows,

Dried Fruits: Phytochemicals and Health Effects
by Cesarettin Alasalvar (Editor), Fereidoon Shahidi

Bio-Nanotechnology: A Revolution in Food, Biomedical and Health Sciences
by Debasis Bagchi (Editor), Manashi Bagchi, Hiroyoshi Moriyama, Fereidoon Shahidi

Cereals and Pulses: Nutraceutical Properties and Health Benefits
by Liangli L. Yu (Editor), Rong Tsao (Editor), Fereidoon Shahidi (Editor)

Functional Food Product Development
by Jim Smith (Editor), Edward Charter (Editor)

Nutrigenomics and Proteomics in Health and Disease: Food Factors and Gene Interactions
by Yoshinori Mine (Editor), Kazuo Miyashita (Editor), Fereidoon Shahidi (Editor)

Dietary Fiber Functionality in Food and Nutraceuticals

From Plant to Gut

*Edited by Farah Hosseinian, B. Dave Oomah
and Rocio Campos-Vega*

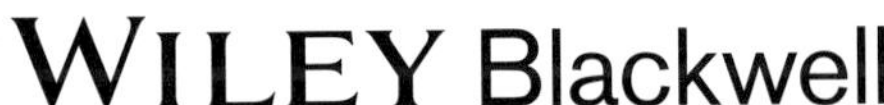

This edition first published 2017 © 2017 by John Wiley & Sons Ltd

Registered office:
John Wiley & Sons Ltd, The Atrium, Southern Gate, Chichester, West Sussex, P019 8SQ, UK

Editorial offices: 9600 Garsington Road, Oxford, OX4 2DQ, UK
The Atrium, Southern Gate, Chichester, West Sussex, P019 8SQ, UK
111 River Street, Hoboken, NJ 07030–5774, USA

For details of our global editorial offices, for customer services and for information about how to apply for permission to reuse the copyright material in this book please see our website at www.wiley.com/wiley-blackwell.

The right of the author to be identified as the author of this work has been asserted in accordance with the UK Copyright, Designs and Patents Act 1988.

Library of Congress Cataloging-in-Publication Data

Names: Hosseinian, Farah, 1960, Oomah, B. Dave, and Campos-Vega, Rocio, editors
Title: Dietary fiber functionality in food & nutraceuticals : from plant to gut / [edited] by Farah Hosseinian.
Other titles: Dietary fiber functionality in food & nutraceuticals | Dietary fibre functionality in food and nutraceuticals | Functional food science and technology series.
Description: Chichester, UK ; Hoboken, NJ : John Wiley & Sons, 2017. | Series: Functional foods science & technology series | Includes bibliographical references and index.
Identifiers: LCCN 2016039780 (print) | LCCN 2016053505 (ebook) | ISBN 9781119138051 (cloth) | ISBN 9781119138075 (pdf) | ISBN 9781119138082 (epub)
Subjects: LCSH: Food–Fiber content–Analysis. | Fiber in human nutrition. | Functional foods.
Classification: LCC TX553.F53 D54 2017 (print) | LCC TX553.F53 (ebook) | DDC 613.2/63–dc23
LC record available at https://lccn.loc.gov/2016039780

A catalogue record for this book is available from the British Library.

Wiley also publishes its books in a variety of electronic formats. Some content that appears in print may not be available in electronic books.

Cover images: Alaettin YILDIRIM/Shutterstock (center);
Science Photo Library/Shutterstock (bottom-right);
SCIEPRO/gettyimages (bottom-left)

Set in 10/12pt WarnockPro by SPi Global, Chennai, India
Printed and bound in Malaysia by Vivar Printing Sdn Bhd
1   2017

Contents

List of Contributors

Maritza Alonzo-Macías
Escuela de Ingeniería y Ciencias
Tecnologico de Monterrey
Querétaro
Mexico

Nawal Alsadi
Faculty of Medicine
University of Ottawa
Ottawa
Ontario
Canada

Rocio Campos-Vega
Programa de Posgrado en Alimentos
del Centro de la República (PROPAC)
Universidad Autónoma de Querétaro
Querétaro
Mexico

Anaberta Cardador-Martínez
Escuela de Ingeniería y Ciencias
Tecnologico de Monterrey
Querétaro
Mexico

Anoma Chandrasekara
Department of Applied Nutrition
Wayamba University of Sri Lanka
Makandura
Gonawila
Sri Lanka

María Teresa Espino-Sevilla
Universidad de Guadalajara
Centro Universitario de la Ciénega
Ocotlán
Mexico

Anthony Fardet
INRA, UMR 1019, UNH, CRNH
Auvergne, Clermont-Ferrand and
Clermont Université
Université d'Auvergne
Unité de Nutrition Humaine
Clermont-Ferrand
France

Antoni Femenia
Department of Chemistry
University of the Balearic Islands
Balearic Islands
Spain

Marcela Gaytan-Martinez
Programa de Posgrado en Alimentos
del Centro de la República (PROPAC)
Research and Graduate Studies in
Food Science, School of Chemistry
Universidad Autónoma de Querétaro
Querétaro
Mexico

Émilie A. Graham
Faculty of Health Sciences
University of Ottawa
Ottawa
Ontario
Canada

Aynur Gunenc
Food Science and Nutrition
Department of Chemistry
Carleton University
Ottawa
Ontario
Canada

Farah Hosseinian
Food Science and Nutrition
Department of Chemistry
Carleton University
Ottawa
Ontario
Canada

Majed Jambi
Faculty of Medicine
University of Ottawa
Ottawa
Ontario
Canada

Guadalupe Loarca-Piña
Programa de Posgrado en Alimentos
del Centro de la República (PROPAC)
Research and Graduate Studies in
Food Science, School of Chemistry
Universidad Autónoma de Querétaro
Querétaro
Mexico

Diego A. Luna-Vital
Programa de Posgrado en Alimentos
del Centro de la República (PROPAC)
Research and Graduate Studies in
Food Science
School of Chemistry
Universidad Autónoma de Querétaro
Querétaro
Mexico

Maria Elena Maldonado
Escuela de Nutrición y Dietética
Universidad de Antioquia
Medellín
Colombia

Jean-François Mallet
Faculty of Medicine
University of Ottawa
Ottawa
Ontario
Canada

Sandra T. Martín del Campo
Escuela de Ingeniería y Ciencias
Tecnologico de Monterrey
Querétaro
Mexico

Chantal Matar
Faculty of Health Sciences and Faculty
of Medicine
University of Ottawa
Ottawa
Ontario
Canada

José Rafael Minjares-Fuentes
Department of Chemistry
University of the Balearic Islands
Balearic Islands
Spain

Luis Mojica
Department of Food Science and
Human Nutrition
University of Illinois at
Urbana-Champaign
Urbana
USA

B. Dave Oomah
Retired
Formerly with Pacific Agri-Food
Research Centre
Agriculture and Agri-Food Canada
Summerland
British Columbia
Canada

Aurea K. Ramírez-Jiménez
Programa de Posgrado en Alimentos
del Centro de la República (PROPAC)
Research and Graduate Studies in
Food Science, School of Chemistry
Universidad Autónoma de Querétaro
Querétaro
Mexico

Fereidoon Shahidi
Department of Biochemistry
Memorial University of
Newfoundland
St. John's
NL
Canada

Luz Amparo Urango
Escuela de Nutrición y Dietética
Universidad de Antioquia
Medellín
Colombia

Haydé A. Vergara-Castañeda
Nucitec
S.A. de C.V.
Querétaro
Mexico

Preface

Dietary fiber is an essential component of most dietary guidelines and regulations although the vast majority of the population consume less than the recommended amount. Individuals with total fiber intake of over 26 g per day have an 18% lower risk of developing diabetes compared to those consuming less than 19 g total fiber per day according to an 11-year diabetes study. Moreover, every daily 10 g increase in overall fiber intake reduces the risk of dying by 15% over the 9 year follow-up period. A high intake of whole grains (210–225 g/day as a fiber source) has also been associated with reduced risk of coronary heart disease, cardiovascular disease, total cancer, and all-cause mortality, as well as mortality from respiratory disease, infectious disease, diabetes, and all non-cardiovascular, non-cancer causes. Regular cereal fiber consumption can reduce the risk of all-cause (19%), heart disease-related (up to 18%), and cancer (15%) mortality. The importance of dietary fiber intake on gut health has been demonstrated in the Belgian Flemish Gut Flora Project (FGFP), where individuals preferring low fiber bread as the major carbohydrate source had reduced microbiome diversity. This is in line with the marketing focus of the function and advantages of dietary fibers in gastrointestinal health benefits, cancer prevention, diabetes risk reduction, cholesterol-lowering effects, and weight management.

It is estimated that the global dietary fiber market volume will reach 465 128.3 metric tons by 2019, with a projected cumulative annual growth rate of 10.4% from 2014 to 2019. Novel fibers are projected to drive this growth, although conventional fibers still dominate the market. Thus, developments and technology of unearthing new fiber sources may boost the demand for dietary fibers, create opportunities for the novel fiber segment, and extend end-use beyond established sectors, particularly for certain segments of the population.

This book presents a large volume of new data. The reader is directed to the table of contents, which illustrates the wide coverage of subjects related to dietary fibers. Knowledge of the physical structure and physicochemical characteristics of dietary fiber on human health (Chapter 1) is essential in providing key restraints/requirements for novel dietary fiber end-use. Phytochemicals often associated with fiber and their interactions (Chapters 2 and 8) may account for the various protective roles of dietary fiber in health. Niche applications are explored (Chapter 3) in the ever-expanding beverage sector with both conventional and novel fiber types. The various fiber fortified foods (Chapter 4) provide a proactive approach towards increasing daily dietary fiber intake in improving human health. The mechanisms of the purported benefits of dietary fibers (Chapters 5, 6, 7, and 8) are explored for specific diseases. Novel fibers (Chapters 5 and 9) may be the launching pad for new types of products that cross over various market segments.

This book should give researchers, nutritionists, health professionals, chemists, and industry professionals interested in dietary fibers useful and up-to-date information to advance the field.

Farah Hosseinian
B. Dave Oomah
Rocio Campos-Vega

1

Do the Physical Structure and Physicochemical Characteristics of Dietary Fibers Influence their Health Effects?

Anthony Fardet

INRA, JRU 1019, UNH, CRNH Auvergne, F-63000 Clermont-Ferrand & Clermont Université, Université d'Auvergne, Unité de Nutrition Humaine, BP 10448, F-63000, Clermont-Ferrand, France

Studies on humans, animals, and *in vitro* have clearly shown that the way dietary fiber is degraded and fermented throughout the digestive tract depends on both its physical and chemical structure (intrinsic properties such as crystallinity and particle size) and its interaction with the closed environment of the gut (i.e., physical–chemical properties such as porosity, water-holding capacity, and solubility) (Guillon and Champ, 2000). For example, cellulose, which has a compact structure, is only partially fermented whereas soluble pectin is fully fermented, due to its much greater porosity (Fardet *et al.*, 1997; Salvador *et al.*, 1993). Thus, a greater porosity enables enzymes to access their substrate and degrade it more efficiently. This illustrates the interaction between factors such as porosity, solubility, and water-holding capacity.

Although much is known about factors influencing the fermentation of dietary fiber, less is known about the influence of a change in fiber structure, either isolated or within a complex food matrix, on human health. For example, is an increase in the porosity of fibers in a food beneficial? What are the consequences of higher fiber porosity on the short-chain fatty acid (SCFA) profiles generated during fermentation in the colon? Increasing porosity probably increases the rate of fermentation within the colon, yielding a more rapid and massive surge of SCFAs. But does the way the SCFAs are released have any effect on human physiology and health? Do the exact location where SCFAs are released (transverse, ascending, or descending colon) influence human health? These questions are of great interest in terms of the important physiological roles of the main SCFAs: butyric (Blouin *et al.*, 2011), propionic (Hosseini *et al.*, 2011), and acetic (Kondo *et al.*, 2009) acids.

Although today we cannot fully answer these questions, this review will attempt to discuss the physicochemical parameters of fiber that can be modified and their relationship with their effects on human physiology and/or health (e.g., glycemia, cholesterolemia, satiety, microbiota, and fecal bulking). In a recent publication, Monro notably reviewed and discussed the impact of polysaccharide-based structures on nutritional properties in the foregut, focusing on complex foods containing such fiber-based structures (Monro, 2014). This review is more

Dietary Fiber Functionality in Food and Nutraceuticals: From Plant to Gut, First Edition.
Edited by Farah Hosseinian, B. Dave Oomah and Rocio Campos-Vega.

focused on isolated fibers and their structural features; some of the best studied being crystallinity, particle size, solubility, porosity, water-holding capacity, and the ability to adsorb bile acids, complex minerals, and trace elements (Guillon and Champ, 2000).

1.1 Influence of the Chemical and Physical Structure on the Metabolic Effects of Fibers

The intrinsic properties of fibers, their chemical and physical structure, are fundamental to their biological actions. The chemical structure of a fiber greatly influences the rate and extent of its fermentation in the colon. Thus, pectins, hemicelluloses, cellulose, lignin, and resistant starch (all included in the definition of fiber) are not all fermented at the same speed and the same extent. Cellulose has a compact structure, whereas hemicellulose is much more porous and more accessible to bacterial enzymes. Hence, hemicelluloses are almost completely degraded in the colon, but cellulose is only partially fermented and is excreted in the feces. Lignins are almost undegraded in humans (Holloway *et al.*, 1978; Slavin *et al.*, 1981).

Interestingly, Eastwood *et al.* (1986) showed that there is no obvious correlation between the chemical composition, structure, molecular size, shape, and physical properties of a fiber and its physiological effects in humans. For example, wheat bran and gum tragacanth have very different chemical structures but they have similar physiological effects. However, these findings are only valid for the physiological properties tested: the weight of stool, serum cholesterol levels, and the excretion of hydrogen. From this study, other physiological parameters have been tested.

It is hardly surprising that the chemical structure of a fiber influences its physiological effects, as each type of fiber is a complex mixture of carbohydrates (including pentoses and hexoses). A review has focused on the relationships between the molecular structure of cereal fibers and their physiological effects in humans (Gemen *et al.*, 2011). There appears to be a clear link between the chemical structure of a fiber and blood glucose and insulin responses and satiety. However, the authors emphasize that information on the molecular structure are rarely given in the literature and there are no obvious trends in the relationship between the molecular structures of fibers and their fermentation profiles in humans (Gemen *et al.*, 2011).

1.1.1 Changing the Molecular Weight

Some of the results appear contradictory. Some studies have shown that reducing the molecular weight of a fiber, and hence its potential viscosity *in vivo*, has no significant effect on the glycemic response (Ellis *et al.*, 1991; Gatenby *et al.*, 1996). These authors concluded that low molecular weight guar gum can be used in bread instead of a high molecular weight guar gum that is more viscous but less palatable (Ellis *et al.*, 1991). Another study showed that reducing the molecular weight of β-glucan in muffins tended to increase the blood glucose and insulin responses in humans (Tosh *et al.*, 2008). Immerstrand *et al.* (2010) showed that β-glucans with different molecular weights all had the same effect on the plasma cholesterol of mice. However, Kim and White (2010) found that low molecular weight β-glucan from oats produced more volatile fatty acids that did the β-glucan with a higher (4.4 times) molecular weight after fermentation for 24 hours *in vitro*.

An exhaustive review of the literature on cereal fiber suggests that the molecular weight of the fiber must be above a certain value to significantly increase the viscosity of the digestive effluents and to have a significant effect on postprandial glycemic and insulinemic responses. The authors even suggest that the thresholds value should be above 100 kDa for β-glucans and above 20 kDa for arabinoxylans. However, although low molecular weight fibers are more rapidly fermented, just how the molecular characteristics of a fiber influence its fermentation profile remains unclear (Gemen *et al.*, 2011). Nevertheless, viscosifying fibers with high molecular weights increase the viscosity of the digesta more than do lower molecular weights fibers that tend to be fermented faster (Gemen *et al.*, 2011). It has been shown that the molecular weights of fungal β-glucans significantly influence the secretion of interleukin-8 (IL-8) by HT29 cells *in vitro*, with lower molecular weight β-glucans producing more secretion than those of high molecular weight (Rieder *et al.*, 2011). Finally, the prebiotic effect of wheat arabinoxylans increases inversely with their molecular weight in the presence of human feces *in vitro* (Hughes *et al.*, 2007).

The fermentation and prebiotic properties of arabinoses from arabinoxylo-oligosaccharides (AXOS) have also been tested with respect to the degree of polymerization and substitution. Low molecular weight AXOS (average MW <3) produced more acetic and butyric acid and also stimulated an increase in the concentrations of bifidobacteria, whereas the fermentation of higher molecular weight (average MW = 61) AXOS resulted in a lack of the branched volatile fatty acids that are considered to be markers of protein fermentation and had no effect on the production of acetic and butyric acids or on bifidobacteria (Van Craeyveld *et al.*, 2008). The authors used an experimental design that varied both the molecular weight and degree of substitution of arabinose in AXOS and concluded that AXOS with an average molecular weight of 5 and a degree of substitution of 0.27 produces the best effects on intestinal health (Van Craeyveld *et al.*, 2008).

1.1.2 Changing the Degree of Crystallinity

Changes in the crystalline structure of a fiber are best illustrated in cellulose, the most abundant fibrous compounds on Earth. Indeed, like starch, cellulose has a crystalline structure, and by modifying it, it is possible to alter its digestibility/fermentation. This was clearly demonstrated in rats fed celluloses having degrees of crystallinity from 6 to 81%. As expected, the more crystalline the cellulose, the less it was fermented (from 9 to 20%) and the lower the fecal water content (Hsu and Penner, 1989). The degree of crystallinity influenced the accessibility of the cellulose to its cellulase enzyme because of the way it altered the porosity of the substrate (Jeoh *et al.*, 2007).

1.1.3 Modifying Particle Size

Intensive grinding of a fiber can influence the speed at which it passes through the gastrointestinal tract, and may promote hydrolysis of its constituent polysaccharides and, ultimately, their hydration and water-holding capacity (Lewis, 1978). Heller *et al.* (1980) showed that coarse wheat bran had a shorter transit time in humans, with more excreted daily in the feces, which had a higher water content, whereas the degradation/digestibility of the cellulose was low. In contrast, the fibrous components of fine bran were more digestible, probably due to its longer retention time in the colon. These results were later confirmed in humans by comparing coarse and fine wheat bran: the authors state that grinding the bran reduced the amount of feces excreted by reducing the water-holding capacity of the fibrous matrix (Wrick *et al.*, 1983). This effect was called the destruction of "the spongy action of fibrous matrix" by van Dokkum *et al.* (1983), who tested bread composed of fine and coarse brans in humans. The integrity of the fibrous matrix therefore appears to significantly influence the weight of the stool (van Dokkum *et al.*, 1983).

However, others found that the size of wheat bran particles (0.5 or 2 mm) had no effect on the morphology or function of rat's intestine (e.g., fat digestion, water content of feces, or cecum length), except that the fiber in the coarser bran was better digested (Kahlon *et al.*, 2001). In another study, the size of wheat bran particles had no effect on the fermentability of fiber in rats (Nyman and Asp, 1985). Similarly, there was no significant difference in the production of volatile fatty acids from coarse and fine wheat bran in the large intestine of pigs (Ehle *et al.*, 1982).

More recently, a Taiwanese team compared increasing intensity of micronization on some physicochemical properties of the fiber-rich fractions extracted from orange peel and cellulose, and showed that the micronized fibers were able to adsorb glucose and reduce the activities of α-amylase and lipase, which could slow down glucose uptake and reduce the serum concentration of glucose (Chau *et al.*, 2006). They tested the reduction of particle size of orange insoluble fiber in hamsters and concluded that micronized fibers would have a positive effect on the health of hamster intestines by decreasing the amount of harmful ammonia produced, increasing the dry weight of stools, and decreasing the activities of β-D-glucuronidase (associated with a lower incidence of colorectal tumors) and mucinase (leading to increased mucins that protect against bacterial invasion) (Wu *et al.*, 2007).

The apparent differences between the results of these studies may be due to differences in the particle sizes tested. Perhaps large differences in particle size (at least 10-fold) are needed to obtain significant differences in physiological effects. Controlling the size of the fiber particles could therefore help improve the health of the digestive tract, particularly the colon. But further studies are needed to confirm these results in humans.

1.2 Influence of the Physicochemical Properties of Fibers on their Metabolic Effects

The physicochemical properties of fibers determine the way they interact with their environment, in this context, the digestive tract, either the small intestine or the colon. But little is known about the long-term influence of changes in the physicochemical properties of fibers on human health. The most studied effect is probably the influence of the viscosity of fibers such as β-glucans and arabinoxylans on the digestion and metabolic fate of other nutrients (glucose or cholesterol). Viscosity is generally modified by changing the molecular weight of the fiber (Chillo *et al.*, 2011; Regand *et al.*, 2011; Wolever *et al.*, 2010). Thus, incorporating soluble, viscous fiber into starchy products significantly reduces their glycemic index (Fardet, 2015). The main actions of the added fiber are to encapsulate the starch (Brennan and Tudorica, 2008), slow the rate at which α-amylase diffuses to its substrate, and/or the movement of glucose to its intestinal absorption site due to increased viscosity and/or delayed transit (Hlebowicz *et al.*, 2008). Some fibers may also slow the rate of gastric emptying (Hlebowicz *et al.*, 2007; Mastropaolo *et al.*, 1986). In a previous recent review I also discussed the implication of pre-hydrolyzing fiber, either soluble or insoluble, on some physiological functions (e.g., cholesterolemia and glycemia) (Fardet, 2015).

1.2.1 Modifying the Degree of Solubility

The solubility of a fiber depends on the conformation of its polysaccharide components (linear or branched) and its crystallinity, and may be affected by grinding, cooking, and other processes (Lewis, 1978). Thus, increasing the proportion of insoluble fiber from wheat bran (0, 200, and 400 g/kg diet) decreases the retention times of both solid and liquid phases in the small intestine and colon of pigs (Wilfart *et al.*, 2007). Increasing the proportion of soluble fiber in the diet increases the viscosity of the digestive effluent, so slowing intestinal transit and the rates of diffusion and absorption of nutrients by the gastrointestinal mucosa.

In general, soluble fibers such as soluble arabinoxylans and β-glucans are rapidly fermented, whereas insoluble fibers such as cellulose and insoluble arabinoxylans are fermented more slowly (Williams *et al.*, 2011). Each type of fiber (e.g., insoluble barley fiber and soluble beet fiber; Fardet *et al.*, 1997) produces a specific profile of volatile fatty acids that may have different metabolic effects. However, the degree of polymerization of a soluble fiber such as the β-glucans or arabinoxylans, and thus their viscosity, does not significantly influence their rate of fermentation or the amounts of butyric, acetic, and propionic acids produced by fermentation (Williams *et al.*, 2011).

1.2.2 Changing the Water-Holding Capacity

There have been very few studies in humans *in vivo* on the influence of changing the water-holding capacity of a fiber on its digestive and fermentative fate. An early study on potato fibers with different water-holding capacities found that the water-holding capacity had no effect on the stool weight, but that the type of fiber, potato or wheat bran, had a significant effect, with wheat bran producing heavier stools (Eastwood *et al.*, 1983). Another study in the same year found that 12 subjects produced significantly heavier stools after consuming a diet that included bread with coarse bran (>0.35 mm) than they did after eating bread containing fine bran. The authors ascribed this observation to the ability of the larger bran particles to retain water and suggested that the "spongy activity of fibrous matrix" is the main factor involved (van Dokkum *et al.*, 1983). A more recent study in rats fed insoluble fibers of tossa jute (*Corchorus capsularis*) and shiitake fungus (*Lentinula edodes*) found that the viscosity of the rat digesta was negatively correlated with its free water content, which was reduced by fibers that held water and swelled (Takahashi *et al.*, 2009). The authors suggested that insoluble fiber may increase the viscosity of the digesta. Similar changes in the colonic digesta of piglets were obtained when they were fed insoluble fiber such as wheat bran (Molist *et al.*, 2009). Such results are important for human nutrition because of the key influence of viscosity on the rate at which nutrients like glucose and cholesterol are absorbed in the intestine and on the physiology of satiety. For example, human subjects fed two liquid meals with identical compositions that differed only in their viscosities, containing oat bran β-glucans with different molecular weights, experienced different degrees of satiety and hormone-related responses (Juvonen *et al.*, 2009).

It is therefore possible to use the water-holding capacity of a fiber, and hence the rheological properties of ingested foods, to control the absorption of nutrients by the human gastrointestinal tract.

1.2.3 Changing Fiber Porosity

Porosity is another important physicochemical parameter of fibers that determines the surface area of a fiber that is accessible to the enzymes responsible for its fermentation (Chesson *et al.*, 1997). Clearly, the greater the porosity, the easier it will be for hydrolytic enzymes to access their substrate and degrade it, as was shown with cellulose under steam explosion (Wong *et al.*, 1988). Thus, digestion in the small intestine can also increase the porosity of a beet fiber matrix by causing a loss of pectin, resulting in faster fermentation *in vitro* (Fardet *et al.*, 1997). Another *in vitro* study found that fermentation was directly correlated with the porosity of beet fiber, indicating that the pore volume accessible to bacteria controlled fermentation (Guillon *et al.*, 1998). How more rapid fiber fermentation influences metabolism and the resulting effects on health remain to be explored.

1.2.4 Adsorption of Bile Acids

Another property of fibers that has been extensively studied is their ability to bind bile acids, and so influence cholesterol metabolism by reducing blood cholesterol. Thus, low molecular weight oat β-glucan binds more bile acids (4.4 times) than do higher molecular weight oat β-glucans (Kim and White, 2010). The ability of various cereal brans (rice, oats, wheat, and maize) to bind bile acids *in vitro* does not appear to be proportional to their soluble fiber content. This suggests that soluble fiber is probably not involved in this property (Kahlon and Chow, 2000). At first glance, these results seem to contradict the finding that viscosifying soluble fiber can reduce plasma cholesterol. However, while soluble fibers bind less bile acid (precursors of cholesterol) than do insoluble fiber *in vitro*, it is possible that the two act in synergy *in vivo*, with insoluble fiber fixing bile acids and viscosifying soluble fiber decreasing the diffusion of ingested cholesterol.

A study tends to confirm these results. Zacherl *et al.* (2011) studied three types of fiber – cellulose, psyllium, and oat fiber – that had been digested to the same degree as when they arrived in the colon and found that the capacity to bind bile acid was mainly, but not solely, correlated with the viscosity of the digested chyme. Heat damage that caused oat fibers to lose their viscosity did not reduce their capacity to bind bile acids, which was higher than that of cellulose. Binding forces other than viscosity (e.g., hydrophobic interactions) are therefore involved. These other binding forces might be responsible for the capacity of insoluble fiber to bind bile acids, as discussed above.

There is therefore good evidence that the hypocholesterolemic capacity of a fiber can be modified by altering its structure.

1.2.5 The Ability to Complex Minerals and to Increase their Extent of Absorption

The properties of fibers are seemingly paradoxical vis-à-vis mineral absorption: they can both form complexes with them (Bergman *et al.*, 1997; Lopez *et al.*, 2002) and promote their absorption by the intestine. The fermented fibers increase the area for their absorption by causing hypertrophy of colon cells and increasing length of the small intestine (Faraldo Correa *et al.*, 2009; Lopez *et al.*, 2000, 2001a), or by promoting the hydrolysis of phytic acid via increased fermentation and stimulating bacterial enzymes (Lopez *et al.*, 2001b; Callegaro *et al.*, 2010). Phytic acid is well known for its ability to complex minerals (Lopez *et al.*, 2002).

The cation-exchange capacity of fiber is due to the presence of negative charges at their surface. These affect the viscosity of the digesta, but the exact mechanisms involved are still not known (Takahashi *et al.*, 2009).

Again, it is possible to manipulate the quality of dietary fiber to promote mineral absorption to a greater or lesser degree. However, the ability of some fibers to increase mineral absorption in humans remains to be demonstrated.

1.2.6 Fiber Structure and Hindgut Health

Monro and colleagues have extensively studied the influence of fiber structure on hindgut functions (Monro, 2014). They report that beyond providing essential fermentable substrates for bacteria, from a physical viewpoint, polysaccharide-based structures that survive fermentation also make a major contribution to fermentation and large bowel function. They act as supports on which societies ("consortia") of bacteria proliferate as biofilms, in which metabolic interactions between species of bacteria determine the metabolic products, such as the type of short-chain fatty acid produced from fermentable substrates (Macfarlane and Dillon, 2007).

One of the most important effects of fiber within hindgut is notably its fecal bulking effect. In fact, "persistent plant structure in the form of robust cells occupies volume and provides water-bearing cavities" (Monro and Mishra, 2010), leading to removal of stagnant fecal water, reducing the chemical activity of toxins, promoting fecal softening, and distributing pressure (Monro, 2014). In other words, (insoluble) fiber with remaining unfermented structure keeps its ability to hold water, participating in very important health effects such as those described by Monro (i.e., potentially being able to protect from constipation, hemorrhoids, diverticular disease, colitis, and colorectal cancer) (Monro, 2014; Rose *et al.*, 2007). In contrast, fermentable fiber has other health benefits within hindgut more in association with fecal microbiota and production of SCFAs. These different behaviors of fiber, depending on their fermentability, illustrate well the dual characteristics of fiber (i.e., insoluble (that I call *lente* fiber)) and soluble (that I call *rapid* fiber) fibers with different health effects.

Interestingly, Monro and colleagues further developed a fecal bulking index in relation to fiber, and expressed in wheat bran equivalents (Monro, 2001). Briefly, "wheat bran equivalents for fecal bulking are defined as the gram quantity of wheat bran that would augment fecal bulk to the same extent as a given quantity of a specified food" (Monro, 2001).

Finally, minimally processed fibers such as those of swede, broccoli head, broccoli rind, and asparagus exhibited a much higher fecal bulking effect (around 2- to 4-fold) than highly processed or unstructured fibers that are generally either added as isolated ingredients in foods or come from ultraprocessed foods (Monro, 2014). These data showed that processed fiber partially lost their ability to hold water via alteration of their original complex physical structure.

Consequent to the fecal bulking effect, there is also a relation between fiber physicochemical properties and transit time. Thus, Cherbut *et al.* (1991) showed that the water-binding capacity of fibers from wheat bran, sugarbeet, maize, pea hulls, and roasted cocoa might affect the orofecal transit time in healthy volunteers. Fibers were found to act through a mechanical effect if they were not fermented, and the partly degradable fibers also changed the transit time via their products of fermentation (i.e., a large production of propionic and butyric acids).

1.3   The Effect of Fiber Structure on Fermentation Patterns and Microbiota Profiles: Slowly versus Rapidly Fermented Fiber

In vitro data from the literature clearly show that fibers impact SCFA fermentation patterns and microbiota profiles differently, depending on their type or origin and their structure. In addition, dietary fiber fermentation profiles are important in determining optimal fibers for colonic health, and may be a function of structure, processing conditions, and other food components. A greater understanding of the relationships between fermentation rate and dietary fiber structure would allow for development of dietary fibers for optimum colonic health. (Rose *et al.*, 2007)

1.3.1 Fiber Structure and Fermentation Patterns

In their review Rose *et al.* (2007) examined parameters of the fiber chemical and physical structure that may play a role on their fermentation rate and patterns. Briefly, they cited numerous studies emphasizing the importance of arabinoxylan cross-linking (through oxidative dimerization of ferulic acid moieties that are esterified to the arabinoxylan polymer), pectin degree of methylation or polymerization, fiber glycosidic linkages and molecular packing, native versus isolated fiber, resistant starch type, and particle size on fermentation patterns (Rose *et al.*, 2007). However, they underlined that the physical inaccessibility of colon renders such analyses difficult.

In a recent study, Rumpagaporn *et al.* (2015) tried to elucidate the structural properties of cereal arabinoxylans that drive the rate of fermentation. They used predigested residues of arabinoxylan isolates from corn, wheat, rice, and sorghum brans, and showed, using *in vitro* human fecal bacteria, that there was no relationship between molecular mass, arabinose/xylose ratio, or degree of substitution to fermentation rate patterns. However, interestingly, slow fermenting wheat and corn arabinoxylans had much higher amount of terminal xylose in branches than fast fermenting rice and sorghum arabinoxylans. The slowest fermenting wheat arabinoxylan additionally contained a complex trisaccharide side chain with two arabinoses linked at the O-2 and O-3 positions of an arabinose that is O-2 linked to the xylan backbone. (Rumpagaporn *et al.*, 2015)

They concluded that the major structural factor that related to slow fermentation was the type of linkage of the branch constituents, and large amounts of branches with single xylose units. Simpler structures were associated with a rapid initial rate of fermentation that was comparable to that of the fast fermenting fructo-oligosaccharides.

Similarly, with cereal arabinoxylans, Karppinen (2003) divided fiber polysaccharides of rye bran into three groups: (1) fermentable, soluble polysaccharides that are rapidly fermented, (2) fermentable cell wall-associated polysaccharides that are gradually released from the cell wall matrix and then fermented, and (3) polysaccharides and cell wall structures that are not fermented at all. However, in the study by Van Nevel *et al.* (2006) fiber water-holding capacity was surprisingly not correlated with fermentability within contents of pig cecum: it was highest for chicory roots, followed by wheat bran and sugar beet pulp; water-holding capacity was very high for sugar beet pulp (10.05 g H_2O/g dry matter), whereas the lowest value was obtained with wheat bran (3.00 g H_2O/g dry matter) (Van Nevel *et al.*, 2006). Similar results were obtained with oat hull fiber, gum arabic, carboxymethylcellulose, soy fiber, and psyllium (Bourquin *et al.*, 1993a), and also with fibers from broccoli, carrot, cauliflower, celery, cucumber, lettuce, onion, and radish (Bourquin *et al.*, 1993b) for which their water-holding capacity – an indirect measure of fecal bulking potential – was not correlated with SCFA production and organic matter disappearance.

The results of these studies seems to show that water solubility is not a major, or at least not the only, determinant of fermentability and that structural characteristics at the molecular level of fiber would be particularly involved. Other physicochemical features have been shown to be involved in fiber fermentability such as gross porosity, microporosity, particle size, or crystallinity (Guillon *et al.*, 1998). Two sources of sugar beet fibers were submitted to various chemical and then dehydration treatments, resulting mainly in the removal of pectic polysaccharides (9–49% recovery) at the expense of cellulose (80–100% recovery). Following chemical extraction, harsh drying induced a noticeable decrease in the total pore volume (from 14.9 to 6.1 mL/g) and especially in the pore volume accessible to bacteria (from 10.4 to 3.2 mL/g). Drying following chemical extraction did not affect the crystallinity of cellulose in the fiber. Main results showed that neither the particle size, nor the crystallinity of cellulose were major determinant factors in degradability of sugar beet fibers, but that pore volume accessible to bacteria in sugar beet fibers was highly correlated ($r = 0.88$) with its fermentability. Authors concluded that such results "illustrate the importance of matrix physical structure (especially porosity) in the control of the physicochemical behavior of fiber." This conclusion was also supported by the results of the study by Mortensen and Nordgaardandersen (1993), showing with cellulose and dietary fiber in common clinical use that the amounts of soluble nonstarch polysaccharides in the fiber were closely associated with the mean productions of SCFAs after *in vitro* incubation with human fecal homogenates, but also that the mean production of ammonia was inversely related to the soluble fraction of the fiber. The authors concluded that their "findings support that the water solubility determines the degree of fermentability of dietary fiber and thereby the corresponding bacterial assimilation of ammonia."

However, most studies do not go as far as recording the physicochemical properties of fibers with fermentation profiles in the analysis, and they only describe SCFA production patterns according to fiber type. For example, in batch cultures of pig intestinal digesta, while β-glucan-grown cultures yielded the highest level of lactate, flaxseed or fenugreek gum-containing cultures generated a significant amount of acetate, propionate, and butyrate (Lin *et al.*, 2011). In another study, 20 soluble fibers (alginate, apple pectin, arabinogalactan, carrageenan, carboxymethylcellulose, citrus pectin, gellan gum, guar gum, gum arabic, gum ghatti, gum karaya, hydrolyzed guar gum, konjac flour, locust bean gum, methylcellulose, oat β-glucan, psyllium, tomato pectin, tragacanth gum, and xanthan gum) were tested *in vitro* for their fermentation profile using three human fecal inocula (Hussein *et al.*,2008). Although all are soluble, and therefore supposed to be quite highly fermentable, significant differences were observed after 24 hours for dry matter disappearance (between 20% and more than 91%) and gas production, with some fiber having no gas produced. In the same vein, Lu *et al.* (2000) examined the effects of an arabinoxylan-rich fiber extracted from a byproduct of wheat flour processing in the rat colon compared with well-characterized soluble/rapidly fermentable (i.e., guar gum) and insoluble/slowly fermentable (i.e., wheat bran) fibers. The SCFA pool was particularly high with arabinoxylan and guar gum fibers. Otherwise, arabinoxylans fiber was a good source for acetate, whereas guar gum and wheat bran favored propionate and butyrate production, respectively. Finally, fecal output was 7-, 6-, and 5-fold higher, respectively, in the arabinoxylan, guar gum, and wheat bran groups of rats than in the nonfiber groups ($p < 0.01$). Authors concluded that these results suggested that arabinoxylan fiber behaves like a rapidly fermentable, soluble fiber in the rat colon.

In another study, Monsma *et al.* (2000) used ileal digesta collected from swine fed oat or wheat bran fermented for $0-96$ hours in an anaerobic *in vitro* system using inocula prepared from ceca of rats fed the same fiber sources. As in the studies described above, the authors distinguished between slow and rapid fiber. Fermentation of wheat bran digesta was significantly slower than fermentation of oat bran digesta, and oat bran digesta fermentation produced a significantly greater molar proportion of SCFAs as propionate, these latter being produced during fermentation of β-glucan. With regard to particle size, in rats coarse wheat bran gave significantly higher fecal butyrate concentrations than rice brans and fine wheat bran (Folino *et al.*, 1995).

More generally, Salvador *et al.* (1993) assessed the relationship between the disappearance of dietary fiber sugars and the production of individual SCFAs by studying *in vitro* using a human fecal inoculum the bacterial degradation of five dietary fibers whose sugars were quantified. Their results confirm that the nature and associations between the fiber sugars were key variables in the fermentability, and that the nature and the amounts of SCFAs produced were closely related to the *in vitro* fermentation of the main sugars available. Thus, as they concluded: uronic acids seemed to be principally involved in the production of acetic acid whereas the production of propionic acid could be promoted by the fermentation of glucose and, to a lesser extent, by that of xylose and arabinose. Xylose tend to have a greater impact than uronic acids and glucose on the production of butyric acid.

Such results, together with those mentioned previously, suggest that one should be able to predict which SCFA would be specifically produced if the chemical composition and structure of the fiber are known (Salvador *et al.*, 1993).

1.3.2 Fiber Structure and Fecal Microbiota Profiles

Some studies showed that fibers differing in their structure may impact differently on the bacterial community structure. For example, oat β-glucan, flaxseed gum, and fenugreek gum significantly influenced bacterial community structure in batch cultures by pig intestinal digesta (Lin *et al.*, 2011). Significant differences in bacterial species were also observed with fiber from chicory roots, sugar beet pulp, wheat bran, and corn cobs incubated with contents of pig cecum (Van Nevel *et al.*, 2006). In addition, bacterial mass increased and was maintained longer during fermentation of oat bran digesta than the wheat bran digesta in an anaerobic *in vitro* system using inocula prepared from ceca of rats (Monsma *et al.*, 2000).

1.4 Conclusions

The results presented here clearly show that the intrinsic and physicochemical properties of fibers determine the rates at which they are fermented and their consequent health impacts (see brief summary in Figure 1.1). It is therefore no exaggeration to say that, there are *slow* and *rapid* (fermented) fibers, just as there are *slowly* and *rapidly* digested carbohydrates (Englyst *et al.*, 2003), fats (Keogh *et al.*, 2011), and proteins (Boirie *et al.*, 1997). What we do not know is how the kinetics of absorption of volatile fatty acids thus modified in the colon impacts the physiology and modifies the health effects over the long term. Nevertheless, the structure of a fiber can be modified to improve colon health, especially by altering the speed of fermentation, the site of fermentation and then butyrate production, which helps protect against carcinomas and colonic inflammation (Rose *et al.*, 2007). However, although many studies have compared the fermentative

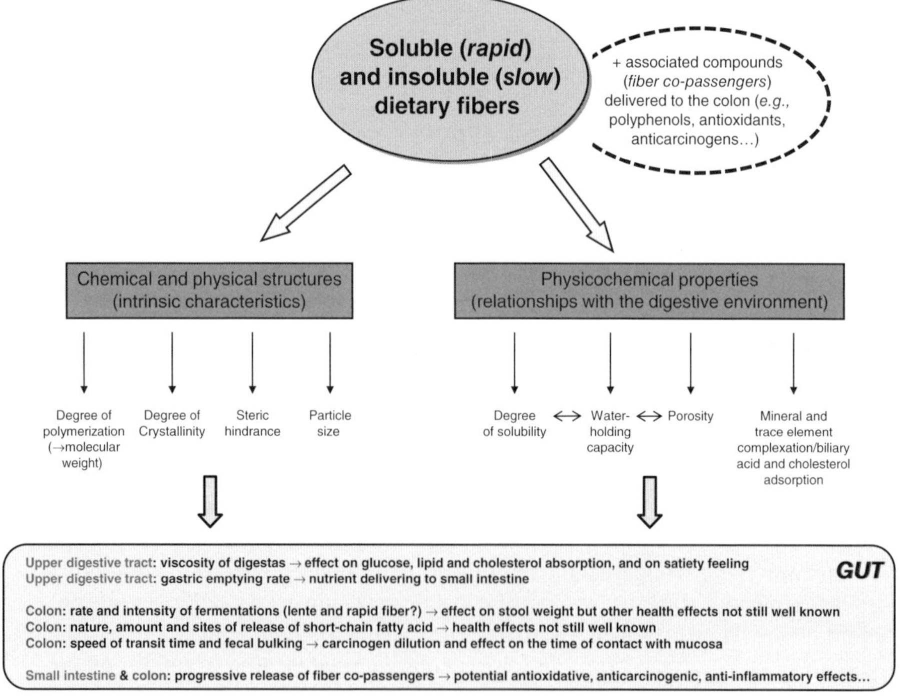

Figure 1.1 Chemical, physical and physicochemical properties of dietary fiber, their digestive fate and potential health effects via the gut.

fate of different types of fibers, few have investigated the relationship between changes in physicochemical parameters of a single given fiber type (i.e., of equal chemical composition) and its implications for human physiology and health. Nevertheless, the development of the fecal bulking index is a promising step in this direction.

It is also worth emphasizing that fibers may act as vectors, delivering compounds associated with their structure in the gastrointestinal tract, notably at colonic level as shown *in vitro*; fruit and vegetable fibers release significantly more polyphenols than cereal fibers, for example (Tabernero *et al.*, 2011). Thus, most of the antioxidants in the colon, such as cereal phenolic acids, are bound to them (Vitaglione and Fogliano, 2010; Vitaglione *et al.*, 2008). Indeed, Vitaglione *et al.* (2008) suggest that fiber-bound antioxidants released at intestinal level by esterases and in the colon by microbiota – as natural free forms of polyphenols – are absorbed into the bloodstream, metabolized in the liver, and then, in conjugated form, exercise antioxidant power vis-à-vis oxidized LDL (low-density lipoproteins), and help to prevent cardiovascular disease. The authors point out that "It is generally accepted that a higher ratio of soluble fiber/insoluble in cereal products means a higher bioavailability of dietary fiber phenolic compounds complex" (Vitaglione and Fogliano, 2010). In addition to delivering antioxidants in the digestive tract, the fibers are also considered a free radical sponge ("A sponge for radicals"), free radicals participating in an increased oxidative stress that is damaging to numerous body metabolic functions (Vitaglione and Fogliano, 2010). Thus, the concept of "dietary fiber's co-passengers" – they may exceed 200 000 – is now increasingly emphasized (Jones, 2010).

Therefore, beyond its mere chemical composition, dietary fiber may indirectly affect health through physical characteristics, the physicochemical structure of its matrix, and its ability to carry other compounds (e.g., as vectors of antioxidants), and to release them more or less quickly depending on their digestive and fermentative fate. Another research field of interest is undoubtedly the ability of fermentable fiber, notably as a result of changing their physicochemical properties, to modify gut microbiota and to further impact human health. Little is known about such an issue. Today, there is still a notable lack of studies in humans, probably because the intestine is difficult to access and still remain a "black box."

References

Bergman CJ, Gualberto DG, Weber CW (1997) Mineral binding capacity of dephytinized insoluble fiber from extruded wheat, oat and rice brans. *Plant Foods Hum Nutr* 51(4):295–310.

Blouin JM, Penot G, Collinet M, Nacfer M, Forest C, Laurent-Puig P, Coumoul X, Barouki R, Benelli C, Bortoli S (2011) Butyrate elicits a metabolic switch in human colon cancer cells by targeting the pyruvate dehydrogenase complex. *Int J Cancer* 128(11):2591–601.

Boirie Y, Dangin M, Gachon P, Vasson MP, Maubois JL, Beaufrere B (1997) Slow and fast dietary proteins differently modulate postprandial protein accretion. *Proc Natl Acad Sci USA* 94(26):14930–5.

Bourquin LD, Titgemeyer EC, Fahey GC, Garleb KA (1993a) Fermentation of dietary fiber by human colonic bacteria – Disappearance of, short-chain fatty-acid production from, and potential water-holding capacity of, various substrates. *Scand J Gastroenterol* 28(3):249–55.

Bourquin LD, Titgemeyer EC, Fahey GC (1993b) Vegetable fiber fermentation by human fecal bacteria – Cell-wall polysaccharide disappearance and short-chain fatty-acid production during invitro fermentation and water-holding capacity of unfermented residues. *J Nutr* 123(5):860–9.

Brennan CS, Tudorica CM (2008) Evaluation of potential mechanisms by which dietary fibre additions reduce the predicted glycaemic index of fresh pastas. *Int J Food Sci Technol* 43(12):2151–62.

Callegaro MGK, Diettrich T, Alves E, Milbradt BG, Denardin CC, Silva LP, Emanuelli T (2010) Supplementation with fiber-rich multimixtures yields a higher dietary concentration and apparent absorption of minerals in rats. *Nutr Res* 30(9):615–25.

Chau C-F, Wen Y-L, Wang Y-T (2006) Effects of micronisation on the characteristics and physicochemical properties of insoluble fibres. *J Sci Food Agric* 86(14):2380–6.

Cherbut C, Salvador V, Barry JL, Doulay F, Delort-Laval J (1991) Dietary fibre effects on intestinal transit in man: involvement of their physicochemical and fermentative properties. *Food Hydrocolloids* 5(1–2):15–22.

Chesson A, Gardner PT, Wood TJ (1997) Cell wall porosity and available surface area of wheat straw and wheat grain fractions. *J Sci Food Agric* 75(3):289–95.

Chillo S, Ranawana DV, Henry CJK (2011) Effect of two barley β-glucan concentrates on in vitro glycaemic impact and cooking quality of spaghetti. *LWT-Food Sci Technol* 44(4):940–8.

Eastwood MA, Robertson JA, Brydon WG, MacDonald D (1983) Measurement of water-holding properties of fibre and their faecal bulking ability in man. *Br J Nutr* 50(3):539–47.

Eastwood MA, Brydon WG, Anderson DM (1986) The effect of the polysaccharide composition and structure of dietary fibers on cecal fermentation and fecal excretion. *Am J Clin Nutr* 44(1):51–5.

Ehle FR, Jeraci JL, Robertson JB, Van Soest PJ (1982) The influence of dietary fiber on digestibility, rate of passage and gastrointestinal fermentation in pigs. *J Anim Sci* 55(5):1071–81.

Ellis PR, Dawoud FM, Morris ER (1991) Blood glucose, plasma insulin and sensory responses to guar-containing wheat breads: effects of molecular weight and particle size of guar gum. *Br J Nutr* 66(3):363–79.

Englyst KN, Vinoy S, Englyst HN, Lang V (2003) Glycaemic index of cereal products explained by their content of rapidly and slowly available glucose. *Br J Nutr* 89(3):329–40.

Faraldo Correa TA, Pissini Machado Reis SM, Costa de Oliveira A (2009) Increase in digestive organs of rats due to the ingestion of dietary fiber with similar solubility to that of common bean. *Arch Latin Nutr* 59(1):47–53.

Fardet A (2015) A shift toward a new holistic paradigm will help to preserve and better process grain product food structure for improving their health effects. *Food Funct* 6(2):363–82.

Fardet A, Guillon F, Hoebler C, Barry JL (1997) In vitro fermentation of beet fibre and barley bran, of their insoluble residues after digestion and of ileal effluents. *J Sci Food Agric* 75(3):315–25.

Folino M, McIntyre A, Young G (1995) Dietary fibers differ in their effects on large bowel epithelial proliferation and fecal fermentation-dependent events in rats. *J Nutr* 125:1521–8.

Gatenby SJ, Ellis PR, Morgan LM, Judd PA (1996) Effect of partially depolymerized guar gum on acute metabolic variables in patients with non-insulin-dependent diabetes. *Diabet Med* 13(4):358–64.

Gemen R, de Vries JF, Slavin J (2011) Relationship between molecular structure of cereal dietary fiber and health effects: focus on glucose/insulin response and gut health. *Nutr Rev* 69:22–33.

Guillon F, Champ M (2000) Structural and physical properties of dietary fibres, and consequences of processing on human physiology. *Food Res Int* 33(3–4):233–45.

Guillon F, Auffret A, Robertson JA, Thibault JF, Barry JL (1998) Relationships between physical characteristics of sugar-beet fibre and its fermentability by human faecal flora. *Carbohydr Polym* 37(2):185–97.

Heller S, Hackler L, Rivers J, Van Soest P, Roe D, Lewis B, Robertson J (1980) Dietary fiber: the effect of particle size of wheat bran on colonic function in young adult men. *Am J Clin Nutr* 33(8):1734–44.

Hlebowicz J, Wickenberg J, Fahlstrom R, Bjorgell O, Almer LO, Darwiche G (2007) Effect of commercial breakfast fibre cereals compared with corn flakes on postprandial blood glucose, gastric emptying and satiety in healthy subjects: a randomized blinded crossover trial. *Nutr J* 6:22.

Hlebowicz J, Darwiche G, Bjorgell O, Almer L-O (2008) Effect of muesli with 4 g oat β-glucan on postprandial blood glucose, gastric emptying and satiety in healthy subjects: A randomized crossover trial. *J Am Coll Nutr* 27(4):470–5.

Holloway WD, Tasman-Jones C, Lee SP (1978) Digestion of certain fractions of dietary fiber in humans. *Am J Clin Nutr* 31(6):927–30.

Hosseini E, Grootaert C, Verstraete W, Van de Wiele T (2011) Propionate as a health-promoting microbial metabolite in the human gut. *Nutr Rev* 69(5):245–58.

Hsu JC, Penner MH (1989) Influence of cellulose structure on its digestibility in the rat. *J Nutr* 119(6):872–8.

Hughes SA, Shewry PR, Li L, Gibson GR, Sanz ML, Rastall RA (2007) In vitro fermentation by human fecal microflora of wheat arabinoxylans. *J Agric Food Chem* 55(11):4589–95.

Hussein HS, Yobi A, Sakuma T, Bollinger LM, Wolf BW, Garleb KA (2008) In vitro fermentation characteristics of native soluble fiber sources by human colonic bacteria. *FASEB J* 22.

Immerstrand T, Andersson KE, Wange C, Rascon A, Hellstrand P, Nyman M, Cui SW, Bergenstahl B, Tragardh C, Oste R (2010) Effects of oat bran, processed to different molecular weights of beta-glucan, on plasma lipids and caecal formation of SCFA in mice. *Br J Nutr* 104(3):364–73.

Jeoh T, Ishizawa CI, Davis MF, Himmel ME, Adney WS, Johnson DK (2007) Cellulase digestibility of pretreated biomass is limited by cellulose accessibility. *Biotechnol Bioeng* 98(1):112–22.

Jones JM (2010) Dietary fibre's co-passengers: is it the fibre or the co-passengers? In *Dietary Fibre: New Frontiers for Food and Health* (eds. JW Van Der Kamp, JM Jones, BV McCleary, DL Topping). Wageningen Academic Publisher, Wageningen.

Juvonen KR, Purhonen AK, Salmenkallio-Marttila M, Lahteenmaki L, Laaksonen DE, Herzig KH, Uusitupa MIJ, Poutanen KS, Karhunen LJ (2009) Viscosity of oat bran-enriched beverages influences gastrointestinal hormonal responses in healthy humans. *J Nutr* 139(3):461–6.

Kahlon TS, Chow FI (2000) In vitro binding of bile acids by rice bran, oat bran, wheat bran, and corn bran. *Cereal Chem* 77(4):518–21.

Kahlon TS, Chow FI, Hoefer JL, Betschart AA (2001) Effect of wheat bran fiber and bran particle size on fat and fiber digestibility and gastrointestinal tract measurements in the rat. *Cereal Chem* 78(4):481–4.

Karppinen S (2003) *Dietary fibre components of rye bran and their fermentation in vitro.* VTT Publications, Finland, 96 pp. www.vtt.fi/inf/pdf/publications/2003/P500.pdf

Keogh JB, Wooster TJ, Golding M, Day L, Otto B, Clifton PM (2011) Slowly and rapidly digested fat emulsions are equally satiating but their triglycerides are differentially absorbed and metabolized in humans. *J Nutr* 141(5):809–15.

Kim HJ, White PJ (2010) In vitro bile-acid binding and fermentation of high, medium, and low molecular weight β-glucan. *J Agric Food Chem* 58(1):628–34.

Kondo T, Kishi M, Fushimi T, Kaga T (2009) Acetic acid upregulates the expression of genes for fatty acid oxidation enzymes in liver to suppress body fat accumulation. *J Agric Food Chem* 57(13):5982–6.

Lewis BA (1978) Physical and biological properties of structural and other nondigestible carbohydrates. *Am J Clin Nutr* 31(10):S82–S5.

Lin B, Gong J, Wang Q, Cui S, Yu H, Huang B (2011) In-vitro assessment of the effects of dietary fibers on microbial fermentation and communities from large intestinal digesta of pigs. *Food Hydrocolloids* 25(2):180–8.

Lopez HW, Coudray C, Bellanger J, Levrat-Verny MA, Demigne C, Rayssiguier Y, Remesy C (2000) Resistant starch improves mineral assimilation in rats adapted to a wheat bran diet. *Nutr Res* 20(1):141–55.

Lopez HW, Levrat-Verny MA, Coudray C, Besson C, Krespine V, Messager A, Demigne C, Remesy C (2001a) Class 2 resistant starches lower plasma and liver lipids and improve mineral retention in rats. *J Nutr* 131(4):1283–9.

Lopez HW, Krespine V, Guy C, Messager A, Demigne C, Remesy C (2001b) Prolonged fermentation of whole wheat sourdough reduces phytate level and increases soluble magnesium. *J Agric Food Chem* 49(5):2657–62.

Lopez HW, Leenhardt F, Coudray C, Remesy C (2002) Minerals and phytic acid interactions: is it a real problem for human nutrition? *Int J Food Sci Technol* 37(7):727–39.

Lu ZX, Gibson PR, Muir JG, Fielding M, O'Dea K (2000) Arabinoxylan fiber from a by-product of wheat flour processing behaves physiologically like a soluble, fermentable fiber in the large bowel of rats. *J Nutr* 130(8):1984–90.

Macfarlane S, Dillon JF (2007) Microbial biofilms in the human gastrointestinal tract. *J Appl Microbiol* 102(5):1187–96.

Mastropaolo G, Dimario F, Aggio L, Corradini G, Naccarato R (1986) Effects of dietary fiber on gastric-emptying and small-bowel transit. *Dig Dis Sci* 31(10):S73.

Molist F, Gomez de Segura A, Gasa J, Hermes RG, Manzanilla EG, Anguita M, Perez JF (2009) Effects of the insoluble and soluble dietary fibre on the physicochemical properties of digesta and the microbial activity in early weaned piglets. *Anim Feed Sci Technol* 149(3–4):346–53.

Monro JA (2001) Wheat bran equivalents based on faecal bulking indices for dietary management of faecal bulk. *Asia Pac J Clin Nutr* 10(3):242–8.

Monro JA (2014) Polysaccharide-based structures in food plants: gut and health effects. In *Polysaccharides – Natural Fibers in Food and Nutrition* (ed. N. Benkeblia). CRC Press, Boca Raton, FL, pp. 347–66.

Monro J, Mishra S (2010) Digestion-resistant remnants of vegetable vascular and parenchyma tissues differ in their effects in the large bowel of rats. In *Food Digestion*. Springer, New York, pp. 47–56.

Monsma DJ, Thorsen PT, Vollendorf NW, Crenshaw TD, Marlett JA (2000) In vitro fermentation of swine ileal digesta containing oat bran dietary fiber by rat cecal inocula adapted to the test fiber increases propionate production but fermentation of wheat bran ileal digesta does not produce more butyrate. *J Nutr* 130(3):585–93.

Mortensen PB, Nordgaardandersen I (1993) The dependence of the invitro fermentation of dietary fiber to short-chain fatty-acids on the contents of soluble nonstarch polysaccharides. *Scand J Gastroenterol* 28(5):418–22.

Nyman M, Asp N-G (1985) Dietary fibre fermentation in the rat intestinal tract: effect of adaptation period, protein and fibre levels, and particle size. *Br J Nutr* 54(03):635–43.

Regand A, Chowdhury Z, Tosh SM, Wolever TMS, Wood P (2011) The molecular weight, solubility and viscosity of oat beta-glucan affect human glycemic response by modifying starch digestibility. *Food Chem* 129(2):297–304.

Rieder A, Grimmer S, Kolset SO, Michaelsen TE, Knutsen SH (2011) Cereal beta-glucan preparations of different weight average molecular weights induce variable cytokine secretion in human intestinal epithelial cell lines. *Food Chem* 128(4):1037–43.

Rose DJ, Demeo MT, Keshavarzian A, Hamaker BR (2007) Influence of dietary fiber on inflammatory bowel disease and colon cancer: Importance of fermentation pattern. *Nutr Rev* 65(2):51–62.

Rumpagaporn P, Reuhs BL, Kaur A, Patterson JA, Keshavarzian A, Hamaker BR (2015) Structural features of soluble cereal arabinoxylan fibers associated with a slow rate of in vitro fermentation by human fecal microbiota. *Carbohydr Polym* 130:191–7.

Salvador V, Cherbut C, Barry J-L, Bertrand D, Bonnet C, Delort-Laval J (1993) Sugar composition of dietary fibre and short-chain fatty acid production during in vitro fermentation by human bacteria. *Br J Nutr* 70(1):189–97.

Slavin JL, Brauer PM, Marlett JA (1981) Neutral detergent fiber, hemicellulose and cellulose digestibility in human subjects. *J Nutr* 111(2):287–97.

Tabernero M, Venema K, Maathuis AJH, Saura-Calixto FD (2011) Metabolite production during in vitro colonic fermentation of dietary fiber: analysis and comparison of two European diets. *J Agric Food Chem* 59(16):8968–75.

Takahashi T, Furuichi Y, Mizuno T, Kato M, Tabara A, Kawada Y, Hirano Y, Kubo K-y, Onozuka M, Kurita O (2009) Water-holding capacity of insoluble fibre decreases free water and elevates digesta viscosity in the rat. *J Sci Food Agric* 89(2):245–50.

Tosh SM, Brummer Y, Wolever TMS, Wood PJ (2008) Glycemic response to oat bran muffins treated to vary molecular weight of β-glucan. *Cereal Chem* 85(2):211 LP-7.

Van Craeyveld V, Swennen K, Dornez E, Van de Wiele T, Marzorati M, Verstraete W, Delaedt Y, Onagbesan O, Decuypere E, Buyse J, *et al.* (2008) Structurally different wheat-derived arabinoxylooligosaccharides have different prebiotic and fermentation properties in rats. *J Nutr* 138(12):2348–55.

Van Dokkum W, Pikaar NA, Thissen JT (1983) Physiological effects of fibre-rich types of bread. 2. Dietary fibre from bread: digestibility by the intestinal microflora and water-holding capacity in the colon of human subjects. *Br J Nutr* 50(1):61–74.

Van Nevel CJ, Dierick NA, Decuypere JA, De Smet SM (2006) In vitro fermentability and physicochemical properties of fibre substrates and their effect on bacteriological and morphological characteristics of the gastrointestinal tract of newly weaned piglets. *Arch Anim Nutr* 60(6):477–500.

Vitaglione P, Fogliano V (2010) Cereal fibres, antioxidant activity and health. In *Dietary Fibre: New Frontiers for Food and Health* (eds. JW Van Der Kamp, JM Jones, BV McCleary, DL Topping). Wageningen Academic Publisher, Wageningen, pp. 379–393.

Vitaglione P, Napolitano A, Fogliano V (2008) Cereal dietary fibre: a natural functional ingredient to deliver phenolic compounds into the gut. *Trends Food Sci Technol* 19(9):451–63.

Wilfart A, Montagne L, Simmins H, Noblet J, van Milgen J (2007) Digesta transit in different segments of the gastrointestinal tract of pigs as affected by insoluble fibre supplied by wheat bran. *Br J Nutr* 98(1):54–62.

Williams BA, Mikkelsen D, le Paih L, Gidley MJ (2011) In vitro fermentation kinetics and end-products of cereal arabinoxylans and (1,3;1,4)-β-glucans by porcine faeces. *J Cereal Sci* 53(1):53–8.

Wolever TM, Tosh SM, Gibbs AL, Brand-Miller J, Duncan AM, Hart V, Lamarche B, Thomson BA, Duss R, Wood PJ (2010) Physicochemical properties of oat β-glucan influence its ability to reduce serum LDL cholesterol in humans: a randomized clinical trial. *Am J Clin Nutr* 92(4):723–32.

Wong KKY, Deverell KF, Mackie KL, Clark TA, Donaldson LA (1988) The relationship between fiber porosity and cellulose digestibility in steam-exploded *Pinus radiata*. *Biotechnol Bioeng* 31(5):447–56.

Wrick KL, Robertson JB, Van Soest PJ, Lewis BA, Rivers JM, Roe DA, Hackler LR (1983) The influence of dietary fiber source on human intestinal transit and stool output. *J Nutr* 113(8):1464–79.

Wu SC, Chien PJ, Lee MH, Chau CF (2007) Particle size reduction effectively enhances the intestinal health-promotion ability of an orange insoluble fiber in hamsters. *J Food Sci* 72(8):S618–S21.

Zacherl C, Eisner P, Engel K-H (2011) In vitro model to correlate viscosity and bile acid-binding capacity of digested water-soluble and insoluble dietary fibres. *Food Chem* 126(2):423–8.

2

Interaction of Phenolics and their Association with Dietary Fiber

Fereidoon Shahidi[1] and Anoma Chandrasekara[2]

[1] Department of Biochemistry, Memorial University of Newfoundland, St. John's, NL, , Canada
[2] Department of Applied Nutrition, Wayamba University of Sri Lanka, Makandura, Gonawila, , Sri Lanka

2.1 Introduction

According to epidemiological evidences, a diet rich in whole grains, legumes, fruits, and vegetables is beneficial in combatting a number of non-communicable chronic diseases, such as type 2 diabetes, cardiovascular diseases, hypertension, chronic kidney diseases, non-alcoholic fatty liver disease, and many forms of cancers. The current dietary guidelines of the US Department of Agriculture advise daily consumption of a variety of vegetables, especially whole fruits and cereals, with frequent choice of whole grains (US Department of Agriculture, 2015). Plant foods, as well as being sources of macronutrients and micronutrients, such as minerals and vitamins, are contributors of fiber and bioactive phytochemicals, including phenolic compounds. Clarification of the role specific dietary components of plant foods play in the prevention and therapy of degenerative diseases is currently emerging.

Phenolic compounds are a highly diversified groups of phytochemicals and are ubiquitous in plant foods (Shahidi and Naczk, 2004). Phenolics play dual roles as substrates for oxidative browning reactions and as antioxidants in foods and biological systems. They exert their impact on organoleptic and nutritional qualities of foods, affect plant growth and metabolism and, moreover, perform several functions related to their bioactivities in the human body. Phenolic and polyphenolic compounds, such as phenolic acids and their conjugates, flavonoids, and proanthocyanidins are present in many foods. Whole cereal grains, roots and tubers, fruits and vegetables, legumes, nuts and oilseeds contain bioactive phenolics which may provide numerous beneficial health effects (Shahidi, 2002; Shahidi and Naczk, 2004; Liyana-Pathirana *et al.*, 2006; Wijerathne *et al.*, 2006; Naczk and Shahidi, 2006; Shahidi *et al.*, 2007; Madhujith and Shahidi, 2007; Liyana-Pathirana and Shahidi, 2007; Amarowicz and Pegg, 2008; Alasalvar *et al.*, 2009; Chandrasekara and Shahidi, 2011a, 2011b; Zhong *et al.*, 2012; Ezekiel *et al.*, 2013). In addition, beverages, spices, and herbs also contribute a considerable amount of phenolics to the human diet (Shahidi and Ambigaipalan, 2015).

Dietary Fiber Functionality in Food and Nutraceuticals: From Plant to Gut, First Edition.
Edited by Farah Hosseinian, B. Dave Oomah and Rocio Campos-Vega.
© 2017 John Wiley & Sons Ltd. Published 2017 by John Wiley & Sons Ltd.

Since the discovery of free radicals, oxidative stress in biological tissues has been connected as a causative factor in a range of degenerative diseases, such as hypertension, cardiovascular diseases, diabetes, some cancers, aging, as well as brain-associated disorders, such as Alzheimer's disease. In addition to the traditional "trio" of antioxidants – ascorbic acids, β-carotene, and α-tocopherol – phenolic compounds have gained a prominent place in the scientific community due to their abundance in many foods that are consumed on a daily basis. It has been noted that consumption of antioxidant-rich foods such as whole grains, legumes, fruits, and vegetables can decrease levels of oxidative damage *in vivo* in humans (Halliwell *et al.*, 2005). Phenolic compounds interact with macro- as well as micromolecules in foods (Pérez *et al.*, 2009).

In food systems, phenolic compounds interact with starch in order to reduce their hydrolysis. This affects the glycemic index (GI) of foods. The GI of food reflects postprandial blood glucose elevations. Furthermore, the beneficial health effects of phenolic compounds are also influenced by their bioaccessibility and bioavailability. Bioavailability reflects the proportion of a compound that is digested, absorbed, and utilized in normal metabolism, whereas bioaccessibility defines the amount of an ingested compound that is available for absorption in the gut after digestion (Hedren *et al.*, 2002).

As shown in many epidemiological studies, whole grain consumption, especially the bran component, has been independently associated with a number of health benefits (Koh-Banerjee *et al.*, 2004; Erkkila *et al.*, 2005). Although the biochemical mechanism behind the physiological effect of whole grain consumption is provisional, the high content of dietary fiber in the bran fraction is the main focus. The beneficial health effects of dietary fiber are modulated through changes in hunger and satiety status, the glycemic index of the diet, and the prebiotic activity of the dietary fiber (Vitaglione *et al.*, 2008). However, the substantial antioxidant activity of phenolic compounds attached to dietary fiber has led to renewed interest in them as a source of antioxidants. This contribution focuses on the interactions of phenolic compounds with proteins and starch, and their associations with dietary fiber.

2.2 Phenolic Compounds

Phenolic compounds are secondary plant metabolites that fulfill a number of ecological roles for protection from biotic and abiotic stresses, chemical defense of plants against predators, and in plant–plant interferences, among others. Furthermore, the phenolic profile of a plant is unique to the species (MeKeehen *et al.*, 1999) and the level of phenolics of a given plant depends on many factors, such as the cultivar, environmental conditions, cultural practices, post-harvest practices, processing and storage conditions (Shahidi and Naczk, 2004).

Phenolic compounds are derivatives of biosynthetic precursors such as pyruvate, acetate, specific amino acids, acetyl CoA, and malonyl CoA, following the pentose phosphate, shikimate, and phenyl propanoid metabolism pathways (Ryan and Robards, 1998; Randhir *et al.*, 2004). Phenylalanine and, to a lesser

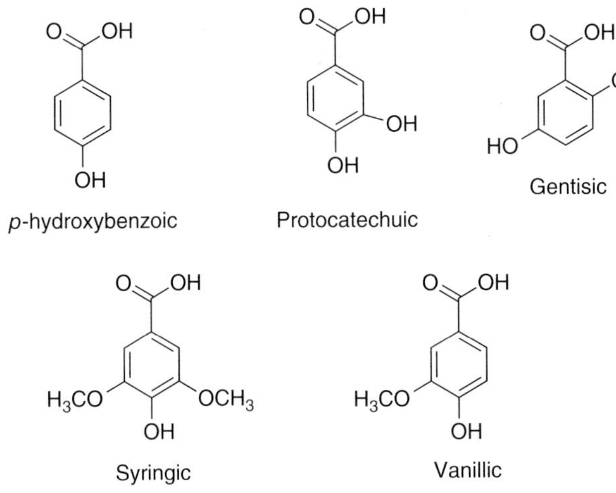

Figure 2.1 Chemical structures of hydroxybenzoic acids.

extent, tyrosine are mainly involved in the synthesis of phenolic compounds in plants (Shahidi, 2002). Abundant phenolic compounds found in plants include simple phenolics, phenolic acids, flavonoids, coumarins, stilbenes, tannins, lignans, and lignins (Naczk and Shahidi, 2006).

Hydroxybenzoic acids and hydroxycinnamic acids are two classes of phenolic acids found in plant materials (Shahidi and Naczk, 2004). Hydroxybenzoic acids include gallic, *p*-hydroxybenzoic, vanillic, gentisic, syringic, and protocatechuic acids (Figure 2.1). Major hydroxycinnamic acids are *p*-coumaric, caffeic, ferulic, and sinapic acids (Figure 2.2). These hydroxycinnamic compounds with a phenyl ring (C_6) and a C_3 side-chain are known as phenylpropanoids and serve as precursors for the synthesis of other phenolic compounds found in foods, beverages, and herbs.

Flavonoids are synthesized by condensation of a phenylpropanoid with three molecules of malonyl coenzyme A. This reaction is catalyzed by the enzyme chalcone synthase, leading to the formation of chalcones. The chalcones are subsequently cyclized under acidic conditions to form flavonoids (Shahidi and Naczk, 2004). There are several different subclasses of flavonoids, including flavones, flavonols, flavonones, flavononols, isoflavones, flavans (catechins and anthocyanidins), and flavonols (Figure 2.3). Flavones and flavonols are present as aglycones in foods and consist of similar C-ring structure with a double bond at the 2–3 positions. However, flavones lack a hydroxyl group at the third position (Shahidi and Naczk, 2004).

By now, it is abundantly clear that phenolic compounds in plant matrices exist in different forms. Phenolics that are extractable into aqueous or aqueous–organic solvent mixtures are soluble phenolics and these include phenolic compounds existing in the non-conjugated form (free) as well as phenolic compounds conjugated to soluble carbohydrates by ester (esterified) and ether (etherified) bonds (Shahidi and Naczk, 2004). The leftover residues after extraction of the soluble phenolics are known as insoluble-bound phenolic compounds.

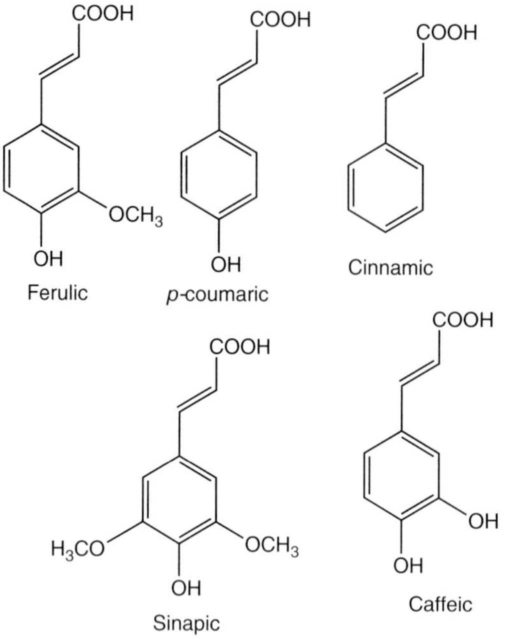

Figure 2.2 Chemical structures of hydroxycinnamic acids.

These include hydroxycinnamic acids, which are mainly esterified to the sugar residues of polysaccharides, providing cross-linking between cell wall polymers (Ishii and Hiroi, 1990). Furthermore, they form ether bonds and C–C linkages with lignins (Grabber *et al.*, 2000). The conjugated and insoluble-bound phenolics can be released at the variable alkaline and acidic gastrointestinal conditions and under colonic fermentation. They may impart health benefits even at local sites, such as the intestinal epithelium and beyond after absorption (Andreasen *et al.*, 2001; Liyana-Pathirana and Shahidi, 2005; Chandrasekara and Shahidi, 2012).

2.3 Bioactivities of Phenolics

Phenolic compounds have been reported to possess a number of biological activities in addition to their conventionally known antioxidant properties. Phenolics are versatile as effective antioxidants and as such possess at least one aromatic ring with one or more hydroxyl groups in addition to other substituents. They neutralize free radicals by donating an electron or a hydrogen atom, thus reducing the rate of oxidation by inhibiting the formation of or deactivating the active species and precursors of free radicals or by direct scavenging of radicals in lipid peroxidation chain reactions or other radicals. Furthermore, emerging evidence suggests that phenolics encompass other bioactivities such as anti-inflammatory, antithrombotic, antibacterial, and anticariogenic effects (Bowden, 1999; Borchardt *et al.*, 2008; Bhattacharya *et al.*, 2010; Palafox-Carlos *et al.*, 2011; Ferrazzano *et al.*, 2011).

Recent work suggests a range of potential mechanisms by which polyphenols may arrest the occurrence of several non-communicable chronic diseases. These

Figure 2.3 Chemical structures of flavonoids.

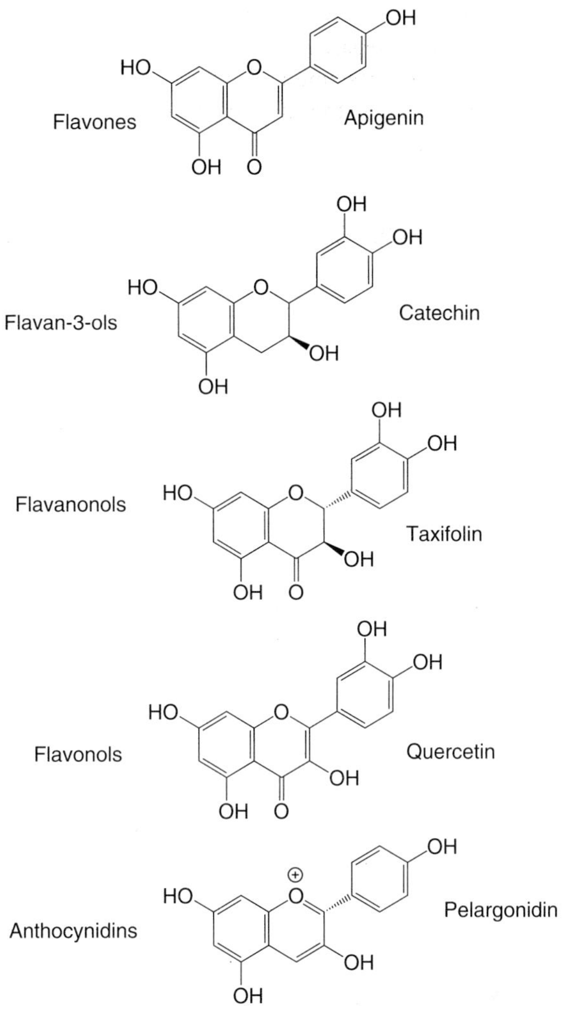

include inhibition of cancer cell proliferation and cholesterol uptake (Leifert and Abeywardena, 2008; Noratto *et al.*, 2009), modulation of enzymes such as telomerase, cycloxygenase, and lipoxygenase (de la Puerta *et al.*, 1999; Schewe *et al.*, 2001; Sadik *et al.*, 2003; Naasani *et al.*, 2003; Hussain *et al.*, 2005; O'Leary *et al.*, 2004), and interaction with several signal transduction pathways (Wiseman *et al.*, 2001; Kong *et al.*, 2000; Spencer *et al.*, 2003; Masella *et al.*, 2004; Rosenblat and Aviram, 2009). In addition, polyphenols may also affect caspase-dependent pathways (Monasterio *et al.*, 2004; Way *et al.*, 2005), cell cycle regulation (Fischer and Lane, 2000), platelet functions (Murphy *et al.*, 2003), and prevent endothelial dysfunctions (Carluccio *et al.*, 2003).

Foods are masticated in the initial step of digestion. Mastication consists of grinding food into small pieces and mixing them with saliva to form a bolus which is ready to be swallowed. The mastication process decreases the particle size, enlarging the surface area available for action by digestive enzymes, thus increasing the overall digestion efficiency (Kulp *et al.*, 2003). Phenolic compounds released from the food matrix by the action of digestive enzymes in the small intestine and by microbial fermentation in the large intestine are bioaccessible in the gut and therefore potentially bioavailable (Saura-Calixto *et al.*, 2007).

2.4 Dietary Fiber

Dietary fibers are non-digestible carbohydrates, in addition to lignin, that are resistant to digestion by human digestive enzymes and pass into the large intestine (Anderson *et al.*, 2009; Jones, 2014). The intake of dietary fibers has been shown to provide a number of health benefits to humans, including reducing the risk of coronary heart disease (Liu *et al.*,1999), stroke (Steffen *et al.*, 2003), hypertension (Whelton *et al.*, 2005), and diabetes (Cummings *et al.*, 2004).

The American Heart Association recommends an intake of 25–30 g dietary fiber per day (Pérez-Jiménez *et al.*, 2008). Furthermore, these complex carbohydrates can directly interact with the compositional components in foods and therefore interfere with their assimilation in the body (Faulks and Southon 2005; Parada and Aguilera 2007; Porrini and Riso 2008; Del Rio *et al.*, 2009; Pérez *et al.*, 2009). Thus, the physical state of the food matrix affects the release, mass transfer, accessibility, and biochemical stability of nutrients and non-nutrient compounds (Aguilera, 2005; Parada and Aguilera, 2007).

Dietary fiber can reduce the bioavailability of macronutrients, such as fat, and some minerals and trace elements present in the human diet. It has been demonstrated that pectin strongly decreases the bioavailability of β-carotene in humans (Rock and Swendseid, 1992). Usually, the main effects of dietary fiber in the foregut include extension of gastric emptying time and retardation of the absorption of nutrients, depending on the physicochemical form of the fiber. There are three main physical forms of dietary fiber in the small intestine: soluble polymer chains in solution, insoluble macromolecular assemblies, and swollen, hydrated, sponge-like networks (Eastwood and Morris, 1992).

In whole grains, dietary fiber is concentrated in the bran and ranges from 18 to 87% of the weight depending on the type and variety of grains (Vitaglione *et al.*, 2008). Depending on their water solubility, cereal dietary fibers are conventionally categorized as soluble dietary fiber (SDF) and insoluble dietary fiber (IDF). Cereal bran of wheat and maize predominantly consist of IDF, whereas oats contain a considerable amount of SDF.

Phenolic compounds are constituents of dietary fiber present in grains, fruits, juices, and other beverages such as beer and wine (Saura-Calixto and Díaz-Rubio, 2007; Díaz-Rubio *et al.*, 2009). Phenolic acids as well as flavonoids are associated with SDF found in fruit juices and beverages. Flavan-3-ols and benzoic acids are associated with dietary fiber in wine (Saura-Calixto *et al.*, 2007). In beer, flavonoids and hydroxycinnamic acids, which are linked to degraded and solubilized arabinoxylans, are present (Díaz-Rubio *et al.*, 2009).

The predominant phenolic acids attached to cell walls in cereals are ferulic acid, diferulic acids, *p*-coumaric acid, sinapic acid, and caffeic acid. Benzoic acid derivatives have also been reported (Bunzel *et al.*, 2005). In plant cell walls, ferulic and *p*-coumaric acids are linked via an ester bond to the arabinoxylans (Hartley *et al.*, 1990) in cereals or to the pectins of dicotyledons such as spinach (Fry, 1982) and sugar beet (Rombouts and Thibault, 1986). In bamboo, hydroxycinnamic acids are esters linked to arabinoxylans as well as xyloglucans (Iiyama *et al.*, 1994). In addition, ferulic and *p*-coumaric acids may also be esterified and etherified to lignin (Iiyama *et al.*, 1990).

The hydroxycinnamic acid moiety attached to dietary fiber determines its structure and physical properties. Cell wall polysaccharides are cross-linked primarily through the formation of diferulates (Bunzel *et al.*, 2001). The main mechanism operating in this process is ferulate dehydrodimerization via radical coupling reactions that leads to the production of a range of different diferulates (Bunzel *et al.*, 2004; Figure 2.4). Diferulates form bridge structures between

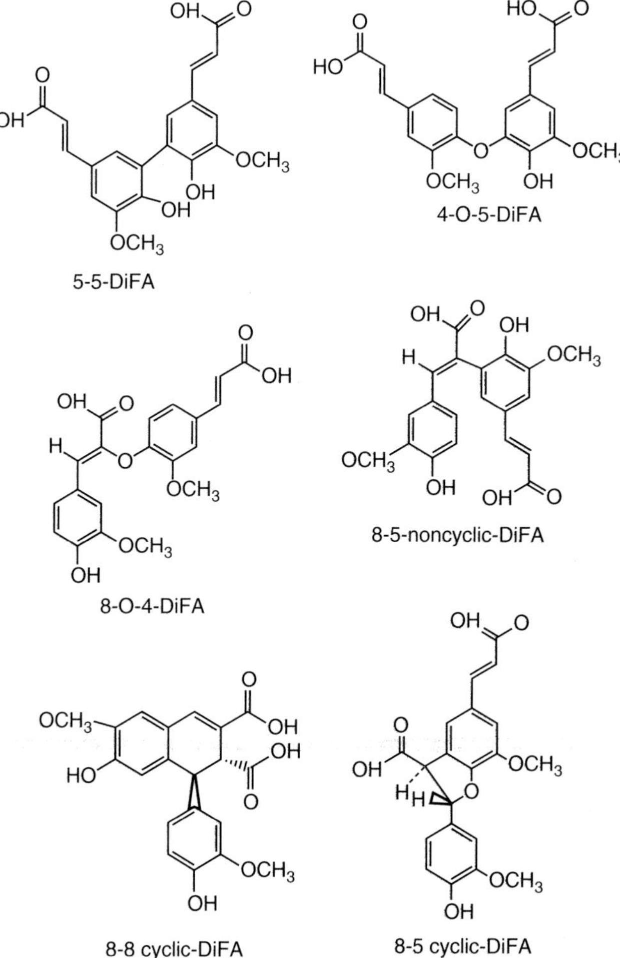

Figure 2.4 Chemical structures of ferulic acid cross-linked compounds.

chains of polysaccharides. The predominant diferulate is the 5,5-diferulic acid (Bunzel *et al.*, 2005). In addition, ferulates are involved in cross-linking polysaccharides to lignin. Thus, they influence the physical parameters of dietary fibers, determining their structure, molecular weight, and water solubility. In general, the levels of diferulates in SDF of cereal are far lower than those in the corresponding IDF (Bunzel *et al.*, 2001). Furthermore, the biological significance of dietary fiber is also influenced by the amounts of diferulates associated with them. Wang *et al.* (2004) hypothesized that the amount of diferulates associated with dietary fiber was inversely related to their fermentability by intestinal microflora.

2.5 Antioxidant Dietary Fiber

In recent years the interest in antioxidant dietary fibers (ADF) has increased gradually due to recognition of their potential health benefits, especially in risk reduction and management of non-communicable chronic diseases. ADFs are natural compounds that scavenge 1,1-diphenyl-2 picrylhydrazyl (DPPH) radicals with at least 50 mg equivalents of vitamin E per gram of ADF and dietary fiber content higher than 50% of dry matter (Saura-Calixto, 1998). Much attention has focused on ADFs in fruit-processing wastes as functional food ingredients (Balasundram *et al.*, 2006). It has been suggested that ADFs could be incorporated into flour used in high dietary fiber bakery goods to give improved color, aroma, taste, and health benefits contributed through their constituent phenolic compounds. Ajila *et al.* (2010) prepared macaroni using mango peel powder to enhance the antioxidant properties of the product. Apple pomace was also incorporated into wheat flour as a fiber source to improve the rheological characteristics of cake (Sudha *et al.*, 2007). Furthermore, grape pomace was mixed with sourdough for the production of rye bread with improved health benefits (Mildner-Szkudlarz *et al.*, 2011). Grape seed flour was used in production of cereal bars, pancakes, and noodles (Rosales Soto *et al.*, 2012).

Sánchez-Tena *et al.* (2013) demonstrated the chemopreventive efficacy of lyophilized red grape pomace containing proanthocyanidin (PA)-rich dietary fiber (GADF) on spontaneous intestinal tumorigenesis in the Apc$^{Min/+}$ mouse model. Feeding a 1% GADF-supplemented diet for 6 weeks reduced intestinal tumorigenesis, reducing the total number of polyps by 76% as well as a considerable reduction in polyp size categories. The comparison of microarray expression profiles of GADF-treated and non-treated mice revealed the molecular mechanisms underlying the inhibition of intestinal tumorigenesis. It was noted that the effects of GADF were due to the induction of a gastrointestinal cell cycle arrest and the downregulation of genes related to the immune response and inflammation (Sánchez-Tena *et al.*, 2013).

2.6 Protein–Phenolic Interactions

Interactions between proteins and phenolic compounds exist in many fruits, vegetables, and beverages such as coffee (Naczk *et al.*, 1996; Clifford, 1999;

Naczk *et al.*, 2006). Hydroxycinnamates, such as ferulic acid and derivatives thereof, interact with proteins in a number of ways. These include interactions with food proteins during food processing, with storage and physiologically active proteins in the plant, with food proteins or enzymes in the course of digestion in the gastrointestinal tract, with blood plasma proteins, and with proteins in target tissues of organs in the human body. The interactions between phenolic compounds and proteins may be non-covalent interactions, which are reversible, or covalent interactions, which are usually irreversible (Rawel and Rohn, 2010). Amino acid sequence and the resulting structural conformation, and external conditions such as pH, temperature, and ionic strength, influence the non-covalent binding of the hydroxycinnamates to proteins (Prigent *et al.*, 2003; Rawel *et al.*, 2005, 2006). Different types of non-covalent interactions exist, such as hydrogen bonds, electrostatic interactions, hydrophobic interactions, van der Waals interactions, and π bonds. The hydrophobic interactions and hydrogen bonds are the major forces for the interaction between the phenolic compounds and proteins. Hydrophobic interactions may take place between phenolic compounds and amino acids, such as alanine, valine, isoleucine, leucine, methionine, phenylalanine, tyrosine, tryptophan, cysteine, and glycine residues. Furthermore, some amino acids, namely lysine, arginine, histidine, asparagine, glutamine, serine, threonine, aspartic acid, glutamic acid, tyrosine, cysteine, and tryptophan, are bound with phenolic compounds by hydrogen bonds, which may occur between their nitrogen or oxygen and hydroxyl groups of phenolic compounds (Rawel and Rohn, 2010).

2.7 Starch–Phenolic Interactions

Phenolic compounds consist of hydroxyl and carboxyl groups which can affect the functional properties of starch by competing for water molecules in the medium, forming inclusion complexes, changing the pH of the starch–water suspensions, and forming non-covalent interactions among phenolic compounds and starch molecules (Beta and Corke, 2004; Zhu *et al.*, 2008, 2009; Barros *et al.*, 2012; Bordenave *et al.*, 2014).

Zhu *et al.* (2009) investigated the effect of various phenolic extracts, namely pomegranate peel, green tea, Chinese hawthorn, and Chinese gall on pasting, thermal, and gel textural properties of wheat starch. All four extracts increased the breakdown values and reduced the final viscosity. The peak viscosity of wheat starch significantly increased upon the addition of pomegranate, green tea, and Chinese gall extracts. Furthermore, peak time and hot paste viscosity was reduced by the addition of pomegranate and Chinese gall extracts. All tested extracts reduced gel hardness and the observed effects were attributed to different phenolic compounds present at varying concentrations in the extracts. Chinese gall extracts are a rich source of gallotannins, whereas green tea contains catechins. The addition of phenolic extracts also reduced the pH of the starch–water suspensions and a positive correlation existed between pH and final viscosity ($R^2 = 0.84$). The presence of phenolic acids, such as gallic and chlorogenic acids, is attributed to reduced pH. As shown by Zhu *et al.* (2009), addition of extracts reduced the final viscosity of starch–water suspensions. Reduced pH as well as the interactions of phenolic compounds with hydrophobic regions of leached amylose and with amylopectin side-chains through hydrogen bonds and van der Waals forces may contribute to this effect. Phenolic compounds interacting with amylose change the properties of the continuous phases, which could weaken the intermolecular interactions between amylose chains. Phenolic extracts changed the textural properties of starch gels. Phenolic extracts reduced the hardness of the gels; Chinese galls showed the greatest effect whereas pomegranate exhibited the least (Zhu *et al.*, 2009).

Earlier, Zhu *et al.* (2008) demonstrated the effect of pure phenolic compounds on pasting properties of wheat starch and reported that 21 out of 25 compounds increased the peak viscosity. However, the extent of effect varied with the structural differences among the phenolic compounds. For instance, gallic acid with three hydroxyl groups caused the highest increase in peak viscosity, whereas 3-hydroxybenzoic acid with one hydroxyl group showed the least. Syringic acid with two methoxy groups resulted in a higher increase in peak viscosity than vanillic acid, which has only one. In addition, syringic and vanillic acids increased peak viscosity to a greater extent than hydroxybenzoic acids devoid of methoxy groups, suggesting a significant influence of methoxy group on the peak viscosity. It was further reported that all hydroxycinnamic acids also increased the peak viscosity, although the influence of the hydroxyl and methoxy groups was found to be different from those of hydroxybenzoic acids (Zhu *et al.*, 2008). Different flavonoids also showed varied effects on peak viscosity of wheat starch. Quercetin (a flavonol) showed the highest increase, whereas catechin (a flavan-3-ol) had the least. These different effects could be attributed to structural differences existing among functional groups of flavonoids.

The addition of ferulic acid and catechin changed the pasting properties of maize and sorghum starches (Beta and Corke, 2004). Furthermore, addition of catechin resulted in a pink-colored paste, whereas ferulic acid had no such effect on the paste color. Ferulic acid and catechin decreased hot paste viscosity (HPV), final viscosity, and setback viscosity of maize and sorghum starch pastes. In addition, both phenolic compounds influenced the peak viscosity (PV) of the sorghum paste. The authors further highlighted that phenolic type as well as pH both significantly influence interactions between phenolics and starch, hence affecting the pasting properties. Changes observed could be due to the formation of starch–phenol complexes that impeded the reassociation of starch molecules. These interactions are pivotal in food matrices where phenolics are added as functional food ingredients (Beta and Corke, 2004).

Wu *et al.* (2009) showed that addition of purified green tea polyphenols may have a reducing effect on starch retrogradation. Rice starch containing 10, 14, or 20% tea polyphenols did not exhibit the retrogradation endotherm on the DSC (differential scanning calorimetry) after 10 days of storage. The authors suggested that this could be due to the hydrogen bonding between hydroxyl groups of tea polyphenols with hydroxyl groups of starch molecules, thus reducing the reassociation of starch polymers during retrogradation. They suggested that this effect may also depend on the strength of the hydrogen bonds between starch and the polyphenolic compounds (Wu *et al.*, 2009).

Later, Xiao *et al.* (2011) showed that green tea phenolics reduced retrogradation of rice starch regardless of their amylose content. The enthalpy of retrogradation of starches containing 10 or 15% of polyphenolics was detected after 20 days of storage. In addition, the degree of retrogradation was significantly reduced. The authors showed that addition of tea phenolics to high amylose rice starch at a concentration of 15% reduced the degree of retrogradation from 79% (control) to 11.7% (Xiao *et al.*, 2011).

2.8 Phenolic Compounds and Starch Digestibility

The attention paid to low glycemic foods has increased as a strategy for risk reduction of non-communicable chronic diseases. A diet rich in digestible starch leads to a high glycemic response which, in turn can cause a number of diseases such as diabetes, cardiovascular ailments, and obesity. Reduction of starch digestibility of products using phenolic compounds is focused on foods with a low glycemic index. Starch digestion involves a number of enzymes, including salivary and pancreatic α-amylases and intestinal α-glucosidases. These are inhibited by phenolic compounds and there are a number of factors that may influence this inhibition. The structure of an enzyme may make it susceptible to different phenolic compounds. For instance, α-amylases may be inhibited by large polyphenolic molecules such as tannins, whereas α-glucosidases tend to be inhibited by smaller phenolic compounds such as phenolic acids. Zajácz *et al.* (2007) demonstrated a mixed type of inhibition of salivary α-amylase by tannin isolated from a gall nut of Aleppo oak when amylose was used as a substrate. However, it was noted that the type of inhibition depended on the concentration of inhibitor: at low concentration of tannin, a competitive inhibition was shown, whereas at high concentration it was non-competitive. Competitive inhibition could be due to the galloylated glucose binding to the active site of salivary α-amylase and interacting with aromatic or subsite residues of the enzyme. In the case of non-competitive inhibition, the tannin molecues may interact with the secondary site of the enzyme or with the substrate (Zajácz *et al.*, 2007). Earlier, McDougall *et al.* (2005) investigated the efficacy of phenolic extracts from different sources on the activity of human salivary α-amylase and porcine pancreatic α-amylase. They demonstrated that strawberry and raspberry extracts were effective inhibitors, followed by blueberry, blackcurrant, and red cabbage for α-amylase from both sources. The effectiveness of inhibition was higher on human salivary α-amylase than on porcine salivary α-amylase, suggesting that the enzyme source also influenced the inhibitory behavior of phenolic compounds. The α-amylase inhibitors of the extracts were soluble, hydrolyzable tannins, which included a mixture of ellagitannins and ellagic acid (McDougall *et al.*, 2005).

Tea polyphenolics appear to inhibit both pancreatic α-amylase and intestinal α-glucosidase. Green tea polyphenolic compounds demonstrated effective enzyme inhibitory activities. The α-amylase was inhibited most effectively, among other digestive enzymes such as pepsin, trypsin, and lipase (He *et al.*, 2007). Molecular weight affected the macromolecular interactions and α-amylase

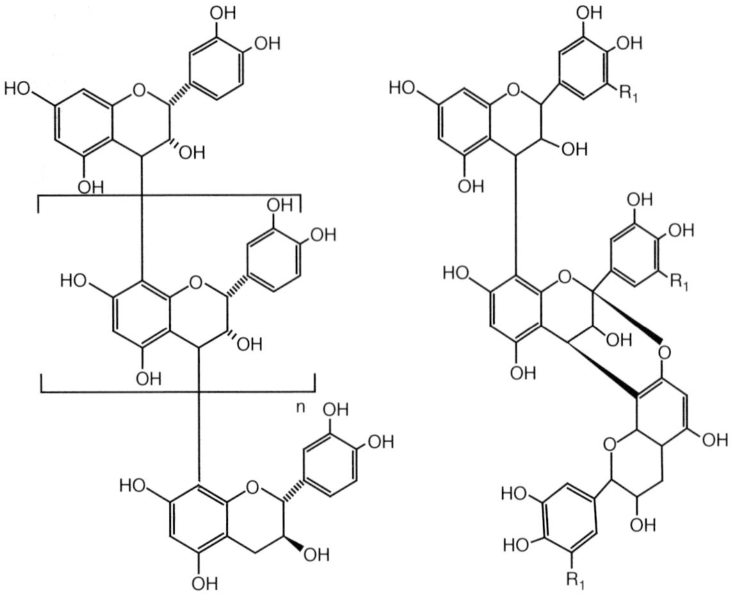

Polyflavan-3-ol with B type interflavan linkages

Heteropolyflavan-3-ols with A- and B-type interflavan linkages
Procyanidin: $R_1 = H$
Prodelphinidin: $R_1 = OH$

Figure 2.5 Structures of proanthocyanidins reported in sorghum.

with highest molecular weight was most susceptible to inhibition. Furthermore, tea phenolics possess hydroxyl and galloyl groups which form hydrogen bonds with polar groups of the enzymes. The number and type of the polar groups may affect the formation and stability of hydrogen bonds between phenolic compounds and enzymes. In addition, phenolics could interact with enzymes through hydrophobic associations (He *et al.*, 2007). Kusano *et al.* (2008) also reported that black tea polyphenolics reduced the activity of α-amylase and lipase. These findings are in agreement with those of Koh *et al.* (2010), who showed that black tea slowed down the digestion of rice noodles. However, phenolic acids, such as cinnamic acids, did not show an inhibitory effect on α-amylase activity (Adisakwattana *et al.*, 2009).

Barros *et al.* (2012) investigated the interactions of sorghum proanthocyanidins (PAs) with starch molecules. PAs decreased setback of normal starch and were poorly extractable after cooking with starches. Furthermore, it was found that pure amylase interacted more effectively with oligomeric and polymeric PA before addition of amylopectin. In addition, PA in sorghum (Figure 2.5) increased the resistant starch content two times more than the monomeric phenolic extract. They further elaborated the fact that sorghum PAs are useful in reducing starch digestibility (Barros *et al.*, 2012).

2.9 Interactions of Phenolic Compounds

Several phenolic compounds are present in foods and each phenolic compound exhibits a different antioxidant capacity depending on its structure, number of aromatic and hydroxyl groups, and their distribution in the structure (Heo *et al.*, 2007). Furthermore, there could be molecular interactions among phenolic compounds found in the food. These interactions between phenolics could be additive, synergistic, or even antagonistic. Therefore, the total antioxidant capacity of the phenolic compounds of a food may not correspond to the sum of individual antioxidant capacity given by isolated antioxidants available in the food. Saura-Calixto (2012) demonstrated individual antioxidant capacity and the interactions of four major phenolic compounds, namely chlorogenic, gallic, protocatechuic, and vanillic acids found in "Ataulfo" mango pulp using the DPPH radical scavenging assay. More than 80% of the phenolic combinations showed synergistic interactions. The arithmetical additive antioxidant capacity value ($47.8 \pm 3.1\%$) was significantly lower ($p \leq 0.05$) than the experimental value ($67.6 \pm 2.8\%$) of the combination of gallic and protocatechuic acids. This indicates that there is a synergistic interaction between gallic and protocatechuic acids, contributing a higher antioxidant capacity compared to a simple additive contribution of each compound (Saura-Calixto, 2012; Figure 2.6).

2.10 Phenolics and Dietary Fiber

Phenolic compounds are found in plant cells, primarily within the vacuole, enclosed by tonoplast and cytoplasmic lipid membranes. Plant cells undergo mechanical and biochemical break down that results in cell rupture, hence allowing the release of phenolic compounds and thus becoming bioaccessible and bioavailable after digestion (Padayachee *et al.*, 2012a, 2012b). Phenolic compounds interact physicochemically with the cell wall polysaccharide–protein matrix as part of cell growth and development (Palafox-Carlos *et al.*, 2011; Padayachee *et al.*, 2012a). These interactions could be either beneficial or detrimental for the bioactivities associated with phenolic compounds.

Studies have shown the nature of interactions existing between different groups of phenolic compounds and the primary components of the cell wall matrix, especially polysaccharide moieties of dietary fiber. According to Renard *et al.* (2001), hydroxycinnamic acids and epicatechin are not bound to the cell walls in apples. In addition, the occurrence of procyanidins is up to 0.6 g per g of cell walls. The cell walls from a number of fruits protect ascorbic acid from oxidation (Motomura and Yoshida, 2002). Apple cell walls have been shown to affect the antioxidant activity of quercetin and L-ascorbic acid (Sun-Waterhouse *et al.*, 2007). Furthermore, Sun-Waterhouse *et al.* (2008) showed that fiber from onions has a favorable interaction only with L-ascorbic acid.

Using cellulose and pectin as cell wall models, it was shown that anthocyanins and phenolic acids interact with both polysaccharides (Padayachee *et al.*, 2012a,

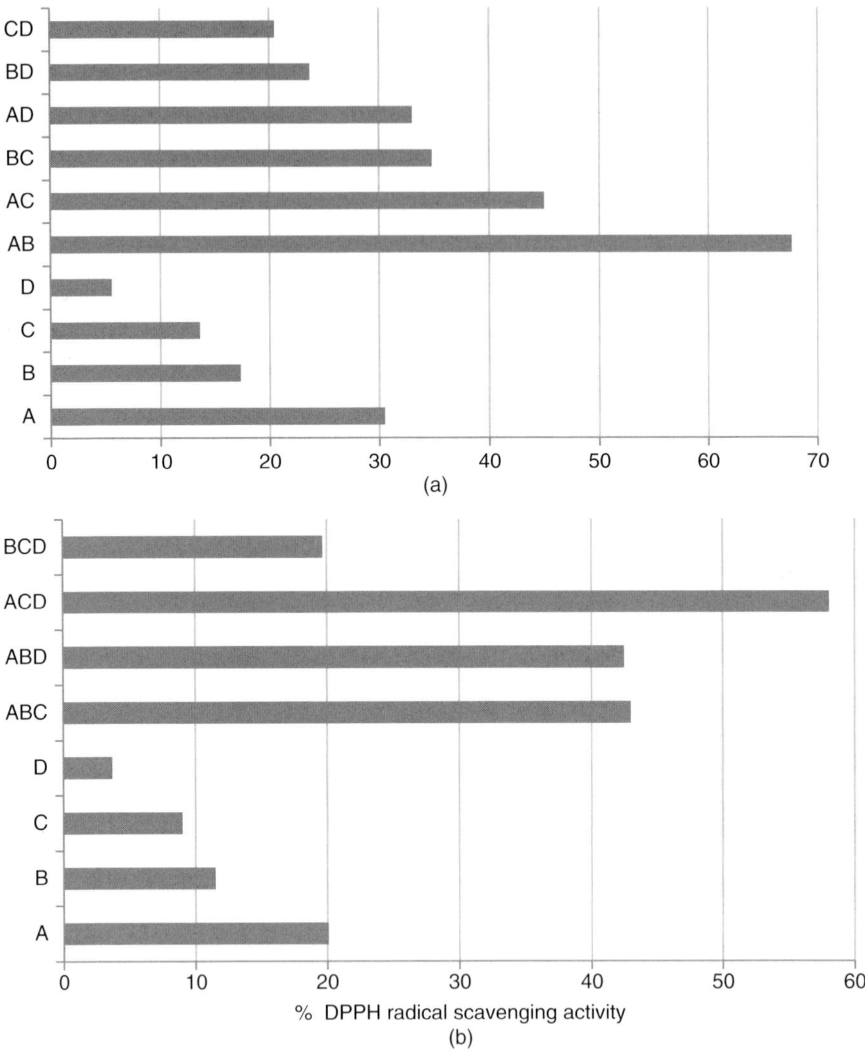

Figure 2.6 Antioxidant capacity of individual phenolic acids and mixtures containing two (a) and three (b) phenolic acids. (A) Gallic acid, (B) protocatechuic acid, (C) chlorogenic acid, (D) vanillic acid. *Source:* Data from Saura-Calixto (2012).

2012b). The interaction between phenolic compounds and dietary fiber components affects the bioaccessibility, bioavailability, and bioactivities of phenolic compounds in foods (Sun-Waterhouse *et al.*, 2008). However, it has been shown that even though phenolic compounds bound to fiber are not available for absorption in the small intestine they could be released by the microbial fermentation in the large intestine. Thus, released phenolic compounds can exert beneficial health effects at the site itself as well as after absorption in the large intestine (Saura-Calixto, 2011; Padayachee *et al.*, 2012a).

Research focused on polyphenolic compounds demonstrates that parent molecules present in food matrices are not transported in the circulatory system and do not reach body tissues to exert bioactivities in the human body (Donovan *et al.*, 2006). Many of the bioactive compounds are metabolites formed in the small intestine and hepatic cells, and low molecular weight catabolic products of the colonic microflora (Del Rio *et al.*, 2009). Hydroxybenzoic and hydroxycinnamic acids in the aglycone form are generally absorbed in the upper part of the gastrointestinal tract (Saura-Calixto *et al.*, 2007). The stomach constitutes an active absorption site for a number of phenolic acids, such as gallic, caffeic, ferulic, coumaric, and chlorogenic acids (Konishi *et al.*, 2006; Lafay *et al.*, 2006; Lafay and Gil-Izquierdo, 2008). This explains the rapid absorption of these compounds, ranging from 1 to 2 hours after intake of fruits and vegetables. It has been shown that aglycone phenolic acids are absorbed to different degrees; absorption of caffeic acid, for example is 19.1% whereas that for ferulic acid is 56.1%. However, when phenolic acids are esterified it decreases the bioavailability to 0.3–0.4% from the original intake because they must be hydrolyzed in the enterocytes before reaching the blood circulation (Lafay *et al.*, 2006).

Recently, Quirós-Sauceda *et al.* (2014) demonstrated that added dietary fiber affects the extracted phenolic content and antioxidant capacity of tropical fruits. This study showed that there were physicochemical interactions between polysaccharides of dietary fiber and methanol extracts of phenolics from tropical fruits. The addition of fruit dietary fiber (FDF) as well as wheat dietary fiber (WDF) to phenolic extracts reduced their total phenolic content (TPC) by 5.9–38.0% (Table 2.1). Furthermore, they showed that addition of fiber to methanolic extracts of phenolic compounds reduced the antioxidant activity as determined by DPPH radical scavenging activity and Trolox equivalent antioxidant capacity (TEAC). In addition it was noted that reduction of TPC as well as antioxidant activity varied with the type of dietary fiber added (Quirós-Sauceda *et al.*, 2014). They further showed that the type of fiber (soluble or insoluble) and the specific components, such as starch available in the food matrix, affected the phenolic content and their antioxidant activities (Quirós-Sauceda *et al.*, 2014). Serrano *et al.* (2009) has previously shown that complex polysaccharides as constituents of dietary fiber form physicochemical interactions with phenolic compounds, thereby preventing their action as antioxidants. According to Palafox-Carlos *et al.* (2011) these interactions may take place either with hydrogen and ester bonds with ferulic and cinnamic acids, or through hydrophobic interactions and covalent bonds. In addition, simple physical entrapment may also lead to an interaction. Overall, the composition, functional group substitution, and physical properties of fibers and phenolic compounds present in the extract affect the type of interaction (Palafox-Carlos *et al.*, 2011).

The discussion here clearly substantiates the importance of dietary fiber in forming an entrapping matrix of phenolic compounds in foods. In the large intestine dietary fiber provides a substrate for fermentation for colonic microflora and upon release phenolic compounds exert systemic as well as local

Table 2.1 Total phenolic content (TPC) of methanolic extracts of tropical fruits and reduction of TPC by adding fruit dietary fiber.

Fruit fiber	TPC before incubation with fiber	TPC after incubation with fruit fiber	Percentage decrease of TPC with fruit fiber	TPC after incubation with wheat fiber	Percentage decrease of TPC with wheat fiber
Pineapple	77.6	69.2	10.8	55.3	28.8
Mango	55.9	42.7	23.7	34.7	38.0
Papaya	51.0	44.3	13.0	35.0	31.3
Guava	222.0	209.0	5.9	186.0	16.2

Source: Data from Quirós-Sauceda *et al.* (2014).

effects. Therefore, emphasis should be placed not only on the total dietary fiber content in the diet but also on the source.

2.11 Conclusion

This contribution demonstrates that the interactions between phenolic compounds and other macromolecules, as well as phenolic–phenolic interactions, impact the physicochemical and nutritional properties of food. The nature of phenolic compounds and their environment in the food matrix influence and change the characteristics associated with food. Starch and phenolic compounds interact to form either inclusion complexes facilitated by hydrophobic effect, or complexes with much weaker binding through hydrogen bonds. This affects the starch functional properties as well as digestibility. Interactions between proteins and phenolic compounds may inhibit the enzymatic activities and availability of amino acids. Antioxidant dietary fiber from by-products of food processing may be used in functional food applications. It would be interesting to investigate the effects of phenolic interactions in foods on the functional properties as well as bioactivities in order to optimize their effects on wellbeing and disease risk reduction.

References

Adisakwattana S., Chantarasinlapin P., Thammarat H., and Yibchok-Anun S. (2009). A series of cinnamic acid derivatives and their inhibitory activity on intestinal alpha-glucosidase. *Journal of Enzyme Inhibition and Medicinal Chemistry*, 24: 1194–1200.

Aguilera J.M. (2005). Why food microstructure? *Journal of Food Engineering*, 67: 3–11.

Ajila C. M., Aalami M., Leelavathi K., and Rao U.J.S.P. (2010). Mango peel powder: A potential source of antioxidant and dietary fiber in macaroni preparations. *Innovative Food Science and Emerging Technologies*, 11: 219–224.

Alasalvar C., Karamac M., Kosinska A., Rybarczyk A., Shahidi F., and Amarowicz R. (2009). Antioxidant activity of hazelnut skin phenolics. *Journal of Agricultural and Food Chemistry*, 57: 4645–4650.

Amarowicz R. and Pegg R.B. (2008). Legumes as a source of natural antioxidants. *European Journal of Lipid Science and Technology*, 110: 865–878.

Anderson J.W., Baird P., Davis Jr., R.H., Ferreri S., Knudtson M., Koraym A., Waters V., and Williams C.L. (2009). Health benefits of dietary fiber. *Nutrition Research*, 67:188–205.

Andreasen M.F., Kroon P.A., Williamson G., and Garcia-Conesa M.T. (2001). Intestinal release and uptake of phenolic antioxidant diferulic acids. *Free Radical Biology and Medicine*, 31: 304–314.

Balasundram N., Sundram K., and Samman S. (2006). Phenolic compounds in plants and agri-industrial by-products: Antioxidant activity, occurrence, and potential uses. *Food Chemistry*, 99: 191–203.

Barros F., Awika J.M., and Rooney L.W. (2012). Interaction of tannins and other sorghum phenolic compounds with starch and effects on in vitro starch digestibility. *Journal of Agricultural and Food Chemistry*, 60: 11609–11617.

Beta T. and Corke H. (2004). Effect of ferulic acid and catechin on sorghum and maize starch pasting properties. *Cereal Chemistry*, 81: 418–422.

Bhattacharya A., Sood P., and Citovsky V. (2010). The roles of plant phenolics in defence and communication during *Agrobacterium* and *Rhizobium* infection. *Molecular Plant Pathology*, 11: 705–719.

Borchardt J.R., Wyse D.L., Sheaffer C.C., Kauppi K.L., Fulcher R.G., Ehlke N.J., Biesboer D.D., and Bey R.F. (2008). Antioxidant and antimicrobial activity of seed from plants of the Mississippi river basin. *Journal of Medicinal Plants Research*, 2: 81–93.

Bordenave N., Hamaker B.R., and Ferruzzi M.G. (2014). Nature and consequences of non-covalent interactions between flavonoids and macronutrients in foods. *Food Functions*, 5: 18–34.

Bowden G.H. (1999). Controlled environment model for accumulation of biofilms of oral bacteria. *Methods in Enzymology*, 310: 216–224.

Bunzel M., Ralph J., Marita J. M., Hatfield R. D., and Steinhart H. (2001). Diferulates as structural components in soluble and insoluble cereal dietary fibre. *Journal of the Science of Food and Agriculture*, 81: 653–660.

Bunzel M., Funk C., and Steinhart H. (2004). Semipreparative isolation of dehydrodiferulic and dehydrotriferulic acids as standard substances from maize bran. *Journal of Separation Science*, 27: 1080–1086.

Bunzel M., Ralph J., and Steinhart H. (2005). Association of non-starch polysaccharides and ferulic acid in grain amaranth (*Amaranthus caudatus* L.) dietary fiber. *Molecular Nutrition and Food Research*, 49: 551–559.

Carluccio M.A., Siculella L., Ancora M.A., Massaro M., Scoditti E., Storelli C., Visioli F., Distante A., and De Caterina R. (2003). Olive oil and red wine antioxidant polyphenols inhibit endothelial activation: Antiatherogenic properties of Mediterranean diet phytochemicals. *Arteriosclerosis, Thrombosis and Vascular Biology*, 23: 622–629.

Chandrasekara, N. and Shahidi, F. (2011a). Antioxidative potential of cashew phenolics in food and biological model systems as affected by roasting. *Food Chemistry*, 129: 1388–1396.

Chandrasekara A. and Shahidi F. (2011b). Determination of antioxidant activity in free and hydrolyzed fractions of millet grains and characterization of their phenolic profiles by HPLC-DAD-ESI-MS^n. *Journal of Functional Foods*, 3: 144–158.

Chandrasekara A. and Shahidi, F. (2012). Bioaccessibility and antioxidant potential of millet grain phenolics as affected by simulated in vitro digestion and microbial fermentation. *Journal of Functional Foods*, 4: 226–237.

Clifford M.N. (1999). Chlorogenic acids and other cinnamates – nature, occurrence and dietary burden. *Journal of the Science of Food and Agriculture*, 79: 362–372.

Cummings J.H., Edmond L.M., and Magee E.A. (2004). Dietary carbohydrates and health: do we still need the fibre concept? *Clinical Nutrition Supplements*, 1: 5–17.

de la Puerta R., Ruiz Gutierrez V., and Hoult, J.R. (1999). Inhibition of leukocyte 5-lipoxygenase by phenolics from virgin olive oil. *Biochemical Pharmacology*, 57: 445–449.

Del Rio D., Costa L.G., Lean M.E.J., and Crozier A. (2009). Polyphenols and health: what compounds are involved? *Nutrition, Metabolism and Cardiovascular Diseases*, 20: 1–6.

Díaz-Rubio M.E., Perez-Jimenez J., and Saura-Calixto F. (2009). Dietary fiber and antioxidant capacity in *Fucus vesiculosus* products. *International Journal of Food Sciences and Nutrition*, 60: 23–34.

Eastwood M.A. and Morris E.R. (1992). Physical properties of dietary fiber that influence physiological function: a model for polymers along the gastrointestinal tract. *American Journal of Clinical Nutrition*, 55: 436–442.

Erkkila A.T., Herrington D.M., Mozaffarian D., and Lichtenstein A.H. (2005). Cereal fibre and whole-grain intake are associated with reduced progression of coronary-artery atherosclerosis in postmenopausal women with coronary artery disease. *American Heart Journal*, 150: 94–101.

Ezekiel R., Singh N., Sharma S., and Kaur A. (2013). Beneficial phytochemicals in potato-a review. *Food Research International*, 50: 487–496.

Faulks R.M. and Southon S. (2005). Challenges to understanding and measuring carotenoid bioavailability. *BBA-Molecular Basis of Disease*, 1740: 95–100.

Ferrazzano G.F., Amato I., Ingenito A., Zarrelli A., Pinto G., and Pollio A. (2011). Plant polyphenols and their anti-cariogenic properties: A Review. *Molecules*, 16:1486–1507.

Fischer P.M. and Lane D.P. (2000). Inhibitors of cyclin-dependent kinases as anti-cancer therapeutics. *Current Medicinal Chemistry*, 7: 1213–1245.

Fry S. (1982). Phenolic components of the primary cell wall. *Biochemical Journal*, 203: 493–504.

Grabber J.H., Ralph J., and Hatfield R.D. (2000). Cross-linking of maize walls by ferulate dimerization and incorporation into lignin. *Journal of Agricultural and Food Chemistry*, 48: 6106–6113.

Halliwell B., Rafter J., and Jenner A. (2005). Health promotion by flavonoids, tocopherols, tocotrienols, and other phenols: direct or indirect effects? Antioxidant or not? *American Journal of Clinical Nutrition*, 81: 268S–276S.

Hartley R.D., Morrison W.H., Himmelsbach D.S., and Borneman W.S. (1990). Cross-linking of cell wall phenolic arabinoxylans in *Graminaceous* plants. *Phytochemistry*, 29: 3705–3709.

He Q., Lv Y., and Yao K. (2007). Effects of tea polyphenols on the activities of alpha-amylase, pepsin, trypsin and lipase. *Food Chemistry*, 101: 1178–1182.

Hedren E., Diaz V., and Svanberg U. (2002). Estimation of carotenoid accessibility from carrots determined by an in vitro digestion method. *European Journal of Clinical Nutrition*, 56: 425–430.

Heo H., Kim Y., Chung D., and Kim D. (2007). Antioxidant capacities of individual and combined phenolics in a model system. *Food Chemistry*, 104: 87–92.

Hussain T., Gupta S., Adhami V.M., and Mukhtar H. (2005). Green tea constituent epigallocatechin-3-gallate selectively inhibits COX-2 without affecting COX-1 expression in human prostate carcinoma cells. *International Journal of Cancer*, 113: 660–669.

Iiyama K., Lam T.B.T., and Stone B.A. (1990). Phenolic acid bridges between polysaccharides and lignin in wheat internodes. *Phytochemistry*, 29: 733–737.

Iiyama K., Lam T.B.T., and Stone B.A. (1994). Covalent cross-links in the cell wall. *Plant Physiology*, 104: 315–320.

Ishii T. and Hiroi T. (1990). Linkage of phenolic acids to cell-wall polysaccharides of bamboo shoot. *Carbohydrate Research*, 206: 297–310.

Jones J.M. (2014). CODEX-aligned dietary fiber definitions help to bridge the 'fiber gap'. *Nutrition Journal*, 13: 34.

Koh L.W., Wong L.L., Loo Y.Y., Kasapis S., and Huang D. (2010). Evaluation of different teas against starch digestibility by mammalian glycosidases. *Journal of Agricultural and Food Chemistry*, 58: 148–154.

Koh-Banerjee P., Franz M., Sampson L., Liu S., Jacobs Jr.,, D.R., Spiegelman, D., Willett W., and Rimm E. (2004). Changes in wholegrain, bran, and cereal fibre consumption in relation to 8-y weight gain among men. *American Journal of Clinical Nutrition*, 80: 1237–1245.

Kong A.N., Yu R., Chen C., Mandlekar S., and Primiano T. (2000). Signal transduction events elicited by natural products: Role of MAPK and caspase pathways in homeostatic response and induction of apoptosis. *Archives of Pharmacal Research*, 23: 1–16.

Konishi Y., Zhao Z., and Shimizu M. (2006). Phenolic acids are absorbed from the rat stomach with different absorption rates. *Journal of Agriculture and Food Chemistry*, 54: 7539–7543.

Kulp K.S., Fortson S.L., Knize M.G., and Felton J.S. (2003). An in vitro model system to predict the bioaccessibility of heterocyclic amines from a cooked meat matrix. *Food and Chemical Toxicology*, 41: 1701–1710.

Kusano R., Andou H., Fujieda M., and Kouno I. (2008). Polymer-like polyphenols of black tea and their lipase and amylase inhibitory activities. *Chemical and Pharmaceutical Bulletin*, 56: 266–272.

Lafay S. and Gil-Izquierdo A. (2008). Bioavailability of phenolic acids. *Phytochemistry Reviews*, 7: 301–311.

Lafay S., Gil-Izquierdo A., Manach C., Morand C., Besson C., *et al.* (2006). Chlorogenic acid is absorbed in its intact form in the stomach of rats. *Journal of Nutrition*, 136: 1192–1197.

Leifert W.R. and Abeywardena M.Y. (2008). Grape seed and red wine polyphenol extracts inhibit cellular cholesterol uptake, cell proliferation, and 5-lipoxygenase activity. *Nutrition Research*, 28: 842–850.

Liu S., Stampfer M.J., Hu F.B., Giovannucci E., Rimm E., Manson J.E., Hennekens C.H., and Willett W.C. (1999). Whole-grain consumption and risk of coronary heart disease: results from the Nurses' Health Study. *American Journal of Clinical Nutrition*, 70: 412–419.

Liyana-Pathirana C. and Shahidi F. (2005). Antioxidant activity of commercial soft and hard wheat (*Triticum aestivum* L.) as affected by gastric pH conditions. *Journal of Agricultural and Food Chemistry*, 53: 2433–2440.

Liyana-Pathirana C.M. and Shahidi F. (2007). Antioxidant and free radical scavenging activities of whole wheat and milling fractions. *Food Chemistry*, 101: 1151–1157.

Liyana-Pathirana C.M., Dexter, J., and Shahidi F. (2006). Antioxidant properties of wheat as affected by pearling. *Journal of Agricultural and Food Chemistry*, 54: 6177–6184.

Madhujith T. and Shahidi F. (2007). Antioxidative and antiproliferative properties of selected barley cultivars and their potential of inhibition of copper induced LDL cholesterol oxidation. *Journal of Agricultural and Food Chemistry*, 55: 5018–5024.

Masella R., Vari R., D'Archivio M., Di Benedetto R., Matarrese P., Malorni W., Scazzocchio B., and Giovannini C. (2004). Extra virgin olive oil biophenols inhibit cell-mediated oxidation of LDL by increasing the mRNA transcription of glutathione-related enzymes. *Journal of Nutrition*, 134: 785–791.

McDougall G.J., Shpiro F., Dobson P., Smith P., Blake A., and Stewart D. (2005). Different polyphenolic components of soft fruits inhibit alpha-amylase and alpha-glucosidase. *Journal of Agricultural and Food Chemistry*, 53: 2760–2766.

Mekeehen J.D., Busch R.H., and Fulcher, R.G. (1999). Evaluation of wheat (*Triticum aestieum* L.) phenolic acids during grain development and their contribution to Fusarium resistence. *Journal of Agricultural and Food Chemistry*, 47: 1476–1482.

Mildner-Szkudlarz S., Zawirska-Wojtasiak R., Szwengiel A., and Pacyński M. (2011). Use of grape by-product as a source of dietary fibre and phenolic compounds in sourdough mixed rye bread. *International Journal of Food Science and Technology*, 46: 1485–1493.

Monasterio A., Urdaci M.C., Pinchuk I.V., Lopez-Moratalla N., and Martinez-Irujo J.J. (2004). Flavonoids induce apoptosis in human leukemia U937 cells through caspase-and caspase-calpain-dependent pathways. *Nutrition and Cancer*, 50: 90–100.

Motomura Y. and Yoshida Y. (2002). Antioxidative ability of cell wall components in fruits against ascorbic acid oxidation. *Paper presented at the XXVI International Horticultural Congress: Issues and Advances in Postharvest Horticulture*, 628.

Murphy K.J., Chronopoulos A.K., Singh I., Francis M.A., Moriarty H., Pike M.J., Turner A.H., Mann N J., and Sinclair A.J. (2003). Dietary flavanols and procyanidin oligomers from cocoa (*Theobroma cacao*) inhibit platelet function. *American Journal of Clinical Nutrition*, 77: 1466–1473.

Naasani I., Oh-Hashi F., Oh-Hara T., Feng W.Y., Johnston J., Chan K., and Tsuruo T. (2003). Blocking telomerase by dietary polyphenols is a major mechanism for limiting the growth of human cancer cells in vitro and in vivo. *Cancer Research*, 63:824–830.

Naczk M. and Shahidi F. (2006). Phenolics in cereals, fruits and vegetables: occurrence, extraction and analysis. *Journal of Pharmaceutical and Biomedical Analysis*, 41: 1523–1542.

Naczk M., Oickle D., Pink D., and Shahidi F. (1996). Protein precipitating capacity of crude canola tannins: effect of pH, tannin, and protein concentrations. *Journal of Agricultural and Food Chemistry*, 44: 2144–2148.

Naczk M., Grant S., Zadernowski R., and Barre E. (2006). Protein precipitating capacity of phenolics of wild blueberry leaves and fruits. *Food Chemistry*, 96, 640–647.

Noratto G., Porter W., Byrne D., and Cisneros-Zevallos L. (2009). Identifying peach and plum polyphenols with chemopreventive potential against estrogen-independent breast cancer cells. *Journal of Agricultural and Food Chemistry*, 57: 5219–5126.

O'Leary K.A., de Pascual-Tereasa S., Needs P.W., Bao Y.P., O'Brien N.M., and Williamson G. (2004). Effect of flavonoids and vitamin E on cyclooxygenase-2 (COX-2) transcription. *Mutation Research*, 551: 245–254.

Padayachee A., Netzel G., Netzel M., Day L., Zabaras D., Mikkelsen D., and Gidley M. (2012a). Binding of polyphenols to plant cell wall analogues – Part 1: Anthocyanins. *Food Chemistry*, 134: 155–161.

Padayachee A., Netzel G., Netzel M., Day L., Zabaras D., Mikkelsen D., and Gidley M. (2012b). Binding of polyphenols to plant cell wall analogues – Part 2: Phenolic acids. *Food Chemistry*, 135: 2287–2292.

Palafox-Carlos H., Ayala-Zavala J.F., and Gonzalez-Aguilar G.A. (2011). The role of dietary fiber in the bioaccessibility and bioavailability of fruit and vegetable antioxidants. *Journal of Food Science*, 76: 6–15.

Palafox-Carlos H., Yahia E., Islas-Osuna M., Gutierrez-Martinez P., Robles-Sanchez M., and Gonzalez-Aguilar G. (2012). Effect of ripeness stage of mango fruit (*Mangifera indica* L., cv. Ataulfo) on physiological parameters and antioxidant activity. *Scientia Horticulturae*, 135: 7–13.

Parada J. and Aguilera J.M. (2007). Food microstructure affects the bioavailability of several nutrients. *Journal of Food Science*, 72: R21–R32.

Pérez-Jiménez J., Arranz S., Tabernero M., Díaz-Rubio M.E., Serrano J., Goñi I., and Saura-Calixto F. (2008). Updated methodology to determine antioxidant capacity in plant foods, oils and beverages: Extraction, measurement and expression of results. *Food Research International*, 41: 274–285.

Pérez J., Serrano J., Tabernero M., Arranz S., Díaz M.E., García L., Goñi I., and Saura-Calixto F. (2009). Bioavailability of phenolic antioxidants associated with dietary fiber: plasma antioxidant capacity after acute and long-term intake in humans. *Plant Foods for Human Nutrition*, 64: 102–107.

Porrini M. and Riso P. (2008). Factors influencing the bioavailability of antioxidants in foods: a critical appraisal. *Nutrition, Metabolism and Cardiovascular Diseases*, 18: 647–650.

Prigent S.P.V.E., Gruppen H., Visser A.J.W.G., Van Koningsveld G.A., De Jong G.A.H., and Voragen A.G.J. (2003). Effects of non-covalent interactions with

5-o-caffeoylquinic acid (chlorogenic acid) on the heat denaturation and solubility of globular proteins. *Journal of Agricultural and Food Chemistry*, 51: 5088–5095.

Quirós-Sauceda A.E., Ayala-Zavala J.F., Sáyago-Ayerdi S.G., Vélez-de la Rocha R., Sañudo-Barajas J.A., and González-Aguilar G.A. (2014). Added dietary fiber affects antioxidant capacity and phenolic compounds content extracted from tropical fruit. *Journal of Applied Botany and Food Quality*, 87: 227–233.

Randhir R., Lin Y., and Shetty K. (2004). Phenolics, their antioxidant and antimicrobial activity in dark germinated fenugreek sprouts in response to peptide and phytochemical elicitors. *Asia Pacific Journal of Clinical Nutrition*, 13: 295–307 .

Rawel H. and Rohn S. (2010). Nature of hydroxycinnamate-protein interactions. *Phytochemistry Reviews*, 9: 93–109.

Rawel H.M., Meidtner K., and Kroll J. (2005). Binding of selected phenolic compounds to proteins. *Journal of Agricultural and Food Chemistry*, 53: 4228–4235.

Rawel H.M., Frey S.K., Meidtner K., Kroll J., and Schweigert F.J. (2006). Determining the binding affinities of phenolic compounds to proteins by quenching of the intrinsic tryptophan fluorescence. *Molecular Nutrition and Food Research*, 50: 705–713.

Renard C.M., Baron A., Guyot S., and Drilleau J.F. (2001). Interactions between apple cell walls and native apple polyphenols: quantification and some consequences. *International Journal of Biological Macromolecules*, 29: 115–125.

Rock C.L. and Swendseid M.E. (1992). Plasma beta-carotene response in humans after meals supplemented with dietary pectin. *American Journal of Clinical Nutrition*, 55: 96–99.

Rombouts F.M. and Thibault J.F. (1986). Feruloylated pectic substances from sugar beet pulp. *Carbohydrate Research*, 154: 177–188.

Rosales Soto M.U., Brown K., and Ross C.F. (2012). Antioxidant activity and consumer acceptance of grape seed flour-containing food products. *International Journal of Food Science and Technology*, 47: 592–602.

Rosenblat M. and Aviram M. (2009). Paraoxonases role in the prevention of cardiovascular diseases. *Biofactors*, 35: 98–104.

Ryan D. and Robards K. (1998). Phenolic compounds in olives. *Analyst*, 123: 31R–44R.

Sadik C.D., Sies H., and Schewe T. (2003). Inhibition of 15-lipoxygenases by flavonoids: Structure-activity relations and mode of action. *Biochemical Pharmacology*, 65: 773–781.

Sánchez-Tena S., Daneida Lizárraga D., Miranda A., Vinardell M.P., García-García F., Dopazo J., *et al.* (2013). Grape antioxidant dietary fiber inhibits intestinal polyposis in ApcMin/+ mice: relation to cell cycle and immune response. *Carcinogenesis*, 34: 1881–1888.

Saura-Calixto F. (1998). Antioxidant dietary fiber product:a new concept and a potential food ingredient. *Journal of Agricultural and Food Chemistry*, 46: 4303–4306.

Saura-Calixto F. (2011). Dietary fiber as a carrier of dietary antioxidants: an essential physiological function. *Journal of Agricultural and Food Chemistry*, 59: 43–49.

Saura-Calixto F. (2012). Concept and health related properties of non-extractable polyphenols: the missing dietary polyphenols. *Journal of Agricultural and Food Chemistry*, 60: 11195–11200.

Saura-Calixto F. and Díaz-Rubio M.E. (2007). Polyphenols associated with dietary fibre in wine: a wine polyphenols gap? *Food Research International*, 40: 613–619.

Saura-Calixto F., Serrano J., and Goñi I. (2007). Intake and bioaccessibility of total polyphenols in a whole diet. *Food Chemistry*, 101: 492–501.

Schewe T., Sadik C., Klotz L.O., Yoshimoto T., Kuhn H., and Sies H. (2001). Polyphenols of cocoa: Inhibition of mammalian 15-lipoxygenase. *Biological Chemistry*, 382: 1687–1696.

Serrano J., Puupponen-Pimia R., Dauer A., Aura A.M., and Saura-Calixto F. (2009). Tannins: current knowledge of food sources, intake, bioavailability and biological effects. *Molecular Nutrition and Food Research*, 53: 310–329.

Shahidi F. (2002). Phytochemicals in oilseeds. In *Phytochemicals in Nutrition and Health*. CRC Press, Boca Raton, Florida, pp. 139–156.

Shahidi F. and Ambigaipalan P. (2015). Phenolics and polyphenolics in foods, beverages and species: Antioxidant activity and health effects: A review, *Journal of Functional Foods*, doi:10.1016/j.jff.2015.06.018.

Shahidi F. and Naczk M. (2004). *Phenolics in Food and Nutraceuticals*. CRC Press, Boca Raton, FL, pp. 1–82.

Shahidi F., Alasalvar C., and Liyana-Pathirana C.M. (2007). Antioxidant phytochemicals in hazelnut (*Corylus avellana* L.) and its by-products. *Journal of Agricultural and Food Chemistry*, 55: 1212–1220.

Spencer J.P., Rice-Evans C., and Williams R.J. (2003). Modulation of pro-survival Akt/protein kinase B and ERK1/2 signaling cascades by quercetin and its in vivo metabolites underlie their action on neuronal viability. *Journal of Biological Chemistry*, 278: 34783–34793.

Steffen L.M., Jacobs D.R., Stevens J., Shahar E., Carithers T., and Folsom A.R. (2003). Associations of whole-grain, refined grain, and fruit and vegetable consumption with risks of all-cause mortality and incident coronary artery disease and ischemic stroke: the Atherosclerosis Risk in Communities (ARIC) Study. *American Journal of Clinical Nutrition*, 78: 383–390.

Sun-Waterhouse D., Melton L.D., O'Connor C.J., Kilmartin P.A., and Smith B.G. (2007). Effect of apple cell walls and their extracts on the activity of dietary antioxidants. *Journal of Agricultural and Food Chemistry*, 56: 289–295.

Sun-Waterhouse D., Smith B.G., O'Connor C.J., and Melton L.D. (2008). Effect of raw and cooked onion dietary fibre on the antioxidant activity of ascorbic acid and quercetin. *Food Chemistry*, 111: 580–585.

Sudha M. L., Baskaran V., and Leelavathi K. (2007). Apple pomace as a source of dietary fiber and polyphenols and its effect on the rheological characteristics and cake making. *Food Chemistry*, 104: 686–692.

US Department of Agriculture (2015) *Dietary Guidelines for Americans 2015–2020* (8th edn.). https://health.gov/dietaryguidelines/2015/guidelines/ (accessed August 17, 2016).

Vitaglione P., Napolitano A., and Fogliano V. (2008). Cereal dietary fibre: a natural functional ingredient to deliver phenolic compounds into the gut. *Trends in Food Science and Technology*, 19: 451–463.

Wang X., Geng, X., Egashira Y., and Sanada H. (2004). Purification and characterization of a feruloyl esterase from the intestinal bacterium *Lactobacillus acidophilus*. *Applied and Environmental Microbiology*, 70: 2367–2372.

Way T.D., Kao M.C., and Lin, J.K. (2005). Degradation of HER2/neu by apigenin induces apoptosis through cytochrome c release and caspase-3 activation in HER2/neu-overexpressing breast cancer cells. *FEBS Letters*, 579: 145–152.

Wijerathne S.S.K., Amarowicz R., and Shahidi F. (2006). Antioxidant activity of almond and their by-products in food model systems. *Journal of the American Oil Chemists' Society*, 83: 223–230.

Wiseman S., Mulder T., and Rietveld A. (2001). Tea flavonoids: Bioavailability in vivo and effects on cell signaling pathways in vitro. *Antioxidants and Redox Signalling*, 3: 1009–1021.

Whelton S.P., Hyre A.D., Pedersen B., Yi Y., Whelton P.K., and He J. (2005). Effect of dietary fiber intake on blood pressure: a meta analysis of randomized, controlled clinical trials. *Journal of Hypertension*, 23: 475–481.

Wu Y., Chen Z., Li X., and Li M. (2009). Effect of tea polyphenols on the retrogradation of rice starch. *Food Research International*, 42: 221–225.

Xiao, H., Lin Q., Liu G-Q., Wu Y., Tian W., Wu W., *et al.* (2011). Effect of green tea polyphenols on the gelatinization and retrogradation of rice starches with different amylose contents. *Journal of Medicinal Plants Research*, 5: 4298–4303.

Zajácz A., Gyemant G., Vitton N., and Kandra L. (2007). Aleppo tannin: structural analysis and salivary amylase inhibition. *Carbohydrate Research*, 342: 717–723.

Zhong Y., Shahidi F., and Naczk M. (2012). Phytochemicals and health benefits of goji berries. In *Composition, Phytochemicals and Health Applications of Dried Fruits* (eds. C. Alasalvar and F. Shahidi). Wiley-Blackwell, Oxford, pp. 133–144.

Zhu F., Cai Y-Z., Sun M., and Corke H. (2008). Effect of phenolic compounds on the pasting and textural properties of wheat starch. *Starch*, 60: 609–616.

Zhu F., Cai Y-Z., Sun M., and Corke H. (2009). Effect of phytochemical extracts on the pasting, thermal, and gelling properties of wheat starch. *Food Chemistry*, 112: 919–923.

3

Dietary Fiber-Enriched Functional Beverages in the Market

Aynur Gunenc[1], Farah Hosseinian[1] and B. Dave Oomah[2]

[1] *Food Science and Nutrition, Department of Chemistry, Carleton University, Ottawa, Ontario, Canada*
[2] *Retired, Formerly with Pacific Agri-Food Research Centre, Agriculture and Agri-Food Canada, Summerland, British Columbia, Canada*

3.1   Introduction

The market for functional foods has increased considerably in recent years because of scientific studies confirming the relationship between food and health. Many of the health benefits mentioned in the literature are attributed to dietary fiber due to their fermentation by gut microbiota and short-chain fatty acid (SCFA) production. Dietary fiber was defined in 1972 by Trowell as "that portion of food which is derived from cell walls of plants which are digested very poorly by human beings." In other words, prebiotic fibers are a food source that helps probiotics to grow and survive in our intestines. These prebiotics are non-digestible oligosaccharides (NDO), specifically fructo-oligosaccharides (FOS) and inulin, commonly recognized as a universal remedy to improve many physiological problems in humans.

There have been many reports about the addition of dietary fiber to food products, including baked goods, confectionary, dairy, soups, and beverages. As a food ingredient, dietary fiber can be added to food to provide function, such as bulking agents, improving/modification of texture, water/fat binding, or increasing viscosity and stability. This chapter focuses on applications of dietary fiber in food products and specifically beverages and non-dairy products, including carbonates, juices, nectars, flavored waters, and powdered drinks. Beverages are hydrating and satiating; bioactives/ingredients added to beverages reach their intended sites faster and are easily digested compared to solid food. However, beverages also impose many limitations to the use of bioactives/ingredients, such as solubility, dispersibility, viscosity, pH environment, shelf stability, and/or other constraints of dietary fiber-containing beverages.

According to a recent study of 187 countries, there are significant differences in current consumption levels for sugar-sweetened beverages, fruit juices, and milk in different countries (Singh *et al.*, 2015). This global analysis shows that consumption of all three categories is lowest in East Asia, whereas intakes of sugar-sweetened beverages is highest in the Caribbean where young (20–39 age

Dietary Fiber Functionality in Food and Nutraceuticals: From Plant to Gut, First Edition.
Edited by Farah Hosseinian, B. Dave Oomah and Rocio Campos-Vega.

group) were found to have the highest average consumption of 3.4 servings of sweetened beverages per day. Furthermore, younger adults consumed the highest levels of sugar-sweetened beverages, whereas older adults consumed more milk. Fortunately, carbonated soft drink consumption has decreased in the past 5 years, whereas the fermented beverage category has experienced the highest annual double-digit growth rates according to recent market research.

3.2   Dietary Fiber Definition and Classification

Dietary fiber includes a mixture of oligosaccharides and polysaccharides such as cellulose, hemicelluloses, gums, resistant starch, inulin, and other non-carbohydrate components (polyphenols, waxes, saponins, cutin, and phytates) (Rodríguez *et al.*, 2006; Yangilar, 2013). Depending on their intestinal solubility, Meyer (2004) defined dietary fiber as insoluble and soluble fiber. Insoluble fibers are lignin, cellulose, and hemicellulose, whereas soluble fibers are pectins, beta-glucans, galactomannans, and a large group of non-digestible oligosaccharides including inulin. Most dietary fiber components are indigestible, but they might be partially exposed to bacterial enzymatic degradation (Heredia *et al.*, 2002). This enzymatic degradation depends on the bacteria type, transit time through the colon, and the dietary fiber components (Kay, 1982; Meyer, 2004). Briefly, degradation starts with extracellular hydrolysis that converts polysaccharides into mono- and disaccharides, followed by intracellular anaerobic glycolysis, releasing acetate, propionate, and butyrate (Saura-Calixto and Goñi, 1993). In the small intestine, the main effect is related to the viscous polysaccharides such as pectins and gums that reduce nutrient incorporation, whereas the insoluble dietary fiber has limited/minimal effects. Bacterial mass is formed from the high fermentable substances, and the less water-holding fermentable substances are responsible for increased fecal bulk (Madar and Odes, 1990). Cereals are the main source of cellulose, lignin, and hemicelluloses, although fruits and vegetables are the principal sources of pectin, gums, and mucilage (Elleuch *et al.*, 2011). Different types and sources of dietary fiber are given in Table 3.1 (Mobley *et al.*, 2013).

3.3   Fiber-Enriched Non-Dairy Beverages

Dietary fiber exists naturally in many different foods, such as whole grain cereals, fruits, and vegetables. It includes polysaccharides, oligosaccharides, lignin, and associated plant substances and exhibits beneficial effects such as laxation (fecal bulking and softening), blood cholesterol and/or blood glucose attenuation. According to the 1994 definition of the National Academy of Sciences, Institute of Medicine, "functional foods are foods that encompass potentially healthful products, including any modified food or food ingredient that may provide a health benefit beyond the traditional nutrient it contains." In the United States, the NLEA (Nutrition Labeling and Education Act) of 1990 allows disease prevention

Table 3.1 The chemical composition and sources of dietary fiber.

Features	Name	Bonds between the subunits	References
Cellulose: fundamental constituent of plant cell walls: abundantly exists in vegetables, fruits, cereals, and legumes; accounts for up to 40% of secondary cell walls	Cellulose	β-(1,4) glucose	Bayer *et al.*, 1998; Tarchevskiĭ and Marchenko, 1991
Hemicellulose: bind to cellulose fibrils through hydrogen bonds; mostly found in cereals, various plants, including legumes, corn, olive, tomato, lettuce, carrot, onion, pepper, liverwort, etc.	β-Glucans	β-(1,4) glucose β-(1,3) glucose	Cui *et al.*, 2013
	Arabinoxylans	β-D-(1,4) xylose	Rose *et al.*, 2010
	Xylans	β-D-(1,4) xylose	Bastawde, 1992
	Mannans	β-D-(1,4) mannose	Hoffman *et al.*, 2005; Kato, 2001
	Inulin	β-(1,2)-D-fructosyl-fructose	Andrieux *et al.*, 1993; Timmermans *et al.*, 1993
	Galactomannans	β-D-(1,4) mannose β-D-(1,4) glucose	Cui *et al.*, 2013; Xing *et al.*, 2013
	Xyloglucans	β-(1,4) glucose	Cao and Ikeda, 2009
Pectin: coexisting with cellulose and hemicelluloses constituting the middle lamella; mostly found in soybean,mustard seed, dehulled rapeseed, honey locust seed, cabbage, and some fruits (e.g., apple, grapes)	Homogalacturonan	α-(1,4)-D-galacturonic acid	Vidal *et al.*, 2003
	Rhamnogalacturonan-I	(1−4) galacturonic acid, (1,2) rhamnose and 1-,2-,4-rhamnose	Oechslin *et al.*, 2003; L. Yu *et al.*, 2010
	Rhamnogalacturonan-II	α-(1,4) galacturonic acid	Yapo *et al.*, 2007
	Arabinanes	α-(1,5)-L-arabinofuranose	Aspinall and Cottrell, 1971
	Galactanes	β-(1,4)-D-galactopyranose	Pollard *et al.*, 2008
	Arabinogalactanes-I	β-(1,4)-D-galactopyranose	X. Zhang *et al.*, 2009
	Arabinogalactanes-II	β-(1,3)-and β-(1,6)-D-galactopyranose	Will and Dietrich, 1992
	Xylogalacturonan	α-(1,4) galacturonic acid	Mort *et al.*, 2008
Gums: hydrocolloids, increasing viscosity; vegetables are the primary sources; also found in oatmeal, haricot bean, legumes	Carrageenan	Sulfato-galactose	Préchoux *et al.*, 2013
	Alginate	β-(1,4)-D-mannuronic acid or α-(1,4)-L-guluronic acid	Agulhon *et al.*, 2012

claims but only a few claims are allowed after US Food and Drug Administration (FDA) requirements are met. Four types of claims are allowed: nutrient content, health, structure–function, and special dietary advantage claims (Prosky, 2000). The beneficial effects can be increased by increasing dietary fiber intake. Some examples are partially hydrolyzed guar gum (PHGG), Fibersol-2 (an indigestible dextrin made from corn starch), inulin, and BeFlora (a fructo-oligosaccharide and transgalactosylated oligosaccharides).

Today, many fiber ingredients are more suitable for use in beverages than traditional cereal or fruit-based fibers, due to their higher solubility and clarity in solution. With the extraction and manufacture of fiber from alternative sources, fortifying drinks have become a reality, making beverages a valid dietary fiber source (Kendall *et al.*, 2010). Adding fibers to beverages is becoming popular because of new soluble fiber ingredients and the potential consumer benefits. These benefits include improving the nutritional profile by reducing the sugar content of the product per serving. Moreover, concentrated and processed fruit juice products often have decreased levels of fiber from their starting material. Therefore, fruit juices made from concentrate are good candidates for producing fiber-fortified beverages (Viscione, 2013). The technical, functional, physical, and nutritional characteristics of dietary fiber are important variables to be considered in the development of new beverages.

3.3.1 Addition of Dietary Fiber into Beverages

Product composition and process parameters for beverage production directly affect texture and stability. Hence, the planned characteristic for the final beverage product dictates the choice of the most appropriate dietary fiber to use in production. Processing conditions such as homogenization, heat treatment, and filling temperature are also important parameters. Moreover, the physical properties, digestive tolerance, and nutritional composition are critical factors that can determine consumer appeal and therefore the choice of fiber for fortification.

In powdered drinks, the physical properties such as particle size, bulk density, particle shape, and hygroscopicity of fibers need to fit with the proposed drink, whereas in ready-to-drink (RTD) beverages, solubility, dispersibility, acid stability, and clarity/transparency are more important characteristics (Viscione, 2013). The stability requirements for beverage productions depend on the quality of ingredients, process, and product shelf life. For instance, instability in acidic conditions of RTD beverages can result in hydrolysis of the fiber ingredient. Depending on the source of dietary fiber, a dramatic loss in fiber content can occur in the drink, resulting in it not fulfilling its nutritional product claim throughout its proposed shelf life. Any instability in the product is undesirable and may cause many physical changes, such as increased sweetness level over time, loss of mouthfeel, stability, texture, and increase in color or fiber precipitation.

Another parameter to consider when formulating a beverage is digestive tolerance, a complex and important issue. It depends on the product matrix, its viscosity, drinking occasion, price, and marketing angle. However, a beverage has the potential to be consumed in fairly large quantities in a very short time; it might put the consumer at risk of overconsumption, and the undesirable consequences of this situation are unacceptable. The physical properties of dietary fiber mentioned above subsequently affect the digestion of a product. In addition, the dose in the product, the drink matrix, consumption time and frequency, other food consumed with the drink, and individual sensitivities should be considered (Marteau and Flourié, 2001). Some of the adverse effects of consuming too much dietary fiber are laxation and gastrointestinal effects, such as abdominal discomfort, flatus, and diarrhea, especially at higher or excessive intakes. It should be emphasized that this unacceptability level is very individual and not easy to define. In general, there is an adjustment period at the beginning and tolerance improves over time when ingesting low-digestible carbohydrates (Grabitske and Slavin, 2009).

3.4 Suitable Dietary Fiber Types for Fortifying Non-Dairy Drinks

3.4.1 β-Glucans

Although β-glucans are mainly present in cereals, including wheat, rye, barley, and oats, they are commercially available from oats or barley in significant amounts. Both oat and barley extracts can be used in beverage formulations. Beta-glucans are linear polysaccharides consisting of β-(1−3)- and β-(1−4)-linked glucosidyl subunits. Their physical properties are controlled by the molecular structure, which is responsible for the technological features and potential of the β-glucans ingredient. Commercially available β-glucans vary greatly from each other in terms of content, viscosity, flavor, and residual materials (Wood *et al.*, 1991). Impaired glucose metabolism is a growing problem in the world, and foods that attenuate the glycemic response are being recognized as beneficial in controlling the metabolic syndrome, coronary heart disease, and type 2 diabetes (Brand-Miller *et al.*, 2003). Oat products have been reported to elicit low postprandial glycemic responses and this effect has been attributed to the presence of the soluble fiber β-glucans (Behall *et al.*, 2005). β-Glucan-enriched beverages have been extensively investigated for their health benefits (Table 3.2). These studies demonstrate that beverages containing β-glucan enhance satiety, reduce hunger, and improve lipid metabolism by reducing serum total and LDL cholesterols and glycemic parameters. Some of the observed responses varied depending on β-glucan dose and molecular weight.

3.4.2 Inulin

Inulin and related products such as fructo- or galacto-oligosaccharides (FOS or GOS) exert satiety benefits from other prebiotic fibers. For example, a recent study indicated that increased doses of alpha-GOSs led to increased effects on food intakes and appetite measurements, as well as levels of the inflammatory biomarkers, lipopolysaccharide (LPS), and C-reactive protein (CRP) (Morel *et al.*, 2015). Inulin is naturally found in many fruits and vegetables, including bananas, artichokes, and chicory (Tungland, 2003). It can be used to modify the rheology

Table 3.2 β-Glucan-enriched beverage intake studies and related health benefits.

Fiber source	Subjects	Design	Results	Reference
Oat bran (4 g β-glucan)	30 healthy females (24 years)	Crossover, single-blind	Enhanced satiety when added to juice	Pentikäinen *et al.*, 2014
High β-glucan extruded oat bran flour; drink powder (30 g)	12 diabetic patients (66 ± 7 years)	Randomized, controlled, repeated measures design	Reduced postprandial glycemic response of external glucose given simultaneously	Tapola *et al.*, 2005
Fermented oat milk	62 free-living subjects with high plasma cholesterol		Reduced total cholesterol (6%, $p = 0.022$)	Mårtensson and Öste, 2004
Oat or barley β-glucan beverage; daily intake of 5 or 10 g β-glucan per 500 mL	89 free-living hypercholesterolaemic adults (mean age 53–59 years)	8 weeks (with 3 weeks run in) single-blind, randomized dose-controlled study; 5 parallel groups	Oat β-glucan (5 g) in a beverage improved lipid (7.4% serum cholesterol reduction) and glucose metabolism; barley β-glucan had no significant effect.	Biorklund *et al.*, 2005
Oat milk (0.5 g β-glucan/100 g); 70 mL/day	52 men with moderate hypercholesterolemia	5-week randomized, controlled, double-blind study with 5 weeks washout period	Oat milk significantly reduced serum total serum and LDL cholesterols (6%)	Önning *et al.*, 1999
Oat β-glucan (5 g) enriched fruit drink	47 adults (18 male/29 female)	Placebo-controlled, double-blind parallel design	β-Glucan reduced serum total and LDL cholesterol	Naumann *et al.*, 2006
Barley β-glucan (BBG) beverage (3 or 6 g/day)	44 healthy adults with baseline hyperglycemia (mean age 56 years)	12 weeks randomized, double-blind, placebo-controlled, parallel group intervention	6 g BBG/day consumed in a beverage improved insulin sensitivity (glycemic parameters) (reduced postprandial glycemia and insulinemia)	Bays *et al.*, 2011

Soup containing 3.5 g oat β-glucan (80 kDa)/day for 8 weeks	53 (21 female/31 men) mildly obese (BMI 30 kg/m^2) diabetic subjects (mean age 62 years)	Parallel, placebo-controlled, blind, randomized trial	Blood lipid profile and glucose control remained unchanged	Cugnet-Anceau *et al.*, 2010
Barley β-glucan 6 g/day (low or high molecular weight)	90 hypercholesterolemic adults (mean age 45 years)	Randomized, double-blind parallel group design	High molecular weight BBG consumption for 6 weeks reduced hunger and body weight and exhibited hypocholesterolemic effects	Smith *et al.*, 2008
Isoenergetic and isovolumic high-fiber oat bran beverage differing in viscosity (mPas); low (<250) or high (>3000)	20 (16 female/4 male) healthy young adults (mean age 22.6 years)	Single-blind, randomized, crossover design	High-viscosity oat bran induced smaller postprandial glucose and insulin responses than low-viscosity beverage.	Juvonen *et al.*, 2009
Beverage with added oat fiber ingredient (DF = 0, 5, and 10 g)	29 (18 female/11 male) healthy young adults (19 – 39 years)	Measurement of subjective perceptions was performed during a 180-min period after ingestion of the sample	β-Glucan rich oat ingredient added to beverage curbed hunger and increased satiety	Lyly *et al.*, 2010
Isoenergetic SDF liquid (oat β-glucan 7.5 g, 500 mL, 500 Kcal)	30 (13 female/17 male) type 2 diabetic adults (mean age 66 years)	Prospective, randomized crossover study	SDF improved postprandial glycemia by delaying gastric emptying	Yu *et al.*, 2014

(*continued overleaf*)

Table 3.2 (Continued)

Fiber source	Subjects	Design	Results	Reference
Juice enriched with oat β-glucan (OatWell 22% β-glucan, 0.38 g/100 mL) or β-glucan/xanthan gum (0.23/0.09 g/100 mL)	14 healthy non-smoking male subjects (mean age 32 years)	Randomized crossover design, each subject consumed 4 juices	β-Glucan alone or in xanthan gum mixture attenuated the incremental glucose peak	Paquin *et al.*, 2012
Oat drink (6 g β-glucan in 150 mL water + 300 mL glucose drink [Glucodex])	11 (5 male/6 female) healthy adults (mean age 34 years)	Randomized, double-blind crossover study	High-viscosity oat β-glucan improves postprandial glycaemic control	Panahi *et al.*, 2007
Beverage supplemented with purified high (580 kg/mol) or low (145 kg/mol) molecular weight oat β-glucan (4 g) in 250 or 600 mL	15 (8 female/7 male) healthy adults (mean age 37 years)	Randomized, controlled block design with repeated measures	Glycemic response depended on β-glucan dose and molecular weight.	Kwong *et al.*, 2013
Soup containing barley β-glucan with high (650 kDa) or low (150 kDa) molecular weight	15 (12 female/3 male) healthy adults (mean age 28 years)	Randomized, balanced, controlled crossover, single-blind repeated measures design	High molecular weight (650 kDa) barley β-glucan delayed gastric emptying due to high viscosity	Thondre *et al.*, 2013

BBG, barley β-glucan; SDF, soluble dietary fiber.

and texture of food products since combined with other ingredients it can compete with other polysaccharides for binding water molecules. If inulin concentration exceeds 15%, it can form a gel or cream (Coussement and Franck, 2001). Inulin is relatively heat stable under normal conditions, however under high temperatures combined with low pH and/or longer processing conditions, loss can occur. For instance at low pH (3.0–4.0) values in soft drinks, inulin products have a tendency to be susceptible to acid hydrolysis and may break down to fructose during shelf life (Klewicki, 2007). At higher pH (>4), breakdown to fructose is limited. The degree of hydrolysis is dependent on pasteurization time and temperature.

Inulin has gained most attention as a fiber source in dairy products since its well-known prebiotic effect on the growth of probiotic bifidobacteria in the colon (Granato *et al.*, 2010). Inulin from chicory can be hydrolyzed to make short chains or fractionated into short-chain and long-chain fractions. The short-chain oligofructose (FOS) is more soluble and sweeter than native inulin, whereas the long-chain inulin is more viscous in solution. Long-chain inulin is also reported to have fat-replacing potential because of its capacity to form aggregates of microcrystals. This property has led to inulin being added to ice cream, yogurts, beverages, and some desserts (Villegas and Costell, 2007).

Inulin digestion has been very well studied and is found to be well tolerated at doses around 20 g/day with only minor digestive complaints. This statement has been supported by other studies (Ellegård *et al.*, 1997; Van Dokkum *et al.*, 1999). The addition of inulin into products fulfills a role in nutritional content and has potential health benefits.

Inulin is a natural food fiber found in more than 30,000 plants, including fruits and vegetables. The inulin from chicory root is one of the best-researched fibers in the world. Over 20 years of nutrition research on chicory root fiber inulin has resulted in 133 human intervention studies, delivering strong evidence for seven distinct physiological benefits: prebiotic effect, bowel function, satiety/energy intake, body weight and blood glucose management, mineral, particularly calcium absorption, and blood glucose postprandial. Some of these physiological benefits have been demonstrated in beverages (Table 3.3).

Inulin, often referred as chicory root fiber, is highly soluble and known in the industry as "the invisible fiber." Furthermore, it can be added to prebiotics without a large impact on the product's functionality or appearance, improving the taste and texture by serving as a fat mimetic and sugar substitute. It is now available in liquid form, making it more convenient to use in beverage processing.

3.4.3 Flaxseed Dietary Fiber

Flaxseed (*Linum usitatissimum* L.) is one of the most important oilseed crops, the third in production after canola and soybean in Canada. It is rich in soluble and insoluble dietary fiber compared to other oilseeds and cereals such as wheat, barley, oat, and soybean (Dhingra *et al.*, 2012). The total dietary fiber of whole flaxseed is ~28%, with ~5–8% soluble dietary fiber, often referred to as flaxseed gum or mucilage. The acidic fraction from flaxseed mucilage is composed of rhamnogalacturonan-I (RG-I) (Qian *et al.*, 2012). Flaxseed hull contains the

Table 3.3 Inulin-enriched beverage intake studies and related health benefits.

Fiber source	Subjects	Design	Results	Reference
Tea containing α-GOSs (6, 12, or 18 g/day for 2 weeks), or a control substance (glucose syrup). Plasma lipopolysaccharide (LPS) and C-reactive protein were evaluated	88 overweight adults (50% men and 50% women; 18–60 years old; BMI 25–28 kg/m^2)	Double-blind, randomized, placebo-controlled trials	Consumption of α-GOSs dose-dependently reduced appetite, food intake, and inflammation in overweight adults. α-GOSs appear to promote long-term weight loss and mitigate metabolic disorders	Morel *et al.*, 2015
Enteral formula containing 50 g/L fiber blend (50:50 insoluble/soluble; pea hull fiber + inulin + FOS+ gum acacia)	20 (10 male/10 female) healthy adults average age 26 years	Randomized, double-blind, crossover design, 14 days with a 4-week washout	Fiber blend exerted prebiotic effect, increased fecal weight, and unaffected the overall gastrointestinal quality-of-life scores	Koecher *et al.*, 2015
ITF (inulin/oligofructose 50/50 mix) 16 g (8 g twice daily) added in warm drinks (coffee, tea, hot chocolate, or dairy products)	30 obese (BMI >30 kg/m^2) women, average age 47 ± 9 years	Randomized, double-blind, placebo-controlled intervention	ITF intervention modulated gut microbiota incurring favorable changes in fat mass, serum LPS levels and metabolism	Dewulf *et al.*, 2012
Chicory root extract (0.25 g inulin/100 mL) 300 mL daily for 4 weeks	47 (8 male/39 female) healthy adults (average age 53 ± 12 years)	Randomized, double-blind, placebo-controlled study	Chicory root extract improved hyperglycemia and bowel movement	Nishimura *et al.*, 2015
Coffee MOS (4 g/day) twice daily for 12 weeks	54 (20 male/34 female) healthy overweight adults (average age 47 years, BMI 30 kg/m^2)	Randomized, double-blind, placebo-controlled design	MOS reduced total body volume and weight in men	Salinardi *et al.*, 2010
Inulin FOS (0.4 g/100 mL)-enriched prebiotic infant formula	56 healthy preterm (maximum gestational age 36 weeks) infants; 36 (16 male/17 female) in the FOS group; maltodextrin placebo 20 (8 male/12 female) infants	Randomized, prospective, double-blind study for 14 days	Inulin stimulated bifidobacteria in the gut while decreasing pathogenic micoorganisms	Kapiki *et al.*, 2007

Highly branched cyclic dextrin (HBCD)	7 male triathletes in 2 duathlon races separated by 1 month	Randomized, double-blind, placebo-controlled, crossover design	HBCD-based drink reduced urinary cytokine levels following exhaustive exercise and may attenuate stress hormone response	Suzuki *et al.*, 2014
High-energy beverages containing 3 soluble fibers: dextrin, polydextrose, and corn fiber (12 g/370 g)	36 (14 male/22 female) healthy young (20–34 years) adults completed 6 testing over 6 weeks	Latin square design, double-blind study	Soluble fiber dextrin reduced energy intake significantly compared to polydextrose or soluble corn fiber relative to isoenergic control.	Monsivais *et al.*, 2011
Agave fructans (0.5 g/100 mL) infant formula	600 healthy term babies (20 ± 7 days), weight ≥2 490 g	Randomized, double-blind, clinical controlled trial	Agave fructans in infant formula was safe and well tolerated similar to human milk	López-Velázquez *et al.*, 2013
Enteral tube fed formula containing FOS (10.6 g fiber + 7 g FOS/liter) for 8 weeks	6 (5 male/1 female) stable head and neck cancer tube-fed patients, average age 55.5 years	Prospective, randomized, double-blind pilot study	FOS stimulated bifidobacteria growth and improved gastrointestinal quality of life	Wierdsma *et al.*, 2009
Maltodextrin Fibersol-2, 0, 5, or 10 g in tea	19 (9 male/10 female) healthy adults (average age 36 ± 16 years; mean BMI 25 kg/m^2)	Randomized, double-blind, placebo-controlled crossover design	10 g of Fibersol-2 delayed hunger and increased satiety significantly by regulating appetite hormones	Ye *et al.*, 2015
Konjack-mannan or guar gum/xanthan gum (0.82 or 0.69 g/300 mL) in apple juice	20 healthy young (28 ± 7 years) men	Randomized, crossover study	Fiber-enriched juice reduced postprandial appetite without affecting glucose homeostasis	Paquet *et al.*, 2014
Agave fructans (3–30 degree of polymerization; 5 g/day in 300 mL H$_2$O)	38 (19 male/19 female) healthy adults (average age 35 years, BMI 24 kg/m^2)	Randomized, double-blind, placebo-controlled, crossover study for 3 weeks followed by a 2-week washout period	Agave fructans modulated gut bacteria and their fermentation profiles with profound effects on bowel habits	Ramnani *et al.*, 2015

major insoluble fiber fractions cellulose, hemicellulose, and lignin (Johnsson *et al.*, 2000).

Flaxseed is the richest plant-based source of alpha-linolenic acid (ALA) in the North American diet and is a functional supplement for people at risk of cardio-vascular diseases, diabetes, and constipation, with a cholesterol-lowering effect (Edel *et al.*, 2015). It is also a crucial ingredient in gluten-free and vegetarian diets (Morris, 2001).

Flaxseed polysaccharides have shown promise as novel food ingredients, but little is known about their effects when added to food emulsions. The major monosaccharides are L-galactose, D-xylose, L-rhamnose, and D-galacturonic acid. Some other constituents such as L-arabinose, D-glucose, and L-fucose are also present in the gum but in smaller amounts (Oomah *et al.*, 1995). Many epidemiological studies and animal and human clinical trials suggest a role for flax in the prevention and treatment of chronic diseases such as heart diseases (Zhao *et al.*, 2007), diabetes (Hilpert *et al.*, 2007), cancers (Lord *et al.*, 2002), and osteoporosis (Griel *et al.*, 2007). Studies with flaxseed dietary fiber-enriched beverages (Table 3.4) demonstrate their blood cholesterol-lowering, increased fat excretion, appetite-suppressing and metagenomic-modulating effects in humans.

3.5 Contributions of Beverages in Dietary Studies

Beverages are excellent carriers for ingredients with nutraceutical potential, such as soluble fiber or herbal extracts, and are an essential part of a healthy diet, since adequate fluid intake is a prime requirement for optimal urinary, gastrointestinal, and cognitive function and maintaining blood glucose homeostasis. According to the Institute of Medicine, total fluid requirement is defined as consuming 1 mL liquid per 1 kcal food, whereby beverages provide 10–14% of food energy (Duffey and Davy, 2015). However, the contribution of beverages is generally not taken into account in most dietary recalls and/or calculations in clinical studies, thereby underestimating the physiological benefits of beverage constituents. Furthermore, fluid intake from beverages may have a synergistic effect with dietary fiber intake, and increasing dietary liquid intake is considered the most important modifiable factor in improving chronic constipation in a population-based study (Markland *et al.*, 2013).

Dietary fiber is essential, particularly when beverages are the only food source, for example in infant and enteral feeding, and the intestinal microbiota is important in health and disease. Beverages are the sole food source for preterm infants/neonates, whose immature gut must acquire a healthy complement of commensal bacteria. The inulin-like fructans short-chain galacto-oligosaccharides (scGOS) and long-chain fructo-oligosaccharides (lcFOS) are prebiotics that are widely used in infant feeding due to their commercial availability as infant milk formulas.

A recently updated review and meta-analysis, which included a total of seven studies with 417 preterm babies, concluded that the use of the prebiotic oligosaccharides (GOS and/or FOS) enhanced beneficial commensal

Table 3.4 Flaxseed-enriched beverage intake studies and related health benefits.

Fiber source	Subjects	Design	Results	Reference
Flaxseed oil (2.5, 5, and 10 mL/kg) and flaxseed mucilage (10 and 20 mg/kg)	Male Wistar rats (165–250 g) were fasted 36 hours before starting the experiments. Animals randomly divided into 5 groups of 6 rats	A rat model of ethanol-induced gastric ulcer	Pretreatment of rats with flaxseed oil and flaxseed mucilage significantly reduced the number and length of gastric ulcer induced by ethanol	Dugani *et al.*, 2008
Flaxseed oil (30 and 70 mg/kg, orally) and flaxseed mucilage (1 and 2.5 g/kg, orally)	BALB-C mice (20–25 g), local breed rabbits (1–1.5 kg), and guinea-pigs (300–400 g), of either gender	20 mice were divided into 4 groups. The test was performed using increasing doses	Flaxseed oil and mucilage exhibit laxative activity, mediated primarily through cholinergic pathway with weak histaminergic effect component evident in flaxseed oil	Hanif Palla and Gilani, 2015
Flaxseed gum (5 g) was incorporated in wheat flour chapattis	60 patients of type 2 diabetes were fed a daily diet for 3 months, along with 6 wheat flour chapattis containing flaxseed gum	Blood biochemistry profiles monitored before starting the study and at monthly intervals	Results showed a decrease in low-density lipoprotein cholesterol from 110 ± 8 mg/dL to 92 ± 9 mg/dL ($p = 0.02$)	Thakur *et al.*, 2009
A low fiber diet (control), a diet with flaxseed fiber drink (3/day) (flax drink), and a diet with flaxseed fiber bread (3/day) (flax bread)	17 young subjects (10 women and 7 men), total fat and energy excretion was measured in feces, blood samples were collected before and after each period	Double-blind randomized crossover study	Both flax drink and flax bread resulted in decreased plasma total and LDL cholesterol and increased fat excretion. Viscous flaxseed dietary fibers may be a useful tool for lowering blood cholesterol	Kristensen *et al.*, 2012
A daily intake of either *L. paracasei* F19 (9.4 log colony-forming units), flaxseed mucilage (10 g) or placebo	58 obese postmenopausal women, metagenomic analysis of fecal DNA to identify the changes in the gut microbiota	Randomized to a single-blind, parallel-group intervention of 6-week duration	A reduction in serum C-peptide, improved insulin sensitivity, gut microbiota composition with flaxseed mucilage showed alterations in abundance of 33 metagenomic species	Brahe *et al.*, 2015
(I) Control (300 mL) vs. flax drink (control drink with 2.5 soluble fiber); and (II) flax drink vs. flax tablet (2.5 g soluble fiber)	24 and 20 subjects were exposed to one of the treatments after an overnight fast, rated appetite sensation for 120 min using visual analog scales (VAS)	Two single-blind randomized crossover acute studies	Flaxseed fiber significantly suppresses appetite, and flaxseed fibers administered as drinks or tablets produce similar responses	Ibrügger *et al.*, 2012

bacterial growth and can potentially restore a healthy balance of gut microbiota (Srinivasjois *et al.*, 2013). The number of pathogenic microorganisms (*E.coli* and enterococci) decreases simultaneously due to the bifidogenic effects of these dietary fiber. Fructans derived from agave also exert safe and effective prebiotic effects in terms of gastrointestinal health in infant formula similar to those of GOS and FOS (López-Velázquez *et al.*, 2013). Fructo-oligosaccharides (containing 10.6 g fiber [4.5 g oat, 3.6 g soy polysaccharides, 1.7 g gum arabic, and 0.8 g carboxymethylcellulose] and 7 g FOS per liter) positively benefited intestinal flora by stimulating bifidobacterial growth of tube-feeding-dependent home-living adult patients in a randomized, double-blind study (Wierdsma *et al.*, 2009). Fiber-blend (50:50 insoluble:soluble mixture of fructo-oligosaccharides and inulin, pea hull fiber, and gum acacia) fortified enteral formula (15 g/L) increased fecal weight and moderated decreases in total bacteria and bifidobacteria (prebiotic effect/gut microbiota) compared with fiber-free formula in healthy adults ($n = 20$; 10 male + 10 female, 26 years old). The fiber-blend fortification did not affect the overall gastrointestinal quality of life scores for subjects consuming formula diets (Koecher *et al.*, 2015).

Dietary fiber intake is of prime importance in the elderly, who are generally known to have reduced bifidobacteria, resulting in decreased immunity. This demographic is also affected by a high incidence of constipation because of dietary habits and often have poor swallowing/chewing ability and so often rely on easily ingestible beverages. Prebiotic fiber (1:1 oligofructose:inulin 8 g/day for 16 weeks) also increases satiety response and reduces energy intake, body fat, and the risk of co-morbidities in overweight and obese children (7–12 years) (Hume *et al.*, 2015).

3.6 The Functional Beverage Market

The functional beverage market has grown due to consumer demand for convenience, preference for natural ingredients, healthy diet and novel innovations, and developments such as "juiceceuticals" – fruit–yogurt beverages that enables fiber supplementation/addition to the diet. Beverages generally contribute appreciably to soluble dietary fiber intake, which is estimated to be 2.13 g/person/day in the Spanish Mediterranean diet (Diaz-Rubio and Saura-Calixto, 2011). Soluble dietary fiber in beverages ranges from 0.8 g/L in white wine to 9.01 g/L in instant coffee, and 4.7–7.5 g/L in brewed coffee rich in antioxidant phenolics (0.87–1.05 mg/L of brewed coffee); its omission may lead to underestimated dietary fiber intakes. Commercial brands of dairy drinks and milks purchased from supermarkets in Recife, Brazil contained 0.65–3.33 g/100 g and 1.50–9.52 g/100 g dietary fiber, respectively (Silva *et al.*, 2013). Inulin was the most common dietary fiber used in these dairy products, followed by GOS/FOS and gums (acacia, xanthan), probably because fructans, inulin, and FOS are by far the most studied prebiotics. In fact, inulin or oligofructose have been found to be the most successful applications in dairy products such as skim milk-based drinks and/or fermented milk/drink due primarily to improved viscosity, mouthfeel, and prebiotic effects. The sweet taste of FOS has made it useful in fortification of pineapple, mango, and orange juice beverages (0.345–0.379 g FOS per liter) (Renuka *et al.*, 2009).

Solubility is the quintessential functional characteristic enabling the use of dietary fiber in beverages. It leads to increased viscosity that reduces the reabsorption of bile acids responsible for the well-known cholesterol-lowering effect of β-glucans. Sometimes, emulsion functionality (capacity and stability) enhance and extend the use of dietary fiber in ensuring thermodynamic stability and targeted delivery in the gastrointestinal tract. For example, inulin has been hydrophobically modified to improve its emulsifying performance under biorelevant conditions of the human gastric and intestinal digestion (Meshulam *et al.*, 2014). The anionic low methoxy pectin inhibits large dense flocs formation in caseinate-stabilized oil-in-water emulsion, thereby modulating the gastrointestinal fate and digestion of emulsified lipids (Zhang *et al.*, 2015). Thus, soluble dietary fiber can slow gastric emptying, thereby reducing postprandial glucose response, total cholesterol, and low-density lipoproteins. Common beverages also contain polyphenols bound to dietary fiber (constituting 2.9–62.8% of soluble dietary fiber in apple juice and red tea, respectively); these polyphenols determine the physiological properties of dietary fiber in humans, since they form the fermentable substrate for bacterial microflora in the colon (Goñi *et al.*, 2009). Cereal beverages have been produced by lactobacilli fermentation, with those formulated with *Lactobacillus plantarum* exhibiting greatest acceptance and highest acetaldehyde concentration (Salmerón *et al.*, 2015). In fact *L. plantarum* cultures (LP09 and A28) have often been used to ferment oat flakes (25%, w/w) or oat flour (5.5%), producing a yogurt-like beverage or oat drink providing over 3 g/day of β-glucan, fulfilling the European Food Safety Authority (EFSA) criteria for products containing β-glucan (Angelov *et al.*, 2006; Luana *et al.*, 2014). Consumption of fermented oat-based product (co-fermented with an exopolysaccharide-producing strain, *Pediococcus damnosus* 2.6) for 5 weeks reduced cholesterol level and stimulated the bifidobacteria flora in the gastrointestinal tract of free-living volunteers with high plasma cholesterol levels (Mårtensson and Öste, 2004). Regulations and health claims relating to intake of β-glucan have also spurred developments of beverages that can reasonably supply the daily requirements and modify physiological response.

Dietary fiber from novel sources has been used in beverages. For example, partially hydrolyzed galactomannan (1.5 g/100 g) from the seed of *Caesalphinia pulcherrima*, a plant from the Fabaceae family, largely found in Brazil, increased total dietary fiber content (>2.5×) of goat-dairy beverages containing fruit (guava or soursoup 15 g/100 g) pulp (Buriti *et al.*, 2014). However, the source of dietary fiber can have variable health effects. This was elegantly demonstrated in a randomized, single-blind crossover study comparing the modulating effects of fiber addition from three sources (oat bran, flaxseed, and unripe banana flour) to shakes (Cândido *et al.*, 2015). The isocaloric shakes increased dietary fiber intake but exerted no hypoglycemic effect, except for unripe banana flour that reduced postprandial glycemic response of shakes by nearly half (43%) due to high resistant starch (17.5%) content. These authors surmised that gut transit time of liquid meals may not be adequate to increase viscosity of soluble fibers responsible for the hypoglycemic effect. Fiber substrate was strongly associated with dynamic changes in the composition of gut bacteria, differentiating the effect of galacto-oligosaccharides, lactulose, apple fiber, and sugar beet pectin in an *in vitro* fermentation study with human colonic microbiota of lean (BMI 23 kg/m^2) and obese (BMI 33 kg/m^2) healthy subjects (Aguirre *et al.*, 2014).

Beverage is a good delivery functional system for dietary fiber targeted for digestion. This has been elegantly described by contrasting two studies where consumption of a small amount (4 g) of non-caloric soluble psyllium fiber with water suppressed postprandial plasma ghrelin concentrations in healthy subjects. By contrast, postprandial ghrelin (a gut hormone) did not decrease after the ingestion of a 300 kcal solid meal enriched with a substantial (23 g) amount of psyllium fiber (Salmenkallio-Marttila *et al.*, 2009). Table 3.5 summarizes examples of fiber available for use in beverages (www.preparedfoods.com). Ingredient suppliers are finding niche markets for drinks, primarily fruit juices or enhanced waters with added soluble fiber. For example, Tropicana orange juice is enriched with 3 g FiberSol-2 soluble fiber per 8-ounce (240 mL) serving.

3.7 Fiber-Enriched Dairy Products

Dairy products, such as beverages, puddings, yogurts, and frozen desserts, can be suitable carriers for fiber enrichment, and consumers are interested in consuming such products for health benefits. Polysaccharides, including guar, locust bean gum, sodium alginate, sodium carboxymethyl cellulose, and xanthan, have been added to dairy products for many years as thickeners and gelling agents. Soluble fibers reduce the risk of developing cardiovascular diseases primarily by lowering blood cholesterol levels, decreasing carbohydrate absorption rate from the small intestine and from fermentation in the large intestine producing SCFAs (acetate, propionate, and butyrate), and promoting healthy balance of colonic microflora (Tungland and Meyer, 2002; Viuda-Martos *et al.*, 2010). It is well documented that the gastrointestinal microbiota impacts overall health and the types as well as quantity of microbiota can be changed by dietary factors, especially prebiotics and probiotics (Douglas, 2008). This also affects consumers' decisions in buying probiotic-containing foods for relief of specific conditions or to improve overall health (Tulk *et al.*, 2013).

Dairy beverages contain low-fat milks (1–2%), sweeteners, thickening agents, and flavors. Sweeteners are added to develop a sweetness equivalent to 4–6% sucrose, and thickening agents such as cellulose gum or guar gum are added at 0.35–0.60% concentration, as well as emulsifiers such as mono- and diglycerides. Vanilla, chocolate, and banana flavors are popular choices for dairy beverages. Acidified dairy products are one of the oldest types of food products but all of them are low in dietary fiber. To improve the health benefits of these products, enrichment with dietary fiber seems an attractive solution. For instance, Nutrinova has developed Caromax, an insoluble dietary fiber derived from the pulp of the carob tree (*Ceratonia siliqua*) as an ingredient that enables manufacturers to capitalize on consumers' concern for health and wellbeing. This

Table 3.5 Industrial fibers used in beverages (www.preparedfoods.com)

Industrial ingredient/ source	Formulations	Benefits	Company
Fibersol® (corn-based, soluble fiber)	Reduce sugar and calories, meet clean label goals, create products that help promote digestive tract health or simply boost the fiber content of a food or beverages	Minimal viscosity; no added flavor, taste, or color and low hygroscopicity in dry formulations, it may help support structure–function claims in qualifying finished products	ADM/Mtsutani LLC
Tea brewer and formulator	Create better testing, better looking teas that are easy to manufacture, deliver consistency of product from batch	Beautiful finished product clarity, ease of use, robust brewed flavor profiles, authentic color and mouth feel	Amelia Bay
Wellmune (a proprietary strain of yeast, β 1,3/1,6 glucan	Provide consumers the immune health benefits	Help to strengthen the immune system, making it easier for consumers to be well and stay well	Biothera
PROFI (vegetable protein solution containing all 9 essential amino acids in proper proportions and fiber)	No flavor masking required	Available in a variety of formulations and gluten-free	Dealers Ingredients Inc.
Prolactal/Rovita	Optimize the texture and sensory experience	Functional ingredients	ICL Food Specialties
Jungbunzlauer (renewable carbohydrate raw materials derived from corn)	Improve flavor and texture	Combination of consistency and taste	Jungbunzlauer

(*continued overleaf*)

Table 3.5 (Continued)

Industrial ingredient/ source	Formulations	Benefits	Company
Sunmalt®-S (from enzymatic processing of starch)	Mask both off-flavors and odors, while retaining flavor quality during shelf life	Prevents starch retrogradation, enhances flavors in food systems	Nagase
Fibregum, Floracia, Equacia, Nexira (natural acacia gum)	Emulsifiers, stabilizer, texturizers	Prebiotic properties and health benefits	Nexira Inc.
Frutalose®SFP (chicory root fiber)	Effective sugar replacer, mask high-intensity sweeteners such as stevia and sucralose	Functional benefits, easy way to increase dietary fiber and improve nutritional profile, prebiotic fiber	Sensus America Inc.
Gum Gurus (guar plant)	Advanced texture and stabilization solutions	Improve the texture, stability, consistency, nutritional profile and shelf life	Tic Gums
Chia seeds	Supports digestive health, strengthens immune systems	Prebiotic in a symbiotic smoothie	Kunahcia
Drinkable savory yogurt	Over 30% more vegetable puree	Easy way to boost vegetable consumption	Blue Hill
Fructo-oligosaccharide/sugar cane/soy protein	Functional, tasteless	Blended solution for vegetarian protein, fiber fortification	ProFi
Peanut milk	Smooth, slightly creamery mouthfeel	All natural ingredients, taste similar to cow's milk	National Peanut Board

Table 3.6 Fiber-enriched dairy beverage intake studies and related health benefits.

Fiber source	Subjects	Design	Results	Reference
High/low-energy-density (0.9/0.4 kcal/g) yogurt beverage (472 mL) containing 6 g inulin	38 (18 male/20 female) healthy young (18–35 years) adults/participants completed 6 test sessions spaced 1 week apart	A within-subject preload design with repeated measures	Inulin increased postprandial satiety power of low-energy-density yogurt	Perrigue *et al.*, 2009
Fiber-enriched (polydextrose 3 g/200 mL) milk consumed on 3 non-consecutive study days	26 (10 male/16 female) healthy adults (age range 25–64; mean BMI 24.6)	Randomized response profile block design	Fiber-enriched milk reduced insulin response and equalized glucose response	Lummela *et al.*, 2009b
200 g/day of yogurt with (synbiotic) or without (control) added probiotics (*Bifidobacterium lactis* Bb12, *Lactobacillus acidophilus* La5, *Lactobacillus casei* CRL431) and 4 g inulin for two 15-day treatment periods	65 healthy adults GI transit time (GTT), duration of color (DOC), GI symptoms and dietary intake were assessed	Randomized crossover double-blind study	GTT and DOC were not different between synbiotic and control. Consuming 200 g/day of synbiotic yogurt did not significantly alter GTT in healthy adults, but was well tolerated and helped to reduce overall energy intake	Tulk *et al.*, 2013

(continued overleaf)

Fiber source	Subjects	Design	Results	Reference
(1) A lactose-free milk drink, (2) a novel fiber-enriched, fat-and lactose-free milk drink and (3) normal fat-free milk	26 healthy volunteers ingested 200 mL of one of these drinks on three non-consecutive days, serum glucose and insulin levels were measured (20, 40, 60, 120, and 180 minutes after ingestion)	Randomized block design	The insulin response was significantly lower for the fiber-enriched milk drink than it was for the other milk products	Lummela *et al.*, 2009a
The incorporation of *Lactobacillus acidophilus*, *Lactobacillus casei* 475, and *Bifidobacterium bifidum* together with lemon (LF) and orange (OF) fibers obtained from juice by-products were tested	A model system: (i) fiber enriched with each probiotic bacteria and (ii) evaluation of populations of probiotic bacteria in fermented milks formulated with citrus fibers	Yogurt starter bacteria in probiotic fermented milks favored the growth and survival of *L. acidophilus* and *B. bifidum.*	Citrus fiber enriched fermented milk have good acceptability and are good vehicles for a variety of commercial probiotics but survival of *B. bifidum* will need to be improved	Sendra *et al.*, 2008
Flaxseed gum and soy-soluble polysaccharides	12 healthy males, a glucose reference, glucose solutions containing soy-soluble polysaccharides (6%), flaxseed gum (0.7%), or guar gum (0.23%)	Randomized crossover postprandial study, Blood samples were collected at fasting and up to 2 hours for glucose and insulin concentrations	No significant differences were observed between the fiber-fortified fluid and gelled dairy-based study treatments and no significant differences were observed in terms of the insulin	Au *et al.*, 2013

tree is generally found in the Mediterranean region, but also grows in Arizona, Australia, and some parts of Latin America. Application studies showed that around 3–5 g of carob fiber can be used in an 8-ounce (240 mL) dairy drink (Van Mol, 2003).

People with diets either high in dairy calcium or high in fiber (low glycemic index) tend to be less obese than those with low dairy calcium and low fiber (high glycemic index) diets according to epidemiological studies. Controlled studies show that diets high in dairy calcium are beneficial for weight loss during calorie restriction periods (Thompson *et al.*, 2005). In that study a combined high-dairy/high-fiber diet (500 kcal/day) was investigated for weight-loss effects in obese subjects compared with normal diet. The results showed that diets high in dairy calcium and high in fiber are beneficial in weight loss, but the lack of significant differences may be due to high calorie restriction (Thompson *et al.*, 2005).

Table 3.6 provides an overview of some example applications of dietary fibers in dairy products and their potential health benefits. Combination of different prebiotic fibers (inulin and dextrin) with whey protein in a coffee beverage significantly reduced hunger and increased satiety compared to control in a large (269 people) human study (Singer *et al.*, 2016). Fermented milk beverages such as kefir have long been popular in Eastern and Central European countries, where they are consumed as part of traditional culture. In this regard we have investigated several sources of dietary fibers such as flaxseed flour and mucilage, faba bean flour, carob pod, pulp, seed flours, and pulp crude mucilage addition to kefir (HadiNezhad *et al.*, 2013; Boudjou *et al.*, 2014; Mahtout *et al.*, 2016). Pulse ingredients (pea fiber, chickpea flour, and lentil flour) have also been investigated in the development of orange and apple juice supplemented beverages (Zare *et al.*, 2015). The study showed that the pulse ingredients can be used at 1–2% level supplementation based on their physical, technical, and sensory properties. Another novel cold-pressed dairy-free beverage made from raw cacao beans (RAU) is a low/no-sugar drink that looks like chocolate milk and contains 9 g of dietary fiber per 8-ounce (240 mL) serving (Watson, 2016). It is also rich in phenolics, with an indulgent flavor profile for the benefit of health-focused consumers.

References

Aguirre, M., Jonkers, M.A., Troost, F.J., Roeselers, G., and Venema, K. (2014). In vitro characterization of the impact of different substrates on metabolite production, energy extraction and composition of gut microbiota from lean and obese subjects. *PLoS One*, 9(11), e113864.

Agulhon, P., Robitzer, M., David, L., and Quignard, F. (2012). Structural regime identification in ionotropic alginate gels: influence of the cation nature and alginate structure. *Biomacromolecules*, 13(1), 215–220. doi: 10.1021/bm201477g

Andrieux, C., Lory, S., Dufour-Lescoat, C., de Baynast, R., and Szylit, O. (1993). Inulin fermentation in germ-free rats associated with a human intestinal flora from methane or non-methane producers. In Studies in Plant Science, *Vol. 3* (ed. A. Fuchs). Elsevier, Amsterdam, pp. 381–384

Angelov, A., Gotcheva, V., Kuncheva, R., and Hristozova, T. (2006). Development of a new oat-based probiotic drink. *International Journal of Food Microbiology*, 112(1), 75–80. doi: 10.1016/j.ijfoodmicro.2006.05.015

Aspinall, G.O. and Cottrell, I.W. (1971). Polysaccharides of soybeans. *VI. Neutral polysaccharides from cotyledon meal. Canadian Journal of Chemistry*, 49(7), 1019–1022. doi: 10.1139/v71-169

Au, M.M.C., Goff, H.D., Kisch, J.A., Coulson, A., and Wright, A.J. (2013). Effects of soy-soluble fiber and flaxseed gum on the glycemic and insulinemic responses to glucose solutions and dairy products in healthy adult males. *Journal of the American College of Nutrition*, 32(2), 98–100. doi: 10.1080/07315724.2013.767579

Bastawde, K.B. (1992). Xylan structure, microbial xylanases, and their mode of action. *World Journal of Microbiology and Biotechnology*, 8(4), 353–368. doi: 10.1007/bf01198746

Bayer, E.A., Chanzy, H., Lamed, R., and Shoham, Y. (1998). Cellulose, cellulases and cellulosomes. *Current Opinion in Structural Biology*, 8(5), 548–557. doi: 10.1016/S0959-440X(98)80143-7

Bays, H., Frestedt, J.L., Bell, M., Williams, C., Kolberg, L., Schmelzer, W., and Anderson, J.W. (2011). Reduced viscosity barley β-glucan versus placebo: a randomized controlled trial of the effects on insulin sensitivity for individuals at risk for diabetes mellitus. *Nutrition and Metabolism*, 8, 58–58. doi: 10.1186/1743-7075-8-58

Behall, K.M., Scholfield, D.J., and Hallfrisch, J. (2005). Comparison of hormone and glucose responses of overweight women to barley and oat. *Journal of the American College of Nutrition*, 24, 182–118.

Biorklund, M., van Rees, A., Mensink, R.P., and Onning, G. (2005). Changes in serum lipids and postprandial glucose and insulin concentrations after consumption of beverages with [beta]-glucans from oats or barley: a randomised dose-controlled trial. *European Journal of Clinical Nutrition*, 59(11), 1272–1281.

Boudjou, S., Zaidi, F., Hosseinian, F., and Oomah, B.D. (2014). Effects of faba bean (*Vicia faba* L.) flour on viability of probiotic bacteria during kefir storage. *Journal of Food Research*, 3(6), 13–22.

Brahe, L.K., Le Chatelier, E., Prifti, E., Pons, N., Kennedy, S., Blædel, T., *et al.* (2015). Dietary modulation of the gut microbiota – a randomised controlled trial in obese postmenopausal women. *British Journal of Nutrition*, 114(3), 406–412. doi: 10.1017/s0007114515001786

Brand-Miller, J., Hayne, S., Petocz, P., and Colagiuri, S. (2003). Low-glycemic index diets in the management of diabetes: a meta-analysis of randomized controlled trials. *Diabetes Care*, 26, 2261–2267.

Buriti, F.C.A., Freitas, S.C., Egito, A.S., and dos Santos, K.M.O. (2014). Effects of tropical fruit pulps and partially hydrolysed galactomannan from *Caesalpinia pulcherrima* seeds on the dietary fibre content, probiotic viability, texture and sensory features of goat dairy beverages. *LWT – Food Science and Technology*, 59(1), 196–203. doi: 10.1016/j.lwt.2014.04.022

Cândido, F.G., Ton, W.T.S., and Alfenas, R.C.G. (2015). Addition of dietary fiber sources to shakes reduces postprandial glycemia and alters food intake. *Nutrición Hospitalaria*, 31(1), 299–306.

Cao, Y. and Ikeda, I. (2009). Antioxidant activity and antitumor activity (in vitro) of xyloglucan selenious ester and surfated xyloglucan. *International Journal of Biological Macromolecules*, 45(3), 231–235. doi: 10.1016/j.ijbiomac.2009.05.007

Coussement, P. and Franck, A. (2001). In *Handbook of Dietary Fiber* (eds. S. S. Cho and M. Dreher). Marcel Dekker, FL, pp. 721–736

Cugnet-Anceau, C., Nazare, J.-A., Biorklund, M., Le Coquil, E., Sassolas, A., Sothier, M., *et al.* (2010). A controlled study of consumption of β-glucan-enriched soups for 2 months by type 2 diabetic free-living subjects. *British Journal of Nutrition*, 103(03), 422–428. doi: 10.1017/S0007114509991875

Cui, S.W., Wu, Y., and Ding, H. (2013). The range of dietary fibre ingredients and a comparison of their technical functionality. In *Fibre-rich and Wholegrain Foods: Improving Quality* (eds. J.A. Delcour and K. Poutanen). Woodhead Publishing (Elsevier), UK, pp. 96–115.

Dewulf, E.M., Cani, P.D., Claus, S.P., Fuentes, S., Puylaert, P.G.B., Neyrinck, A.M., *et al.* (2012). Insight into the prebiotic concept: lessons from an explaratory, double blind intervention study with inulin-type fructans in obese women. *Gut*, 1–10. doi: 10.1136/gutjnl-2012-303304

Diaz-Rubio, M.E. and Saura-Calixto, F.D. (2011). Beverages have an appreciable contribution to the intake of soluble dietary fibre: a study in the Spanish diet. *International Journal of Food Sciences and Nutrition*, 62(7), 715–718. doi: 10.3109/09637486.2011.579950

Dhingra, D., Michael, M., Rajput, H., and Patil, R.T. (2012). Dietary fibre in foods: a review. *Journal of Food Science and Technology*, 49(3), 255–266.

Douglas, L.C. (2008). Probiotics and prebiotics in dietetics practice. *Journal of the American Dietetic Association*, 108(3), 510–521. doi: 10.1016/j.jada.2007.12.009

Duffey, K.J. and Davy, B.M. (2015). The Healthy Beverage Index is associated with reduced cardiometabolic risk in US adults: a preliminary analysis. *Journal of the Academy of Nutrition and Dietetics*, 115(10), 1682–1689. doi: 10.1016/j.jand.2015.05.005

Dugani, A., Auzzi, A., Naas, F., and Megwez, S. (2008). Effects of the oil and mucilage from flaxseed (*Linum usitatissimum*) on gastric lesions induced by ethanol in rats. *Libyan Journal of Medicine*, 3(4), 166–169. doi: 10.4176/080612

Edel, A.L., Rodriguez-Leyva, D., Maddaford, T.G., Caligiuri, S.P.B., Austria, J.A., Weighell, W., *et al.* (2015). Dietary flaxseed independently lowers circulating cholesterol and lowers it beyond the effects of cholesterol-lowering medications alone in patients with peripheral artery disease. *Journal of Nutrition*, 145(4), 749–757.

Ellegård, L., Andersson, H., and Bosaeus, I. (1997). Inulin and oligofructose do not influence the absorption of cholesterol, or the excretion of cholesterol, Ca, Mg, Zn, Fe or bile acids but increases energy excretion in ileostomy subjects. *European Journal of Clinical Nutrition*, 51(1), 1–5.

Elleuch, M., Bedigian, D., Roiseux, O., Besbes, S., Blecker, C., and Attia, H. (2011). Dietary fibre and fibre-rich by-products of food processing: Characterisation, technological functionality and commercial applications: A review. *Food Chemistry*, 124, 411–442.

Goñi, I., Díaz-Rubio, M.E., Pérez-Jiménez, J., and Saura-Calixto, F.D. (2009). Towards an updated methodology for measurement of dietary fiber, including associated polyphenols, in food and beverages. *Food Research International*, 42(7), 840–846. doi: 10.1016/j.foodres.2009.03.010

Grabitske, H.A., and Slavin, J. L. (2009). Gastrointestinal effects of low-digestible carbohydrates. *Critical Reviews in Food Science and Nutrition*, 49(4), 327–360. doi: 10.1080/10408390802067126

Granato, D., Branco, G.F., Cruz, A.G., Faria, J.D.A.F., and Shah, N.P. (2010). Probiotic dairy products as functional foods. *Comprehensive Reviews in Food Science and Food Safety*, 9(5), 455. doi: 10.1111/j.1541-4337.2010.00120.x

Griel, A.E., Kris-Etherton, P.M., Hilpert, K.F., Zhao, G., West, S.G., and Corwin, R.L. (2007). An increase in dietary n-3 fatty acids decreases a marker of bone resorption in humans. *Nutrition Journal*, 6(1), 2–2. doi: 10.1186/1475-2891-6-2

HadiNezhad, M., Duc, C., Han, N.F., and Hosseinian, F. (2013). Flaxseed soluble dietary fibre enhances lactic acid bacterial survival and growth in kefir and possesses high antioxidant capacity. *Journal of Food Research*, 2(5), 152–163.

Hanif Palla, A. and Gilani, A.-H. (2015). Dual effectiveness of flaxseed in constipation and diarrhea: Possible mechanism. *Journal of Ethnopharmacology*, 169, 60–68. doi: 10.1016/j.jep.2015.03.064

Heredia, A., Jiménez, A., Fernández-Bolaños, J., Guillén, R., and Rodríguez, R. (eds.). (2002). *Fibra Alimentaria.* Biblioteca de Ciencias, Madrid.

Hilpert, K.F., West, S.G., Kris-Etherton, P.M., Hecker, K.D., Simpson, N.M., and Alaupovic, P. (2007). Postprandial effect of n-3 polyunsaturated fatty acids on apolipoprotein B-containing lipoproteins and vascular reactivity in type 2 diabetes. *American Journal of Clinical Nutrition*, 85(2), 369.

Hoffman, M., Jia, Z., Peña, M.J., Cash, M., Harper, A., Blackburn II,, A.R., *et al.* (2005). Structural analysis of xyloglucans in the primary cell walls of plants in the subclass Asteridae. *Carbohydrate Research*, 340(11), 1826–1840. doi: 10.1016/j.carres.2005.04.016

Hume, M., Nicolucci, A., and Reimer, R. (2015). Prebiotic fiber consumption decreases energy intake in overweight and obese children. *FASEB Journal*, 29(1 Supplement).

Ibrügger, S., Kristensen, M., Mikkelsen, M.S., and Astrup, A. (2012). Flaxseed dietary fiber supplements for suppression of appetite and food intake. *Appetite*, 58(2), 490–495. doi: 10.1016/j.appet.2011.12.024

Johnsson, P., Kamal-Eldin, A., Lundgren, L.N., and Aman, P. (2000). HPLC method for analysis of secoisolariciresinol diglucoside in flaxseeds. *Journal of Agricultural and Food Chemistry*, 48(11), 5216–5219. doi: 10.1021/jf0005871

Juvonen, K.R., Purhonen, A.-K., Salmenkallio-Marttila, M., Lähteenmäki, L., Laaksonen, D.E., Herzig, K.L.-H., *et al.* (2009). Viscosity of oat bran-enriched beverages influences gastrointestinal hormonal responses in healthy humans. *Journal of Nutrition*, 139(3), 461–466. doi: 10.3945/jn.108.099945

Kapiki, A., Costalos, C., Oikonomidou, C., Triantafyllidou, A., Loukatou, E., and Pertrohilou, V. (2007). The effect of a fructo-oligosaccharide supplemented formula on gut flora of preterm infants. *Early Human Development*, 83, 335–339.

Kato, Y. (2001). Structure of plant cell walls and implications for nutrient acquisition. In *Plant Nutrient Acquisition* (eds. N. Ae, J. Arihara, K. Okada, and A. Srinivasan). Springer, Tokyo, pp. 276–296.

Kay, R.M. (1982). Dietary fiber. *Journal of Lipid Research*, 23, 221–242.

Kendall, C.W.C., Esfahani, A., and Jenkins, D.J.A. (2010). The link between dietary fibre and human health. *Food Hydrocolloids*, 24(1), 42–48. doi: org/10.1016/j.foodhyd.2009.08.002

Klewicki, R. (2007). The stability of gal-polyols and oligosaccharides during pasteurization at a low pH. *LWT – Food Science and Technology*, 40(7), 1259–1265. doi: 10.1016/j.lwt.2006.08.008

Koecher, K.J., Thomas, W., and Slavin, J.L. (2015). Healthy subjects experience bowel changes on enteral diets: addition of a fiber blend attenuates stool weight and gut bacteria decreases without changes in gas. *Journal of Parenteral and Enteral Nutrition*, 39(3), 337–343.

Kristensen, M., Jensen, M.G., Aarestrup, J., Petersen, K.E., Søndergaard, L., Mikkelsen, M.S., and Astrup, A. (2012). Flaxseed dietary fibers lower cholesterol and increase fecal fat excretion, but magnitude of effect depend on food type. *Nutrition and Metabolism*, 9(1), 8–8. doi: 10.1186/1743-7075-9-8

Kwong, M.G.Y., Wolever, T.M.S., Brummer, Y., and Tosh, S.M. (2013). Increasing the viscosity of oat β-glucan beverages by reducing solution volume does not reduce glycaemic responses. *British Journal of Nutrition*, 110(8), 1465–1471. doi: 10.1017/S000711451300069X

López-Velázquez, G., Díaz-García, L., Anzo, A., Parra-Ortiz, M., Llamosas-Gallardo, B., Ortiz-Hernández, A.A., *et al.* (2013). Safety of a dual potential prebiotic system from Mexican agave "Metlin® and Metlos®", incorporated to an infant formula to term newborn babies: a randomized controlled trial. *Revista de Investigación Clinica*, 65(6), 483–490.

Lord, R.S., Bongiovanni, B., and Bralley, J.A. (2002). Estrogen metabolism and the diet-cancer connection: rationale for assessing the ratio of urinary hydroxylated estrogen metabolites. *Alternative Medicine Review*, 7(2), 112–129.

Luana, N., Rossana, C., Curiel, J.A., Kaisa, P., Marco, G., and Rizzello, C.G. (2014). Manufacture and characterization of a yogurt-like beverage made with oat flakes fermented by selected lactic acid bacteria. *International Journal of Food Microbiology*, 185, 17–26. doi: 10.1016/j.ijfoodmicr0.2014.05.004

Lummela, N., Kekkonen, R.A., Jauhiainen, T., Pilvi, T.K., Tuure, T., Järvenpää, S., *et al.* (2009a). Effects of a fibre-enriched milk drink on insulin and glucose levels in healthy subjects. *Nutrition Journal*, 8(1), 45–45. doi: 10.1186/1475-2891-8-45

Lummela, N., Kekkonen, R.A., Jauhiainen, T., Pilvi, T.K., Tuure, T., Järvenpää, S., *et al.* (2009b). Effects of a fibre-enriched milk drink on insulin and glucose levels in healthy subjects. *Nutrition*, 8(1), 1–7. doi: 10.1186/1475-2891-8-45

Lyly, M., Ohls, N., Lähteenmäki, L., Salmenkallio-Marttila, M., Liukkonen, K.H., Karhunen, L., and Poutanen, K. (2010). The effect of fibre amount, energy level and viscosity of beverages containing oat fibre supplement on perceived satiety. *Food and Nutrition Research*, 54(21), 2149.

Madar, Z. and Odes, H.S. (eds.) (1990). *Dietary Fibre in Metabolic Diseases.* Karger, Basel.

Mahtout, R., Zaidi, F., Saadi, L.O., Boudjou, S., Oomah, B.D., HadiNezhad, M., *et al.* (2016). Carob (*Ceratonia silique* L.) supplementation affects kefir quality and antioxidant capacity during storage. *International Journal of Engineering and Techniques*, 2(2), 168–177.

Markland, A.D., Palsson, O., Goode, P.S., Burgio, K.L., Busby-Whitehead, J., and Whitehead, W.E. (2013). Association of low dietary intake of fiber and liquids with constipation: evidence from the National Health and Nutrition Examination Survey. *American Journal of Gastroenterology*, 108(5), 796–803.

Marteau, P. and Flourié, B. (2001). Tolerance to low-digestible carbohydrates: symptomatology and method. *British Journal of Nutrition*, 85(1), 17–21.

Mårtensson, O. and Öste, R. (2004). Changes in plasma lipids and faecal *Bifidobacterium* spp. in humans after consumption of fermented oat-based products for 5 weeks. In *Proceedings 7th International Oat Conference* (eds. P Peltonen-Sainio and M. Topi-Hulmi). Agrifood Research Reports 51. MTT Agrifood Research, Finland, p. 103.

Meshulam, D., Slavuter, J., and Lesmes, U. (2014). Behavior of emulsions stabilized by a hydrophobically modified inulin under bio-relevant conditions of the human gastro-intestine. *Food Biophysics*, 9(4), 416–423. doi: 10.1007/s11483-014-9353-4

Meyer, P.D. (2004). Nondigestible oligosaccharides as dietary fiber. *Journal of the Association of Official Analytical Chemists*, 87(3), 718–726.

Mobley, A.R., Slavin, J.L., and Hornick, B.A. (2013). The future of grain foods recommendations in dietary guidance. *Journal of Nutrition*, 143(9), 1–6.

Monsivais, P., Carter, B.E., Christiansen, M., Perrigue, M.M., and Drewnowski, A. (2011). Soluble fiber dextrin enhances the satiating power of beverages. *Appetite*, 56(1), 9–14. doi: 10.1016/j.appet.2010.10.010

Morel, F.B., Dai, Q., Ni, J., Thomas, D., Parnet, P., and Fança-Berthon, P. (2015). New data from University of Nantes illuminate findings in inflammation (alpha-galacto-oligosaccharides dose-dependently reduce appetite and decrease inflammation in overweight adults). *Journal of Nutrition*, 145, 75–83.

Morris, D.H. (2001). Essential nutrients and other functional compounds in flaxseed. *Nutrition Today*, 36(3), 159–162. doi: 10.1097/00017285-200105000-00012

Mort, A., Zheng, Y., Qiu, F., Nimtz, M., and Bell-Eunice, G. (2008). Structure of xylogalacturonan fragments from watermelon cell-wall pectin. Endopolygalacturonase can accommodate a xylosyl residue on the galacturonic acid just following the hydrolysis site. *Carbohydrate Research*, 343(7), 1212–1221. doi: org/10.1016/j.carres.2008.03.021

Naumann, E., van Rees, A.B., Önning, G., Öste, R., Wydra, M., and Mensink, R.P. (2006). β-Glucan incorporated into a fruit drink effectively lowers serum LDL-cholesterol concentrations. *American Journal of Clinical Nutrition*, 83(3), 601–605.

Nishimura, M., Ohkawara, T., Kanayama, T., Kitagawa, K., Nishimura, H., and Nishihira, J. (2015). Effects of the extract from roasted chicory (*Cichorium intybus* L.) root containing inulin-type fructans on blood glucose, lipid metabolism, and fecal properties. *Journal of Traditional and Complementary Medicine*, 5(3), 161–167. doi: 10.1016/j.jtcme.2014.11.016

Oechslin, R., Lutz, M.V., and Amadò, R. (2003). Pectic substances isolated from apple cellulosic residue: structural characterisation of a new type of rhamnogalacturonan I. *Carbohydrate Polymers*, 51(3), 301–310. doi: 10.1016/S0144–8617(02)00214-X

Önning, G., Wallmark, A., Persson, M., Åkesson, B., Elmståhl, S., and Öste, R. (1999). Consumption of oat milk for 5 weeks lowers serum cholesterol and LDL cholesterol in free-living men with moderate hypercholesterolemia. *Annals of Nutrition and Metabolism*, 43(5), 301–309.

Oomah, B.D., Kenaschuk, E.O., Cui, W., and Mazza, G. (1995). Variation in the composition of water-soluble polysaccharides in flaxseed. *Journal of Agricultural and Food Chemistry*, 43(6), 1484–1488. doi: 10.1021/jf00054a013

Panahi, S., Ezatagha, A., Temelli, F., Vasanthan, T., and Vuksan, V. (2007). β-Glucan from two sources of oat concentrates affect postprandial glycemia in relation to the level of viscosity. *Journal of the American College of Nutrition*, 26(6), 636–644.

Paquet, É., Bédard, A., Lemieux, S., and Turgeon, S.L. (2014). Effects of apple juice-based beverages enriched with dietary fibers and xanthan gum on the glycemic response and appetite sensations in healthy men. *Bioactive Carbohydrates and Dietary Fibre*, 4, 39–47.

Paquin, J., Bédard, A., Lemieux, S., Tajchakavit, S., and Turgeon, S.L. (2012). Effects of juices enriched with xanthan and β-glucan on the glycemic response and satiety of healthy men. *Applied Physiology, Nutrition, and Metabolism*, 38(4), 410–414. doi: 10.1139/apnm-2012-0207

Pentikäinen, S., Karhunen, L., Flander, L., Katina, K., Meynier, A., Aymard, P., *et al.* (2014). Enrichment of biscuits and juice with oat β-glucan enhances postprandial satiety. *Appetite*, 75, 150–156. doi: 10.1016/j.appet.2014.01.002

Perrigue, M.M., Monsivais, P., and Drewnowski, A. (2009). Added soluble fiber enhances the satiating power of low-energy-density liquid yogurts. *Journal of the American Dietetic Association*, 109(11), 1862–1868. doi: 10.1016/j.jada.2009.08.018

Pollard, A., St. Michael, F., Connor, L., Nichols, W., and Cox, A. (2008). Structural characterization of *Haemophilus parainfluenzae* lipooligosaccharide and elucidation of its role in adherence using an outer core mutant. *Canadian Journal of Microbiology*, 54(11), 906–917. doi: 10.1139/w08-082

Préchoux, A., Genicot, S., Rogniaux, H., and Helbert, W. (2013). Controlling carrageenan structure using a novel formylglycine-dependent sulfatase, an endo-4S-iota-carrageenan sulfatase. *Marine Biotechnology*, 15(3), 265–274. doi: 10.1007/s10126-012-9483-y

Prosky, L. (2000). When is dietary fiber considered a functional food? *BioFactors*, 12, 289–297.

Qian, K.Y., Cui, S.W., Wu, Y., and Goff, H.D. (2012). Flaxseed gum from flaxseed hulls: Extraction, fractionation, and characterization. *Food Hydrocolloids*, 28(2), 275–283. doi: 10.1016/j.foodhyd.2011.12.019

Ramnani, P., Costabile, A., Bustillo, A.G.R., and Gibson, G.R. (2015). A randomised, double-blind, cross-over study investigating the prebiotic effect of agave fructans in healthy human subjects. *Journal of Nutritional Science*, 4, e10.

Renuka, B., Kulkarni, S.G., Vijayanand, P., and Prapulla, S.G. (2009). Fructooligosaccharide fortification of selected fruit juice beverages: Effect on the quality characteristics. *LWT – Food Science and Technology*, 42(5), 1031–1033. doi: 10.1016/j.lwt.2008.11.004

Rodríguez, R., Jiménez, A., Fernández-Bolaños, J., Guillén, R., and Heredia, A. (2006). Dietary fibre from vegetable products as source of functional ingredients. *Trends in Food Science and Technology*, 17(1), 3–15. doi: 10.1016/j.tifs.2005.10.002

Rose, D.J., Patterson, J.A., and Hamaker, B.R. (2010). Structural differences among alkali-soluble arabinoxylans from maize (*Zea mays*), rice (*Oryza sativa*), and wheat (*Triticum aestivum*) brans influence human fecal fermentation profiles. *Journal of Agricultural and Food Chemistry*, 58(1), 493–499.

Salinardi, T.C., Rubin, K.H., Black, R.M., and St-Onge, M.P. (2010). Coffee mannooligosaccharides, consumed as part of a free-living, weight-maintaining diet, increase the proportional reduction in body volume in overweight men. *Journal of Nutrition*, 140, 1943–1948.

Salmenkallio-Marttila, M., Due, A., Gunnarsdottir, I., Karhunen, L., Saarela, M., and Lyly, M. (2009). *Satiety, Weight Management and Foods*. Literature review. Nordic Innovation Centre, Oslo, Norway. Accessed via http://nordicinnovation.org/ (1 August 2016).

Salmerón, I., Thomas, K., and Pandiella, S.S. (2015). Gram-positive bacteria; Findings from University of Sunderland in the area of Lactobacillus reported (Effect of potentially probiotic lactic acid bacteria on the physicochemical composition and acceptance of fermented cereal beverages). Food Weekly News, 69.

Saura-Calixto, F.D., and Goñi, I. (eds.) (1993). *Dietary Fibre Intakes in Europe*. Commission of the European Communities, Brussels.

Sendra, E., Fayos, P., Lario, Y., Fernández-López, J., Sayas-Barberá, E., and Pérez-Alvarez, J.A. (2008). Incorporation of citrus fibers in fermented milk containing probiotic bacteria. *Food Microbiology*, 25(1), 13–21. doi: 10.1016/j.fm.2007.09.003

Silva, T.M., Melo, J.F.H., and Lima, V.L.A.G. (2013). Content of soluble fibers present in dairy products marketed in Recife-PE, Brazil. *Revista de Alimentacao Human*, 19(3), 93–101.

Singer, J., Grinev, M., Silva, V., Cohen, J., and Singer, P. (2016). Safety and efficacy of coffee enriched with inulin and dextrin on satiety and hunger in normal volunteers. *Nutrition*, 32(7), 754–760.

Singh, G.M., Micha, R., Khatibzadeh, S., Shi, P., Lim, S., Andrews, K.G., *et al.* (2015). Global, regional, and national consumption of sugar-sweetened beverages, fruit juices, and milk: A systematic assessment of beverage intake in 187 countries. *PLoS One*, 10(8), e0124845.

Smith, K.N., Queenan, K.M., Thomas, W., Fulcher, G., and Slavin, J.L. (2008). Physiological effects of concentrated barley beta glucan in mildly hypercholesterolemic adults. *Journal of the American College of Nutrition*, 27(3), 434–440.

Srinivasjois, R., Rao, S., and Patole, S. (2013). Prebiotic supplementation in preterm neonates: updated systematic review and meta-analysis of randomised controlled trials. *Clinical Nutrition (Edinburgh, Scotland)*, 32(6), 958–965. doi: 10.1016/j.clnu.2013.05.009

Suzuki, K., Shiraishi, K., Yoshitani, K., Sugama, K., and Kometani, T. (2014). Effect of a sport drink based on highly-branched cyclic dextrin on cytokine responses to exhaustive endurance exercise. *Journal of Sports Medicine and Physical Fitness*, 54(4), 622–630.

Tapola, N., Karvonen, H., Niskanen, L., Mikola, M., and Sarkkinen, E. (2005). Glycemic responses of oat bran products in type 2 diabetic patients. *Nutrition,*

Metabolism and Cardiovascular Diseases, 15(4), 255–261. doi: 10.1016/j.numecd.2004.09.003

Tarchevskiĭ, I.A. and Marchenko, G.N. (1991). *Cellulose: Biosynthesis and Structure.* Springer-Verlag, Berlin, New York.

Thakur, G., Mitra, A., Pal, K., and Rousseau, D. (2009). Effect of flaxseed gum on reduction of blood glucose and cholesterol in type 2 diabetic patients. *International Journal of Food Sciences and Nutrition*, 60(s6), 126–136. doi: 10.1080/09637480903022735

Thompson, W.G., Rostad, H.N., Janzow, D.J., Slezak, J.M., Morris, K.L., and Zemel, M.B. (2005). Effect of energy-reduced diets high in dairy products and fiber on weight loss in obese adults. *Obesity Research*, 13, 1344–1353.

Thondre, P.S., Shafat, A., and Clegg, M.E. (2013). Molecular weight of barley β-glucan influences energy expenditure, gastric emptying and glycaemic response in human subjects. *British Journal of Nutrition*, 110(12), 2173–2179. doi: 10.1017/S0007114513001682

Timmermans, J.W., Leeflang, B.R., and Tournois, H. (1993). Structure analysis of small inulin oligosaccharides by 1D- and 2D-NMR. In Studies in Plant Science, *Vol. 3* (ed. A. Fuchs). Elsevier, New York, pp. 129–134.

Tulk, H.M.F., Blonski, D.C., Murch, L.A., Duncan, A.M., and Wright, A.J. (2013). Daily consumption of a synbiotic yogurt decreases energy intake but does not improve gastrointestinal transit time: a double-blind, randomized, crossover study in healthy adults. *Nutrition Journal*, 12(1), 87–87. doi: 10.1186/1475-2891-12-87

Tungland, B.C. (2003). Fructooligosaccharides and other fructans: Structures and occurrence, production, regulatory aspects, food applications and nutritional health significance. In *Oligosaccharides in Food and Agriculture* (eds. G. Eggleston and G.L. Cote). ACS Symposium Series, American Chemical Society, Washington, DC, pp. 135–152.

Tungland, B.C. and Meyer, D. (2002). Nondigestible oligo- and polysaccharides (dietary fiber): Their physiology and role in human health and food. *Comprehensive Reviews in Food Science and Food Safety*, 1, 90–109.

Van Dokkum, W., Wezendonk, B., Srikumar, T.S., and van den Heuvel, E.G. (1999). Effect of nondigestible oligosaccharides on large-bowel functions, blood lipid concentrations and glucose absorption in young healthy male subjects. *European Journal of Clinical Nutrition*, 53(1), 1–7.

Van Mol, R. (2003). Carob fiber for dairy foods. *Dairy Foods*, 104(3), 56.

Vidal, S., Williams, P., Doco, T., Moutounet, M., and Pellerin, P. (2003). The polysaccharides of red wine: total fractionation and characterization. *Carbohydrate Polymers*, 54(4), 439–447. doi: 10.1016/S0144-8617(03)00152-8

Villegas, B. and Costell, E. (2007). Flow behaviour of inulin–milk beverages. Influence of inulin average chain length and of milk fat content. *International Dairy Journal*, 17(7), 776–781. doi: 10.1016/j.idairyj.2006.09.007

Viscione, L. (2013). Fibre-enriched beverages. In *Fibre-rich and Wholegrain Foods: Improving Quality* (eds. J.A. Delcour and K. Poutanen). Woodhead Publishing (Elsevier), UK, pp. 369–388.

Viuda-Martos, M., López-Marcos, M.C., Fernández-López, J., Sendra, E., López-Vargas, J.H., and Pérez-Álvarez, J.A. (2010). Role of fiber in cardiovascular diseases: a review. *Comprehensive Reviews in Food Science and Food Safety*, 9(2), 240–258. doi: 10.1111/j.1541-4337.2009.00102.x

Watson, E. (2016). From bean to bottle: RAU chocolate starts a cold-pressed cacao revolution. http://www.foodnavigator-usa.com (accessed January 25, 2016).

Wierdsma, N.J., van Bodegraven, A.A., Uitdehaag, B.M.J., Arjaans, W., Savelkoul, P.H.M., Kruizenga, H.M., and van Bokhorst-de van der Schueren, M.A.E. (2009). Fructo-oligosaccharides and fibre in enteral nutrition has a beneficial influence on microbiota and gastrointestinal quality of life. *Scandinavian Journal of Gastroenterology*, 44(7), 804–812. doi: 10.1080/00365520902839675

Will, F. and Dietrich, H. (1992). Isolation, purification and characterization of neutral polysaccharides from extracted apple juices. *Carbohydrate Polymers*, 18(2), 109–117. doi: 10.1016/0144-8617(92)90132-A

Wood, P.J., Weisz, J., and Mahn, W. (1991). Molecular characterisation of cereal β-glucans. II. Size-exclusion chromatography for comparison of molecular weight. *Cereal Chemistry*, 68, 530–536.

Xing, X., Cui, S.W., Nie, S., Phillips, G.O., Goff, H.D., and Wang, Q. (2013). A review of isolation process, structural characteristics, and bioactivities of water-soluble polysaccharides from Dendrobium plants. *Bioactive Carbohydrates and Dietary Fibre*, 1(2), 131–147.

Yangilar, F. (2013). The application of dietary fibre in food industry: structural features, effects on health and definition, obtaining and analysis of dietary fibre: A review. *Journal of Food and Nutrition Research*, 1(3), 13–23.

Yapo, B.M., Lerouge, P., Thibault, J.F., and Ralet, M.C. (2007). Pectins from citrus peel cell walls contain homogalacturonans homogenous with respect to molar mass, rhamnogalacturonan I and rhamnogalacturonan II. *Carbohydrate Polymers*, 69(3), 426–435. doi: 10.1016/j.carbpol.2006.12.024

Ye, Z., Arumugam, V., Haugabrooks, E., Williamson, P., and Hendrich, S. (2015). Soluble dietary fiber (Fibersol-2) decreased hunger and increased satiety hormones in humans when ingested with a meal. *Nutrition Research*, 35(5), 393–400. doi: 10.1016/j.nutres.2015.03.004

Yu, K., Ke, M.-K., Li, W.-H., Zhang, S.-Q., and Fang, X.-C. (2014). The impact of soluble dietary fibre on gastric emptying, postprandial blood glucose and insulin in patients with type 2 diabetes. *Asia Pacific Journal of Clinincal Nutrition*, 23(2), 210–218.

Yu, L., Zhang, X., Li, S., Liu, X., Sun, L., Liu, H., *et al.* (2010). Rhamnogalacturonan I domains from ginseng pectin. *Carbohydrate Polymers*, 79(4), 811–817. doi: 10.1016/j.carbpol.2009.08.028

Zare, F., Orsat, V., and Boye, J. I. (2015). Functional, physical and sensory properties of pulse ingredients incorporated into orange and apple juice beverages. *Journal of Food Research*, 4(5), 143–156.

Zhang, R., Zhang, Z., Zhang, H., Decker, E.A., and McClements, D.J. (2015). Influence of emulsifier type on gastrointestinal fate of oil-in-water emulsions containing anionic dietary fiber (pectin). *Food Hydrocolloids*, 45, 175–185. doi: 10.1016/j.foodhyd.2014.11.020

Zhang, X., Yu, L., Bi, H., Li, X., Ni, W., Han, H., *et al.* (2009). Total fractionation and characterization of the water-soluble polysaccharides isolated from Panax ginseng C. *A. Meyer. Carbohydrate Polymers*, 77(3), 544–552. doi: 10.1016/j.carbpol.2009.01.034

Zhao, G., Etherton, T.D., Martin, K.R., Gillies, P.J., West, S.G., and Kris-Etherton, P.M. (2007). Dietary alpha-linolenic acid inhibits proinflammatory cytokine production by peripheral blood mononuclear cells in hypercholesterolemic subjects. *American Journal of Clinical Nutrition*, 85(2), 385.

4

Dietary Fiber as Food Additive: Present and Future

Anaberta Cardador-Martínez[1], María Teresa Espino-Sevilla[2], Sandra T. Martín del Campo[1] and Maritza Alonzo-Macías[1]

[1] *Escuela de Ingeniería y Ciencias, Tecnologico de Monterrey, Querétaro, Mexico*
[2] *Universidad de Guadalajara, Centro Universitario de la Ciénega, Ocotlán, Mexico*

4.1 Dietary Fiber: Definition

The concept and the meaning of the term dietary fiber were first discussed by Hipsley (1953). Although it was then used to designate non-digestible plant cell wall constituents (Cho and Dreher, 2001), the definition is still controversial and several definitions have been suggested. The most commonly used definition is the following: "dietary fibers are oligosaccharides, polysaccharides and the (hydrophilic) derivatives which cannot be digested by the human digestive enzymes to absorbable components in the upper alimentary tract, and this includes lignins" (Thebaudin *et al.*, 1997). Thus dietary fiber is a combination of chemically heterogeneous substances and is conventionally classified into two categories according to its water solubility: insoluble dietary fiber (IDF), such as cellulose, some hemicellulose, and lignin, and soluble dietary fiber (SDF), such as pentosans, pectin, gums, and mucilage (Figure 4.1) (Chawla and Patil, 2010). Total dietary fiber can also be divided into two groups: viscous fiber (pectin, gums, and mucilage, which were previously classified as water-soluble fiber) and non-viscous fiber (cellulose, hemicellulose, and lignin, which were previously classified as water-insoluble fiber) (Riccioni *et al.*, 2012).

In the early days of food science, dietary fiber was promoted for its nutritional properties. Now, it is well known that a diet high in fiber-containing foods is associated with health benefits, but the extent of the benefits can be enhanced or diminished not only by the type and degree of its processing, but also by the influence of various non-dietary factors (e.g., genetic factors, physical activity, stress) (Cho and Dreher, 2001; Gómez *et al.*, 2003). The importance of dietary fiber in the food industry has increased because of the properties it can add to food, such as texture modifications and enhancement of the stability of the food during production and storage (Thebaudin *et al.*, 1997).

Dietary Fiber Functionality in Food and Nutraceuticals: From Plant to Gut, First Edition.
Edited by Farah Hosseinian, B. Dave Oomah and Rocio Campos-Vega.
© 2017 John Wiley & Sons Ltd. Published 2017 by John Wiley & Sons Ltd.

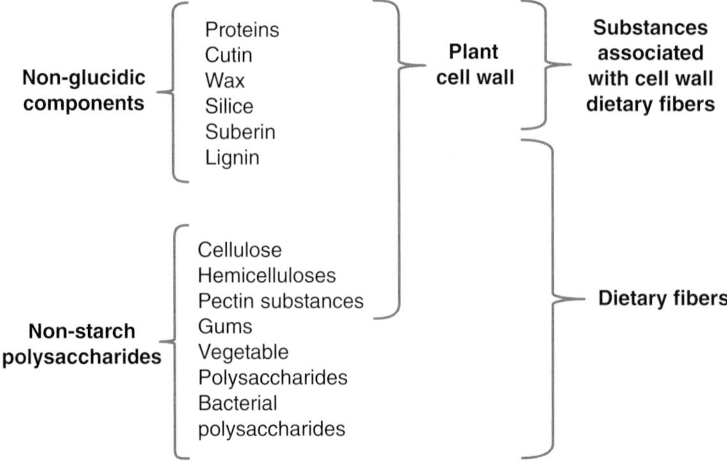

Figure 4.1 Composition of dietary fibers and associated substances. *Source*: Thebaudin *et al.* (1997). Reproduced with permission from Elsevier.

4.2 Chemical Nature of Dietary Fiber Used as Food Additive

Dietary fiber includes polysaccharides, oligosaccharides, lignin, and associated plant substances (Table 4.1) (Chawla and Patil, 2010). Dietary fiber can be classified into soluble (e.g., gums, pectins), insoluble (e.g., cellulose), or mixed (e.g., bran) (Table 4.1), fermentable and non-fermentable. Insoluble, non-fermentable fibers are known for their bulking effect, which decreases transit time and increases fecal mass. The extent of fermentation of soluble fibers depends on their physical and chemical structure. Fermentation decreases intraluminal pH and stimulates proliferation of colonic epithelial cells (Carabin and Flamm, 1999). Insoluble fiber is typically associated with laxation, whereas soluble fiber is linked with reducing cholesterol levels and improving postprandial blood glucose levels. All fibers can function as prebiotics, providing food for gut microorganisms (Brummer *et al.*, 2015).

Fructan is a term used for naturally occurring plant oligo- and polysaccharides and refers to any carbohydrate compound in which one or more fructosyl–fructose links comprise the majority of glycosidic bonds. Fructans are linear or branched fructose polymers which are joined by two types of linkages: $\beta(2-1)$, seen in inulin (Figure 4.2a), or $\beta(2-6)$, in other fructans, such as agavin (Figure 4.2b) (Carabin and Flamm, 1999). Inulin is a carbohydrate consisting mainly of fructose with one terminal glucose. It is included in soluble and fermentable dietary fiber (Brummer *et al.*, 2015).

Chitin is a long, unbranched polymer of N-acetyl-D-glucosamine residues linked through $\beta1-4$ bonds (Figure 4.3). It is found in fungi and is the principal component of arthropod and lower animal exoskeletons, such as insect, crab, and shrimp shells. Because of the abundance of chitin, biotechnological

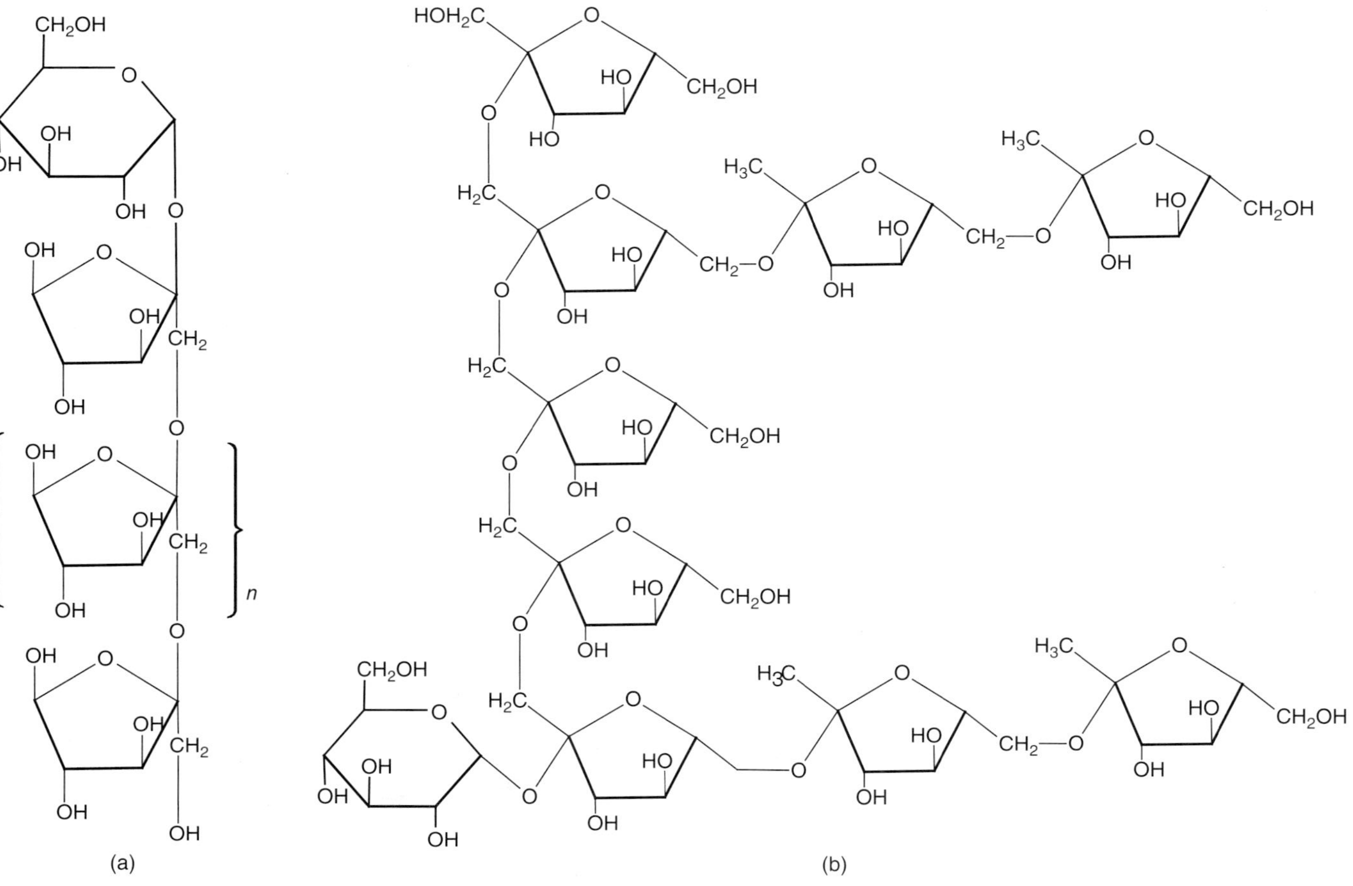

Figure 4.2 Polymers of fructose. (a) Inulin; (b) agavin.

Table 4.1 Classification of dietary fiber according to its water solubility properties.

Soluble	Insoluble
Oligosaccharides	Cellulose
Fructo oligosaccharides	Hemicellulose
Fructans	Lignan
Inulins	
Chitins	
β-Glucans	
Pectins	

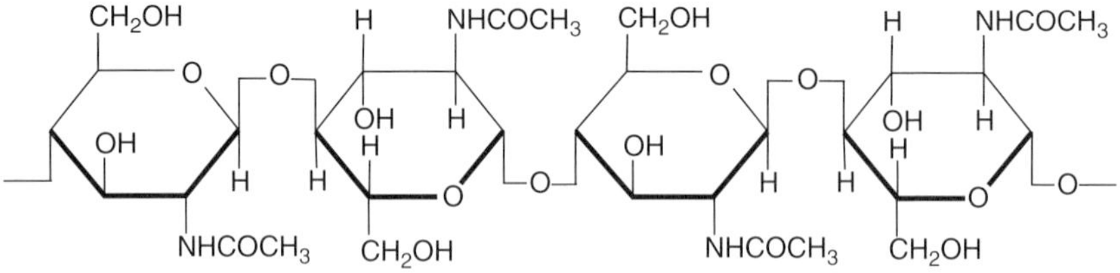

Figure 4.3 Chitin structure.

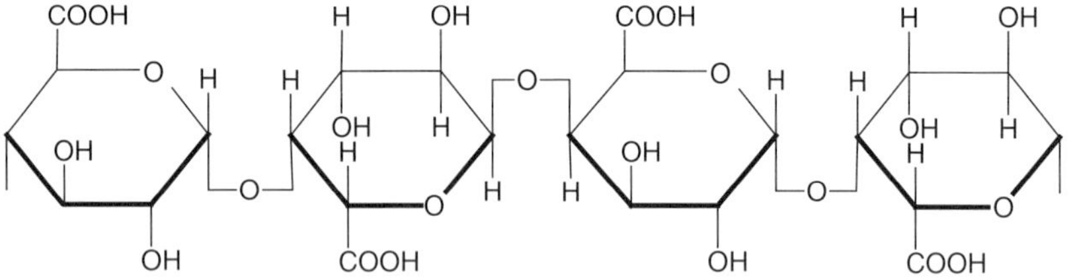

Figure 4.4 Pectin (polygalacturonic acid) structure.

applications are being developed, such as use as additive in food industry (Martínez *et al.*, 2001).

Pectin is a polysaccharide that acts as a strengthening material in the cell walls of all plant tissues. The white portion of the rind of lemons and oranges contains approximately 30% pectin. Pectin is the methylated ester of polygalacturonic acid, which consists of chains of 300–1000 galacturonic acid units joined with α1–4 linkages (Figure 4.4). The degree of esterification affects the gelling properties of pectin. It is an important ingredient of fruit preserves, jellies, and jams because of its functions as a gelling and stabilizing polymer (Mohnen, 2008).

Cellulose is a linear polymer of β-D-glucose, which, in contrast to starch, is oriented with -CH_2OH groups alternating above and below the plane of the cellulose molecule (Figure 4.5). The absence of side-chains allows cellulose molecules to lie close together and form rigid structures. Cellulose is the major structural material of plants. Wood is largely cellulose, and cotton is almost pure cellulose.

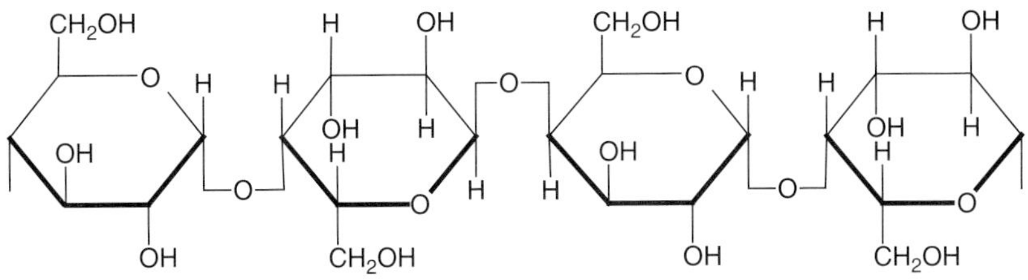

Figure 4.5 Cellulose $(\beta 1-4 \text{ glucose})_n$.

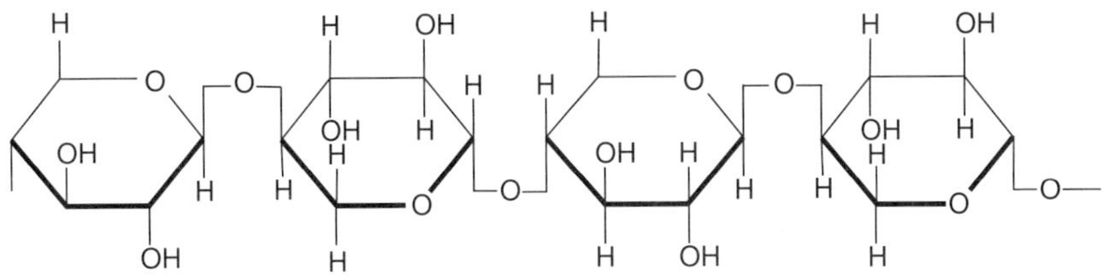

Figure 4.6 Hemicellulose structure.

Hemicelluloses are the polysaccharide components of plant cell walls other than cellulose, or the polysaccharides in plant cell walls that are extractable by dilute alkaline solutions. Hemicelluloses comprise almost one-third of the carbohydrates in woody plant tissue. The chemical structure of hemicelluloses consists of long chains of a variety of pentoses, hexoses, and their corresponding uronic acids (Figure 4.6). Hemicelluloses may be found in fruit, plant stems, and grain hulls. Although hemicelluloses are not digestible, they can be fermented by yeasts and bacteria.

4.3 Sources of Dietary Fiber

That fiber is an important ingredient has been recognized in recent years since its role in health has been demonstrated by several studies. The amount of fiber in the modern human diet has decreased considerably since the pre-industrial era and its effects on health have been felt. In recent years, however, there has been a move within the food industry to reduce the fat in food because of its association with health disorders such as cardiovascular diseases, and fiber has shown its suitability as an ingredient in reducing fat and improving food characteristics.

The increased need on the amount of fiber as an ingredient and not as part of the original food has led to the development of new methods for fiber extraction and research into new sources. Nowadays, there are several industrial sources of fiber, such as cereals, fruits, nuts, vegetables, roots, plants, and even microorganisms. Most of the time, fiber is obtained as an industrial byproduct from other food production industries or by using undervalued products. The composition and technological properties as well as the industrial applications of the obtained fibers are highly dependent on the source and extraction method used. Sometimes fiber is extracted and purified to get a product with specific characteristics, but other times the source is only dried and milled to obtain fiber-rich powders that are used directly.

An important fiber source is cereals, such as wheat, rice bran, barley, and millet. Wheat bran is an agricultural by product with a high availability and low cost. It has been used as a direct source of fiber without extraction (Hemery *et al.*, 2011). In contrast, arabinoxylans have been obtained and purified from de-starched wheat bran with different methods yielding products with different characteristics such as color, residual fat content, carbohydrates composition, polymerization degree, and phytic acid content (Aguedo *et al.*, 2014, Aguedo *et al.*, 2015, Inglett, 1992). Soluble and insoluble dietary fibers have also been extracted from defatted rice bran (Daou and Zhang, 2014). Millet flour has been used as a direct fiber source without fiber purification to increase the proportion of fiber in wheat flour for baking purposes (Aprodu and Banu, 2015).

Fruit or fruit parts have been used as fiber sources because, as industry byproducts, they are often discarded and are an important pollution issue. Usable fiber has been extracted from fruit peel, fruit pulp, seeds, and other fruit parts. Pectins are extracted from various fruits, such as apple, passion fruit and citrus fruits (Chawla and Patil, 2010, de Oliveira *et al.*, 2015). Mango peel powder has been used as a source of fiber without fiber extraction (Ajila *et al.*, 2010, Ajila *et al.*, 2008, Larrauri *et al.*, 1996) but fiber has also been extracted from peels, skins, and fibrous residues (Gourgue *et al.*, 1992). Both soluble and insoluble dietary fibers have been extracted from *Citrus sinensis* L. cv. Liucheng peel (Chau and Huang, 2003) and from wine grape pomace. Lemon albedo has been used as a source of dietary fiber in the food industry (Lario *et al.*, 2004), including for meat products (Fernández-Ginés *et al.*, 2004). In the case of *Mangifera pajang* Kort., pulp fiber was separated from pulp by extracting the juice and washing the obtained pomace (Al-Sheraji *et al.*, 2011). Palm date seeds have been used as fiber source without extraction in bread making and gave results similar to those using wheat bran, depending on the particle size (Almana and Mahmoud, 1994).

Other types of fiber source include nuts, such as hazelnuts. Hazelnut testa has been used as a direct fiber source without extraction in bread making (Anil, 2007).

Vegetables have been also used as fiber source. Dried powdered cladodes from prickly pear (*Opuntia*) were used as a direct fiber source added to wheat flour for bakery (Ayadi *et al.*, 2009) and carrot peel has been shown to be a good source of antioxidant dietary fiber source (Chantaro *et al.*, 2008).

Other plants such as algae and agave (*Agave tequilana*), or plant roots such as those of Jerusalem artichoke (*Helianthus tuberosus*), chicory (*Cichorium intybus*), or root byproducts such as maca (*Lepidium meyenii* Walp.) have been used as fiber sources. Various kinds of algae are used as sources of algal phycocolloids, such as alginate, carrageenan, and agar (Brownlee *et al.*, 2005; Chawla and Patil, 2010). Fructans have also been extracted and purified from agave, Jerusalem artichoke, and chicory (Carabin and Flamm, 1999; Flamm *et al.*, 2001). Dietary fiber has been extracted from maca and liquor residues (Chen *et al.*, 2015) by different methods.

Other sources of fiber are trees exudates considered as gums, such as karaya gum from *Sterculia urens*, tragacanth gum from *Astragalua gummifer*, and Arabic gum from *Acacia senegal* (Chawla and Patil, 2010).

Some microorganisms are also sources of fiber, mostly in the form of hydrocolloids that act as soluble dietary fiber. Xanthan gum is produced by *Xanthomonas compestris* and gellan gum by *Pseudomonas elodea* (Chawla and Patil, 2010),

4.4 Role of Dietary Fiber as a Food Additive

The nutritional and sensory qualities of foods are both important aspects that affect consumers' decisions. Because of this, several authors have studied the best options for consumers, taking both nutritional and sensory criteria into account.

The importance of dietary fiber as a food additive has a positive impact, depending on the product. For example, dietary fiber may interact with other components of the food during processing, and these interactions may lead to changes in bioavailability of nutrients, texture, or flavor or the product (Staffolo *et al.*, 2004). Orange juice, for example, has potential as a source of dietary fiber due to its pectin content and, in addition, it is plentiful and inexpensive. Pectin is effective in bringing down blood cholesterol levels, specifically by decreasing the low density lipoprotein cholesterol fraction without changing the levels of high density lipoprotein cholesterol and triglycerides (Cerda *et al.*, 1988). In addition to its clinical effects, pectin is also used as a food additive because of its properties as a gelling agent (Grigelmo-Miguel and Martín-Belloso, 1998; Schröder *et al.*, 2004).

For bread, dietary fiber usually alters the rheology of dough and thus the quality and sensory properties of the final product. It has pronounced effects on dough properties, increasing water absorption, mixing tolerance, and tenacity, and reducing extensibility in comparison with dough made without the addition of fiber (Almeida *et al.*, 2013; Gómez *et al.*, 2003; Masoodi and Chauhan, 1998).

In the case of partially hydrolyzed guar gum, this can impact various aspects. For example, it can improve the processing of cereals by increasing flowability, providing body and a mellow flavor in most beverages, stabilizing the colloid system of dry and liquid meal replacements, giving a mellow tartness and firm texture to yogurts, stabilizing the foam system of shakes, improving suspension of particulate in soups and dressings, and imparting good eating qualities to baked goods (Yoon *et al.*, 2008).

4.5 Food Products Added with Fiber

The importance of food fibers has led to the development of a large and potential market for fiber-rich products and ingredients and, in recent years, there is a trend to find new sources of dietary fiber that can be used as ingredients in the food industry.

4.5.1 Bread

Nowadays, there is more consumer interest in bakery cereal products enriched with dietary fiber than in ones prepared using non-traditional components. Dietary fiber increases the nutritional value of bread but usually at the same time alters the rheological properties of dough and, ultimately, the quality and sensory properties of the bread (Stoin *et al.*, 2012; Kučerová *et al.*, 2013; Sivam *et al.*, 2010)

Dietary fiber is added in bread making to obtain desired properties such as an increase of dietary fiber content and to prolong freshness during shelf-life, or to manipulate process parameters such as mixing time (Almeida *et al.*, 2013). Table 4.2 summarizes some investigations performed in recent years on the addition of dietary fiber from different sources in bread making and its effect on dough characteristics.

Wheat is the most important cereal crop in the world and wheat bran is the major byproduct of the wheat industry (Manisseri and Gudipati, 2010). Wheat bran amounts to approximately 12–15% of the grain. In general, the literature has reported various detrimental effects on dough handling and bread quality associated with flour replacement by dietary fiber, such as wheat bran and resistant starch, in bread making (Angioloni and Collar, 2011). On the other hand, locust bean gum (LBG) is a hydrocolloid, considered to be dietary fiber, that has demonstrated good results in increasing the technological quality of baked goods (Sharadanant and Khan, 2003), and it could be useful in breads with added wheat bran and resistant starch (Almeida *et al.*, 2013).

Apple fiber improves water-holding capacity better than wheat or oat bran when added to cookies and muffins, without modifying their quality (Masoodi and Chauhan, 1998). Rice straw added to bread increased both water- and oil-holding capacities, as well as particle size and physicochemical characteristics (Sangnark and Noomhorm, 2004). Chia, a prehispanic cereal, has been studied as a source of dietary fiber, both as whole and defatted flour. Bread with chia seeds or flour showed similar technological quality to the control bread, and an increase in specific bread volume. Although a decrease in crumb firmness and changes in crumb color were observed, sensory analysis showed that the inclusion of chia increased overall acceptability by consumers (Iglesias-Puig and Haros, 2013).

Researchers have evaluated the addition of coarse date seed fiber and wheat bran in bread making. The rheological properties obtained were similar in both cases. Bread containing 10% coarse date seed fiber had a higher dietary fiber content and similar sensorial properties to the wheat bran control. Breads containing the fine date seed fiber had higher dietary fiber contents than wheat bran controls, but lower color, flavor, odor, chewing, uniformity, and overall acceptability sensory scores (Hamada *et al.*, 2002).

4.5.2 Breakfast Cereals

Breakfast cereal products were originally sold as milled grains of wheat and oats that required further cooking in the home prior to consumption. In recent decades, in response to efforts to reduce the amount of in-home preparation

Table 4.2 Effect of various dietary fibers added in bread making.

Dietary fiber added	Bread quality characteristics	Characteristics obtained	Reference
Wheat bran (WB) 20%, granular RS2-type corn resistant starch (RS) 20%, and locust bean gum (LBG) 3% Bread type: Pan bread	Loaf apparent volume Crumb color Sensorial evaluation	WB reduced specific volume and crumb, luminosity and increased high-speed mixing time, crumb color, and crumb moisture content LBG reduced crumb luminosity and increased crumb moisture content, but reduced high-speed mixing time RS increased high-speed mixing time, but was a more "inert" fiber source in relation to bread quality characteristics	Almeida *et al..*, 2013
Apple fiber, wheat, and oat bran In bread, cookies and muffins 4, 8, and 12% concentrations	Water-holding capacity (WHC) Bulk density Viscosity Loaf volume Crumb grain	Apple fiber had higher WHC than other fibers Apple fiber is higher in total dietary fiber than wheat and oat brans and may have a potential use in bread baking	Masoodi and Chauhan, 1998
Rice straw in bread	Color Particle density WHC Dough stickiness Loaf volume Crumb color Bread texture Oil-binding capacity (OBC) Dough expansion Sensorial evaluation	Brightness of the straw increased WHC increased significantly Swollen straw volume increased OBC increased	Sangnark and Noomhorm, 2004
Chia (*Salvia hispanica* L) Whole chia flour, semi-defatted	Nutritional quality Specific bread volume Crumb firmness Sensory analysis Crumb color Thermal properties	Levels of protein, lipids, ash, and dietary fiber increased Breads with seeds or ground seeds showed similar technological quality to the control bread	Iglesias-Puig and Haros, 2013

time, breakfast cereal technology has evolved from the simple procedure of milling grains for cereal products that require cooking to the manufacturing of highly sophisticated ready-to-eat products that are convenient and quick to prepare (Jozinović *et al.*, 2013).

Up to now wheat milling byproducts have mainly been used in "all-bran" breakfast extruded products (Eastman *et al.*, 2001). These products contain almost exclusively IDF (the average amount of SDF is about 1.5%) and many recent nutritional studies have stressed that the average dietary intake of SDF is far below the optimum (Cui *et al.*, 1999).

Several studies have shown the noticeable antioxidant activity of cereal products. This activity is mainly due to phenol compounds that can be either the same as those contained in fruits and vegetables, or unique to the specific cereal (Adom *et al.*, 2003). Whole grain bread has an antioxidant activity that is almost double that of white bread (Miller *et al.*, 2000) and can act as free radical scavengers through the entire digestive tract and in colon tissue. It is clear that antioxidants are concentrated in the bran fraction, but it is not clear to what extent both free and carbohydrate-bound compounds are measured by a given assay (Esposito *et al.*, 2005).

In the preparation of pies, cakes, and pastries from fruits, the apple pulp is used as filler and has been used in making bread; this source has gained a strong interest because it contains 36.8% dietary fiber. In fact, researchers have characterized apple pomace fiber and found that this source of fiber is higher quality than that of wheat and oat bran, because the fibers of citrus and apple pomace contain bioactive compounds such as flavonoids, polyphenols, and carotenoids, which are considered higher quality dietary fiber. Furthermore, researchers have reported that polyphenols, which are mainly responsible for the antioxidant activity, are present in apple pomace and hence this could be a cheap and readily available source of dietary antioxidants (Sudha *et al.*, 2007).

4.5.3 Pasta

Pasta is a traditional cereal-based food product that is becoming increasingly popular worldwide because of its convenience, nutritional quality, and palatability. Durum wheat (*Triticum durum*) is the best raw material for pasta products due to its unique color, flavor, and cooking quality (Dexter and Edwards, 1998).

Many researchers have established that the content and composition of proteins, and the gluten strength in particular, are important for the cooking quality of pasta (Grzybowski and Donnelly, 1979). In addition, the physical characteristics of durum wheat, such as test weight, kernel weight, kernel size, and degree of vitreousness, are also known to influence its milling performance and thus also pasta quality directly or indirectly (Dexter *et al.*, 1988, 1994; Troccoli *et al.*, 2000).

The type and amount of added fiber influences the overall quality of both raw and cooked pasta and it has been shown that pasta texture, structure, cooking characteristics, and potential nutritional quality are intrinsically linked to the integration of fiber into pasta systems (Tudorica *et al.*, 2002).

Functional pastas enriched with β-glucans and dietary fiber were produced by substituting 50% of standard durum wheat semolina with β-glucan-enriched barley flour fractions. Although darker than durum wheat pasta, these pastas had good cooking qualities with regard to stickiness, bulkiness, firmness, and total organic matter released in rinsing water (Cleary and Brennan, 2006).

Chitosan, a polysaccharide derived from shellfish, is an important fiber source whose effects has been investigated after its addition to wet noodles. These studies clearly demonstrated that chitosan can be used as an effective preservative in wet noodles due to its antimicrobial activity (No *et al.*, 2007).

4.5.4 Jam and Marmalades

In making of jams and marmalades, the most common added fibers are those consisting of pectin with different degree of esterification, which mainly comes from fruits and are a factor in keeping the stability of the final product. Substitution of pectin by dietary fiber in strawberry jams resulted in jams with acceptable sensory qualities, although they were darker than controls (Grigelmo-Miguel and Martín-Belloso, 1999). Hussein *et al.* (2015) studied the use of carrot peel, apple pomace, banana peel, and mandarin peel in preparing jam with high fiber content.

4.5.5 Beverages

In the case of beverages and drinks, the addition of dietary fiber increases their viscosity and stability. Soluble fiber is the most used because it is more dispersible in water than insoluble fiber. Some examples of these soluble fibers are those from fractions of grains and multi-fruits, pectin, β-glucan, cellulose beetroot fiber, and polydextrose (Dhingra *et al.*, 2012; Mitchell, 2001; Nelson, 2001; Faccin *et al.*, 2009).

Rice bran has been used in beverages and sensory preference tests showed positive results (Faccin *et al.*, 2009).

4.5.6 Dairy Products

In milk products, some types of soluble fibers, such as pectin, inulin, guar gum, and carboxymethyl-cellulose, are utilized as functional ingredients. For example, guar gum, pectin, and inulin are added during cheese processing to decrease its fat percentage without losing its organoleptic characteristics, such as texture and flavor (Noronha *et al.*, 2007). The addition of resistant starch, Novelose 240 (40% granular RS2 starch, derived from high amylose corn starch) to imitation cheese at levels from 21 to 43% resulted in an increase in moisture and decrease in cheese hardness; at the high level of fiber, the cheese maintained acceptable functional properties, and had the added value of lower fat levels than control cheese (Noronha *et al.*, 2007). On the other hand, Escobar *et al.* (2012) demonstrated that addition of fava resistant starch may loosen the protein structure of fresh panela cheese, decreasing its firmness. This effect was attributed to the high water absorption capacity of starch. Addition of this fiber also does not increase the capacity of panela cheese to function as a probiotic carrier.

Yogurt is one of the most common dairy products consumed around the world. The addition of dietary fiber into yogurts and ice-creams improves the stability of these emulsions (Ozcan and Kurtuldu, 2014; Isik *et al.*, 2011). Several kinds of dietary fibers have been used as additive in yogurts, for instance, inulin (Isik *et al.*, 2011; Pimentel *et al.*, 2013; Aryana *et al.*, 2007; Canbulat and Ozcan, 2014), acacia gum (Min *et al.*, 2012), dietary fiber from barley and oat β-glucan (Ozcan and Kurtuldu, 2014; Fernandez-Garcia *et al.*, 1998), and date (Hashim *et al.*, 2009) among others. With regard to sensory acceptability, the prebiotics inulin, soluble corn fiber, and polydextrose added to yogurt were shown to alter the sensory properties of a yogurt drink when incorporated at different levels (Allgeyer *et al.*, 2010). According to Pimentel *et al.* (2013), yogurts with inulin added to reduce fat content had a more intense homogeneous appearance, acid aroma, and fermented milk aroma compared with the traditional full-fat yogurt. β-Glucan in yogurt acts both as a dietary fiber and as a prebiotic, improving the viability and metabolic activity of *B. bifidum* (Ozcan and Kurtuldu, 2014). Oat fiber addition improved the body and texture of unsweetened yogurts, possibly by increasing total solids, but had no effect on fructose-sweetened yogurts (Fernandez-Garcia *et al.*, 1998).

4.5.7 Meat Products

Dietary fiber has also played an important role in the meat industry. Its contribution is that it has the ability to increase the water retention capacity, and its inclusion in the meat matrix contributes to maintaining juiciness, which implies that the volatile compounds responsible for the flavor of the product are released more slowly (Mansour and Khalil, 1999). The fiber sources used in these products are pectin, cellulose, soy, wheat, maize or rice isolates, and beet fiber, which can be used for improving the texture of meat products, such as sausages, pâtés, and salami, and, at the same time, are used to prepare low-fat products, such as dietetic hamburgers and meatballs (Hu and Yu, 2015; Talukder, 2015; Mansour and Khalil, 1999). The rheological and textural properties of meat batters with added vegetable oil and rice bran fiber were modified as compared to the control. In addition, batters supplemented with vegetable oil and rice bran fiber had lower cooking loss and better emulsion stability (Choi *et al.*, 2009).

Rye bran, oat bran, and barley fiber have been compared as additives in low-fat sausages and meatballs. Oat bran has been the best alternative in low-fat sausages due to its gelling ability upon heating. Addition of up to 20% oat bran to meatballs improves their nutritional value and health benefits (Karin *et al.*, 2014). Studies by Hu and Yu (2015) showed a reduction in *trans* fatty acids upon addition of hemicellulose rice bran in meatballs without affecting sensorial characteristics.

4.6 Conclusions

Dietary fiber is the edible parts of plants or analogous carbohydrates that are resistant to digestion and absorption in the human small intestine, with complete or partial fermentation in the large intestine. The use of dietary fiber has increased in recent decades along with the demand for fiber-enriched food products. Concerns about health issues are the main reasons for this increase, because of the recognition that dietary fiber not only increases the bulk of the food and moves it through the gastrointestinal tract more rapidly, but also helps in preventing constipation and possibly some kinds of cancer.

In addition, dietary fiber can be added to a number of products such as bread, cookies, meat, and dairy products, among others. Researchers have reported that the physicochemical and sensorial characteristics of such products are not modified after addition of dietary fiber, and in some cases some features are improved, for instance, fat content.

The use of dietary fiber as a food supplement is likely to increase in the near future not only because of its health attributes but also for the technological characteristics its use provides to a variety of food products.

References

Adom, K. K., Sorrells, M. E., and Liu, R. H. (2003). Phytochemical profiles and antioxidant activity of wheat varieties. *Journal of Agricultural and Food Chemistry*, 51(26), 7825–7834.

Aguedo, M., Fougnies, C., Dermience, M., and Richel, A. (2014). Extraction by three processes of arabinoxylans from wheat bran and characterization of the fractions obtained. *Carbohydrate Polymers*, 105, 317–324.

Aguedo, M., Ruiz, H. A., and Richel, A. (2015). Non-alkaline solubilization of arabinoxylans from destarched wheat bran using hydrothermal microwave processing and comparison with the hydrolysis by an endoxylanase. *Chemical Engineering and Processing: Process Intensification*, 96, 72–82.

Ajila, C. M., Leelavathi, K., and Prasada Rao, U. J. S. (2008). Improvement of dietary fiber content and antioxidant properties in soft dough biscuits with the incorporation of mango peel powder. *Journal of Cereal Science*, 48, 319–326.

Ajila, C., Aalami, M., Leelavathi, K., and Rao, U. P. (2010). Mango peel powder: A potential source of antioxidant and dietary fiber in macaroni preparations. *Innovative Food Science and Emerging Technologies*, 11, 219–224.

Almana, H. A. and Mahmoud, R. M. (1994). Palm date seeds as an alternative source of dietary fiber in Saudi bread. *Ecology of Food and Nutrition*, 32, 261–270.

Almeida, E. L., Chang, Y. K., and Steel, C. J. (2013). Dietary fibre sources in bread: Influence on technological quality. *LWT – Food Science and Technology*, 50, 545–553.

Allgeyer, L., Miller, M., and Lee, S.-Y. (2010). Sensory and microbiological quality of yogurt drinks with prebiotics and probiotics. *Journal of Dairy Science*, 93, 4471–4479.

Al-Sheraji, S. H., Ismail, A., Manap, M. Y., Mustafa, S., Yusof, R. M., and Hassan, F. A. (2011). Functional properties and characterization of dietary fiber from *Mangifera pajang* Kort. fruit pulp. *Journal of Agricultural and Food Chemistry*, 59, 3980–3985.

Angioloni, A. and Collar, C. (2011). Nutritional and functional added value of oat, Kamut, spelt, rye and buckwheat versus common wheat in breadmaking. *Journal of Science and Food Agriculture*, 91, 1283–1292.

Anil, M. (2007). Using of hazelnut testa as a source of dietary fiber in breadmaking. *Journal of Food Engineering*, 80, 61–67.

Aprodu, I. and Banu, I. (2015). Rheological, thermo-mechanical, and baking properties of wheat-millet flour blends. *Food Science and Technology International*, 21, 342–353.

Aryana, K. J., Plauche, S., Rao, R. M., McGrew, P., and Shah, N. P. (2007). Fat-free plain yogurt manufactured with inulins of various chain lengths and *Lactobacillus acidophilus*. *Journal of Food Science*, 72, M79–84.

Ayadi, M., Abdelmaksoud, W., Ennouri, M., and Attia, H. (2009). Cladodes from Opuntia ficus indica as a source of dietary fiber: Effect on dough characteristics and cake making. *Industrial Crops and Products*, 30, 40–47.

Brownlee, I., Allen, A., Pearson, J., Dettmar, P., Havler, M., Atherton, M., and Onsøyen, E. (2005). Alginate as a source of dietary fiber. *Critical Reviews in Food Science and Nutrition*, 45, 497–510.

Brummer, Y., Kaviani, M., and Tosh, S. M. (2015). Structural and functional characteristics of dietary fibre in beans, lentils, peas and chickpeas. *Food Research International*, 67, 117–125.

Canbulat, Z. and Ozcan, T. (2014). Effects of short-chain and long-chain inulin on the quality of probiotic yogurt containing *Lactobacillus rhamnosus*. *Journal of Food Processing and Preservation*, 39(6), 1251–1260.

Carabin, I. G. and Flamm, W. G. (1999). Evaluation of safety of inulin and oligofructose as dietary fiber. *Regulatory Toxicology and Pharmacology*, 30, 268–282.

Cerda, J., Robbins, F., Burgin, C., Baumgartner, T., and Rice, R. (1988). The effects of grapefruit pectin on patients at risk for coronary heart disease without altering diet or lifestyle. *Clinical Cardiology*, 11, 589–594.

Cho, S.S. and Dreher, M. L. (2001). *Handbook of Dietary Fiber*. Marcel Dekker, New York.

Cleary, L. and Brennan, C. (2006). The influence of a $(1 \rightarrow 3)(1 \rightarrow 4)$-β-d-glucan rich fraction from barley on the physico-chemical properties and in vitro reducing sugars release of durum wheat pasta. *International Journal of Food Science and Technology*, 41, 910–918.

Chantaro, P., Devahastin, S., and Chiewchan, N. (2008). Production of antioxidant high dietary fiber powder from carrot peels. *LWT-Food Science and Technology*, 41, 1987–1994.

Chau, C.-F. and Huang, Y.-L. (2003). Comparison of the chemical composition and physicochemical properties of different fibers prepared from the peel of *Citrus sinensis* L. Cv. Liucheng. *Journal of Agricultural and Food Chemistry*, 51, 2615–2618.

Chawla, R. and Patil, G. R. (2010). Soluble dietary fiber. *Comprehensive Reviews in Food Science and Food Safety*, 9, 178–196.

Chen, J., Zhao, Q., Wang, L., Zha, S., Zhang, L., and Zhao, B. (2015). Physicochemical and functional properties of dietary fiber from maca (*Lepidium meyenii* Walp.) liquor residue. *Carbohydrate Polymers*, 132, 509–512.

Choi, Y.-S., Choi, J.-H., Han, D.-J., Kim, H.-Y., Lee, M.-A., Kim, H.-W., *et al.* (2009). Characteristics of low-fat meat emulsion systems with pork fat replaced by vegetable oils and rice bran fiber. *Meat Science*, 82, 266–271.

Cui, W., Wood, P. J., Weisz, J., and Beer, M. U. (1999). Nonstarch polysaccharides from preprocessed wheat bran: carbohydrate analysis and novel rheological properties. *Cereal Chemistry Journal*, 76(1), 129–133.

Daou, C. and Zhang, H. (2014). Functional and physiological properties of total, soluble, and insoluble dietary fibres derived from defatted rice bran. *Journal of Food Science and Technology*, 51, 3878–3885.

De Oliveira, C. F., Giordani, D., Gurak, P. D., Cladera-Olivera, F., and Marczak, L. D. F. (2015). Extraction of pectin from passion fruit peel using moderate electric field and conventional heating extraction methods. *Innovative Food Science and Emerging Technologies*, 29, 201–208.

Dexter, J. and Edwards, N. (1998). *The implications of frequently encountered grading factors on the processing quality of durum wheat*. Canadian Grain Commission, Grain Research Laboratory, Winnipeg, Manitoba

Dexter, J. E., Williams, P. C., Edwards, N. M., and Martin, D. G. (1988). The relationships between durum wheat vitreousness, kernel hardness and processing quality. *Journal of Cereal Science*, 7(2), 169–181.

Dexter, J., Martin, D., Sadaranganey, G., Michaelides, J., Mathieson, N., Tkac, J., *et al.* (1994). Preprocessing: effects on durum wheat milling and spaghetti-making quality. *Cereal Chemistry*, 71(1), 10–15.

Dhingra, D., Michael, M., Rajput, H., and Patil, R. (2012). Dietary fibre in foods: a review. *Journal of Food Science and Technology*, 49, 255–266.

Eastman, J., Orthoefer F., and Solorio, S. (2001). Using extrusion to create breakfast cereal products. *Cereal Food World*, 46, 468–471.

Escobar, M. C., Van Tassell, M. L., Martínez-Bustos, F., Singh, M., Castaño-Tostado, E., Amaya-Llano, S. L., and Miller, M. J. (2012). Characterization of a panela cheese with added probiotics and fava bean starch. *Journal of Dairy Science*, 95, 2779–2787.

Esposito, F., Arlotti, G., Maria Bonifati, A., Napolitano, A., Vitale, D., and Fogliano, V. (2005). Antioxidant activity and dietary fibre in durum wheat bran by-products. *Food Research International*, 38(10), 1167–1173.

Faccin, G. L., Miotto, L. A., Do Nascimento Vieira, L., Barreto, P. L. M., and Amante, E. R. (2009). Chemical, sensorial and rheological properties of a new organic rice bran beverage. *Rice Science*, 16, 226–234.

Fernandez-Garcia, E., McGregor, J. U., and Traylor, S. (1998). The addition of oat fiber and natural alternative sweeteners in the manufacture of plain yogurt. *Journal of Dairy Science*, 81, 655–663.

Fernández-Ginés, J., Fernandez-Lopez, J., Sayas-Barbera, E., Sendra, E., and Perez-Alvarez, J. (2004). Lemon albedo as a new source of dietary fiber: Application to bologna sausages. *Meat Science*, 67, 7–13.

Flamm, G., Glinsmann, W., Kritchevsky, D., Prosky, L., and Roberfroid, M. (2001). Inulin and oligofructose as dietary fiber: a review of the evidence. *Critical Reviews in Food Science and Nutrition*, 41, 353–362.

Gómez, M., Ronda, F., Blanco, C., Caballero, P., and Apesteguía, A. (2003). Effect of dietary fibre on dough rheology and bread quality. *European Food Research and Technology*, 216, 51–56.

Gourgue, C. M., Champ, M. M., Lozano, Y., and Delort-Laval, J. (1992). Dietary fiber from mango byproducts: Characterization and hypoglycemic effects determined by in vitro methods. *Journal of Agricultural and Food Chemistry*, 40, 1864–1868.

Grigelmo-Miguel, N. and Martín-Belloso, O. (1998). Characterization of dietary fiber from orange juice extraction. *Food Research International*, 31, 355–361.

Grigelmo-Miguel, N. and Martín-Belloso, O. (1999). Influence of fruit dietary fibre addition on physical and sensorial properties of strawberry jams. *Journal of Food Engineering*, 41, 13–21.

Grzybowski, R. A. and Donnelly, B. J. (1979). Cooking properties of spaghetti: factors affecting cooking quality. *Journal of Agricultural and Food Chemistry*, 27, 380–384.

Hamada, J., Hashim, I., and Sharif, F. (2002). Preliminary analysis and potential uses of date pits in foods. *Food Chemistry*, 76, 135–137.

Hashim, I. B., Khalil, A. H., and Afifi, H. S. (2009). Quality characteristics and consumer acceptance of yogurt fortified with date fiber. *Journal of Dairy Science*, 92, 5403–5407.

Hemery, Y., Chaurand, M., Holopainen, U., Lampi, A.-M., Lehtinen, P., Piironen, V., Sadoudi, A., and Rouau, X. (2011). Potential of dry fractionation of wheat bran for the development of food ingredients, part I: Influence of ultra-fine grinding. *Journal of Cereal Science*, 53, 1–8.

Hipsley, E. H. (1953). Dietary "fibre" and pregnancy toxaemia. *British Medical Journal*, 2, 420–422.

Hu, G. and Yu, W. (2015). Effect of hemicellulose from rice bran on low fat meatballs chemical and functional properties. *Food Chemistry*, 186, 239–243.

Hussein, A. M., Kamil, M. M., Hegazy, N. A., Mahmoud, K. F., and Ibrahim, M. A. (2015). Utilization of some fruits and vegetables by-products to produce high dietary fiber jam. *Food Science and Quality Management*, 37, 39–45.

Iglesias-Puig, E. and Haros, M. (2013). Evaluation of performance of dough and bread incorporating chia (*Salvia hispanica* L.). *European Food Research and Technology*, 237, 865–874.

Inglett, G. E. (1992). Method of making soluble dietary fiber compositions from cereals. Patent US5082673 A.

Isik, U., Boyacioglu, D., Capanoglu, E., and Nilufer Erdil, D. (2011). Frozen yogurt with added inulin and isomalt. *Journal of Dairy Science*, 94, 1647–1656.

Jozinović, A., Šubarić, D., Ačkar, Đ., Babić, J., Planinić, M., Pavoković, M., and Blažić, M. (2013). Effect of screw configuration, moisture content and particle size of corn grits on properties of extrudates. *Croatian Journal of Food Science and Technology*, 4, 95–101.

Karin, P., Ophélie, G., Ann-Charlotte, E., and Eva, T. (2014). The effect of cereal additives in low-fat sausages and meatballs. Part 2: Rye bran, oat bran and barley fiber. *Meat Science*, 96, 303–508.

Kučerová, J., Šottníková, V., and Nedomová, Š. (2013). Influence of dietary fibre addition on the rheological and sensory properties of dough and bakery products. *Czech Journal of Food Sciences*, 31, 340–346.

Lario, Y., Sendra, E., Garci, Amp, X, A-Pérez, J., Fuentes, C., Sayas-Barberá, E., Fernández-López, J., and Pérez-Alvarez, J. A. (2004). Preparation of high dietary fiber powder from lemon juice by-products. *Innovative Food Science and Emerging Technologies*, 5, 113–117.

Larrauri, J. A., Rupérez, P., Borroto, B., and Saura-Calixto, F. (1996). Mango peels as a new tropical fibre: preparation and characterization. *LWT-Food Science and Technology*, 29, 729–733.

Manisseri, C. and Gudipati, M. (2010). Bioactive xylo-oligosaccharides from wheat bran soluble polysaccharides. *LWT – Food Science and Technology*, 43, 421–430.

Mansour, E. H. and Khalil, A. H. (1999). Characteristics of low-fat beefburgers as influenced by various types of wheat fibres. *Journal of the Science of Food and Agriculture*, 79, 493–498.

Martínez, J. P., Falomir, M. P., and Gozalbo, D. (2001). *Chitin: A structural biopolysaccharide with multiple applications*. In eLS. John Wiley and Sons, Chichester. doi: 10.1002/9780470015902.a0000694.pub3

Masoodi, F. A. and Chauhan, G. S. (1998). Use of apple pomace as a source of dietary fiber in wheat bread. *Journal of Food Processing and Preservation*, 22, 255–263.

Miller, H., Rigelhof, F., Marquart, L., Prakash, A., and Kanter, M. (2000). Whole-grain products and antioxidants. *Cereal Foods World*, 45(2), 59–63.

Min, Y. W., Park, S. U., Jang, Y. S., Kim, Y. H., Rhee, P. L., Ko, S. H., *et al.* (2012). Effect of composite yogurt enriched with acacia fiber and *Bifidobacterium lactis*. *World Journal of Gastroenterology*, 18, 4563–4569.

Mitchell, H. (2001). Fibre-enriched beverages and Litesse: the effect on viscosity, flavour impact, acid and thermal stability of beverages when adding Litesse. *Soft Drinks International*, 25–27.

Mohnen, D. (2008). Pectin structure and biosynthesis. *Current Opinion in Plant Biology*, 11, 266–277.

Nelson, A. L. (2001). *High-fiber Ingredients*. Eagan Press, Thatcham, UK.

No, H., Meyers, S., Prinyawiwatkul, W., and Xu, Z. (2007). Applications of chitosan for improvement of quality and shelf life of foods: a review. *Journal of Food Science*, 72, R87–R100.

Noronha, N., O'Riordan, E., and O'Sullivan, M. (2007). Replacement of fat with functional fibre in imitation cheese. *International Dairy Journal*, 17, 1073–1082.

Ozcan, T. and Kurtuldu, O. (2014). Influence of dietary fiber addition on the properties of probiotic yogurt. *International Journal of Chemical Engineering and Applications*, 5, 397.

Pimentel, T. C., Cruz, A. G.. and Prudencio, S. H. (2013). Short communication: Influence of long-chain inulin and *Lactobacillus paracasei* subspecies *paracasei* on the sensory profile and acceptance of a traditional yogurt. *Journal of Dairy Science*, 96, 6233–6241.

Riccioni, G., Sblendorio, V., Gemello, E., Di Bello, B., Scotti, L., Cusenza, S., and D'Orazio, N. (2012). Dietary fibers and cardiometabolic diseases. *International Journal of Molecular Sciences*, 13, 1524.

Sangnark, A. and Noomhorm, A. (2004). Chemical, physical and baking properties of dietary fiber prepared from rice straw. *Food Research International*, 37, 66–74.

Schröder, R., Clark, C. J., Sharrock, K., Hallett, I. C., and Macrae, E. A. (2004). Pectins from the albedo of immature lemon fruitlets have high water binding capacity. *Journal of Plant Physiology*, 161, 371–379.

Sharadanant, R. and Khan, K. (2003). Effect of hydrophilic gums on the quality of frozen dough: II. Bread characteristics. *Cereal Chemistry Journal*, 80, 773–780.

Sivam, A. S., Sun-Waterhouse, D., Quek, S., and Perera, C. O. (2010). Properties of bread dough with added fiber polysaccharides and phenolic antioxidants: A review. *Journal of Food Science*, 75, R163–R174.

Staffolo, M. D., Bertola, N., Martino, M., and Bevilacqua, Y. A. (2004). Influence of dietary fiber addition on sensory and rheological properties of yogurt. *International Dairy Journal*, 14, 263–268.

Stoin, D., Dogaru, D. V., Cocan, I., Mateescu, C., and Jianu, C. (2012). Studies regarding the obtaining of some bread varieties with a high content of dietary fiber. *Journal of Agroalimentary Processes and Technologies*, 18, 350–357.

Sudha, M. L., Baskaran, V., and Leelavathi, K. (2007). Apple pomace as a source of dietary fiber and polyphenols and its effect on the rheological characteristics and cake making. *Food Chemistry*, 104(2), 686–692.

Talukder, S. (2015). Effect of dietary fiber on properties and acceptance of meat products: a review. *Critical Reviews in Food Science and Nutrition*, 55, 1005–1011.

Thebaudin, J., Lefebvre, A., Harrington, M., and Bourgeois, C. (1997). Dietary fibres: nutritional and technological interest. *Trends in Food Science and Technology*, 8, 41–48.

Troccoli, A., Borrelli, G. M., De Vita, P., Fares, C., and Di Fonzo, N. (2000). Mini review: Durum wheat quality: a multidisciplinary concept. *Journal of Cereal Science*, 32(2), 99–113.

Tudorica, C., Kuri, V., and Brennan, C. (2002). Nutritional and physicochemical characteristics of dietary fiber enriched pasta. *Journal of Agricultural and Food Chemistry*, 50, 347–356.

Yoon, S.-J., Chu, D.-C., and Juneja, L. R. (2008). Chemical and physical properties, safety and application of partially hydrolyzed guar gum as dietary fiber. *Journal of Clinical Biochemistry and Nutrition*, 42, 1.

5

Biological Effect of Antioxidant Fiber from Common Beans (*Phaseolus vulgaris* L.)

Diego A. Luna-Vital[1], Aurea K. Ramírez-Jiménez[1], Marcela Gaytan-Martinez[1], Luis Mojica[2] and Guadalupe Loarca-Piña[1]

[1] *Programa de Posgrado en Alimentos del Centro de la República (PROPAC), Research and Graduate Studies in Food Science, School of Chemistry, Universidad Autónoma de Querétaro, Querétaro, Mexico*
[2] *Department of Food Science and Human Nutrition, University of Illinois at Urbana-Champaign, Urbana, USA*

5.1   Introduction

The common bean (*Phaseolus vulgaris* L.) is a legume of outstanding importance for human nutrition throughout the world (Doria *et al.*, 2010). In 2012, 23 million tonnes were produced globally, the most important consumers regionally being South America (9.3 kg/per capita/year), the Caribbean (9.1 kg/per capita/year), Central America (8.8 kg/per capita/year), and Middle Africa (8.0 kg/per capita/year) (FAO, 2014).

Phaseolus vulgaris is the most important among the 50 species of native *Phaseolus* present in the Americas. Currently, the consumption of this legume is changing due to different factors such as increasing availability of common bean varieties, and regional and cultural changes associated with modern life, such as the lack of domestic time to cook them at home (Rodríguez-Licea *et al.*, 2010).

Today, the importance of beans in the Mexican diet remains critical, mainly due to its nutritional qualities, characterized by the high content of protein substances, carbohydrates, vitamins, minerals, and bioactive compounds. Bean seed composition is influenced by environmental factors but also has a strong genetic component (Hacisalihoglu *et al.*, 2010). Common beans are a remarkable source of carbohydrates and proteins, containing approximately 16–33% protein, and are considered a good source of protein even though they are deficient in sulfur amino acids. In Central and South America, for instance, this legume contributes around 5–6 g/capita/day of protein (FAO, 2014).

Studies related to the nutraceutical potential of legumes have gained prominence in recent years. Recently, the common bean has received functional food status because it contains bioactive phenolic compounds and large amounts of complex carbohydrates and fiber, as well as minerals, specifically iron, phosphorus, magnesium, manganese, zinc, and calcium (Feliciano *et al.*, 2014). Among the major bioactive compounds of beans are enzyme inhibitors, lectins, phytates, phenolic compounds (condensed tannins and flavonoids), and polysaccharides.

Dietary Fiber Functionality in Food and Nutraceuticals: From Plant to Gut, First Edition.
Edited by Farah Hosseinian, B. Dave Oomah and Rocio Campos-Vega.

Phenolic compounds are notable for their importance because they exhibit antimutagenic and antioxidant activity (Cardador-Martínez *et al.*, 2002).

The indigestible polysaccharides, including dietary fiber (soluble and insoluble) and resistant starch, show biological activity when included in the human diet: decreased blood cholesterol levels, decreased risk of colon cancer and cardiovascular diseases, bifidogenic activity (Campos-Vega *et al.*, 2009; Cruz-Bravo *et al.*, 2011), increased fecal volume, and special benefits for people with diabetes (Paredes-López and Valverde, 2006).

5.2 *Phaseolus vulgaris* Generalities

Legumes have become important in the human diet because of their nutritional properties, low cost, and the physiological effects associated with their intake. The major legumes consumed in Latin America are common beans (*Phaseolus vulgaris* L.), which are an inexpensive and important source of protein, complex carbohydrates, minerals, vitamins, and phenolic compounds (Díaz *et al.*, 2010).

5.2.1 Nutritional Properties

The common bean seed is an important source of protein, complex carbohydrates, minerals, and dietary fiber, especially in developing countries. Proteins (16–33%) and carbohydrates are the main compounds present in all genotypes studied (González de Mejía *et al.*, 2005). Campos-Vega *et al.* (2009) reported on four bean cultivars, using raw and cooked seeds: protein ranged from 15% to 19.7% in raw and cooked seeds; lipid content in cooked bean ranged from 0.4% to 1.2%; ash content ranged from 3.7% to 4.7%. Bean protein is characterized by its deficiency in sulfur-containing amino acids such as methionine and cysteine, as well as tryptophan. However, it contains an outstanding level of lysine, sufficient to meet the current requirements for children and adults according to the World Health Organization and the Food and Agriculture Organization of the United Nations (Paredes-López *et al.*, 2006). This is very relevant since, when combined with cereals, the mixture brings high-quality protein to the diet, covering the deficiencies in essential amino acids that they would have separately.

With regard to mineral content, common beans are a good source of calcium, phosphorus, iron, and zinc, and of the water-soluble vitamins thiamin, riboflavin, niacin, vitamin B5, and folic acid. Essential fatty acids such as linoleic and linolenic acids as well as dietary fiber are other components present in this legume (Reyes-Moreno and Paredes-López, 1993; Feliciano *et al.*, 2014).

5.2.2 Nutraceutical Composition

Legumes have become important in the human diet because of their nutritional properties, low cost, and the physiological effects associated with its intake. The major legume consumed in Latin America, the common bean (*Phaseolus vulgaris* L.), is well known as a rich source of phytochemicals, such as flavonoids, polyphenols, and phenolics, which exhibit natural antioxidant properties. The antioxidant properties of phenolic compounds may provide health benefits for consumers. Factors that influence the levels of total phenolics in beans include genotype, environment, maturity at harvest, seed size, seed weight, and seed age

Phenolic compounds have at least one aromatic ring with one or more hydroxyl groups attached and can be classified as phenolic acids, flavones, flavanones, isoflavones, flavonols, flavanols, anthocyanins, and condensed tannins (Del Rio *et al.*, 2013; Valls *et al.*, 2009). These are products of plant secondary metabolism and are mediators of plant stress, including insect and microbial defense (Rocha-Guzmán *et al.*, 2007). The primary phenolic compounds in beans and their hulls are flavonoids, mainly caffeic, *p*-coumaric, ferulic, and sinapic esters. The black beans contain differentiated anthocyanins, specifically delphinidin, petunidin, and malvidin. In addition, kaempferol is found in pinto beans and quercetin and kaempferol in pink beans (Oomah *et al.*, 2010).

Mojica *et al.* (2015) evaluated the nutraceutical composition of 12 varieties of bean (Mexico and Brazil) . They found that the major phenolic compounds were catechin (1.75–5.42%) and epicatechin (3.80–12.48%), which were found in all samples. Flavonols such as catechin, quercetin, myricetin, and kaempferol were present as aglycones. Proanthocyanidin dimers (0.24–0.8%) were found in 10 cultivars. Aparicio-Fernández *et al.* (2005) identified proanthocyanidin monomers, dimers, trimers, tetramers, pentamers, and hexamers in black bean seed coat. Phenolic acids as syringic acid, ferulic acid, p-coumaric acid, and o-coumaric acid, vanillic acid were found in the studied cultivars; those compounds have been reported in common beans (Díaz-Batalla *et al.*, 2006; Luthria and Pastor-Corrales, 2006). Myricetin and kaempferol 3-*O* galactoside were identified only in black beans (1.5%). Vanillin (0.80–7.9%) and daidzin (2.29–1.18%) were found in eight and nine cultivars, respectively.

5.3 Composition of Common Bean Antioxidant Fiber

5.3.1 Definition

Dietary fiber has been well recognized as a potent bioactive compound with protective properties against cardiovascular disease development (Kutos *et al.*, 2003; Pereira *et al.*, 2004), hyperlipidemia (Jenkins *et al.*, 2006; Anderson *et al.*, 2009) and several types of cancer (Aune *et al.*, 2012; Hansen *et al.*, 2012). The concept of dietary fiber has been a popular topic of discussion over the years. The most recent update provided by the Codex Alimentarius Commission defines dietary fiber as carbohydrate polymers that are not hydrolyzed by the endogenous enzymes in the small intestine of humans (Codex, 2015). These include edible carbohydrate polymers naturally occurring in the food as consumed; those that have been obtained from food by physical, enzymatic, or chemical means and that show a physiological health effect generally demonstrated by scientific evidence; and synthetic carbohydrate polymers with physiological effects demonstrated by scientific evidence. A footnote included in 2014 recognizes carbohydrates of 3 to 9 monomeric units, lignin and associated substances as part of the dietary fiber complex (Miller Jones, 2014).

Among the associated substances are compounds such as polyphenols and carotenoids that are commonly bound to dietary fiber (Jiménez-Escrig *et al.*, 2001; Martinez-Tome *et al.*, 2004), conferring to fiber an antioxidant character. The term "antioxidant fiber" was first defined by Saura-Calixto (1998), as a natural product rich in dietary fiber and polyphenolic compounds. In order to be considered a source of antioxidant fiber, plant materials must fulfill the following criteria (Saura-Calixto, 1998): contain at least 50% of dietary fiber in a dry matter basis measured by the AOAC methodology (Prosky *et al.*, 1988); 1 g of dietary fiber should inhibit lipid oxidation equivalent to 200 mg of vitamin E and exert free radical scavenging equivalent to 50 mg of vitamin E; and the antioxidant capacity must be inherent to the plant food.

Regarding the studies done with *Phaseolus vulgaris*, few, if any, meet all the requirements to be considered a source of antioxidant fiber. Instead, the non-digestible fraction (NDF) and their antioxidant associated compounds have been well characterized (Vergara-Castañeda *et al.*, 2012; Feregrino-Pérez *et al.*, 2008; Campos-Vega *et al.*, 2009, Hernández-Salazar *et al.*, 2010; Cruz-Bravo, *et al.* 2011).

The main constituents of NDF comprise polysaccharides such as resistant starch, soluble and insoluble fiber, and non-digestible oligosaccharides (Champ *et al.*, 2003; Hoover and Zhou, 2003). Other associated components present in the NDF from common beans include resistant proteins (Vergara-Castañeda *et al.*, 2012), resistant peptides (Luna-Vital *et al.*, 2014a), and phenolic compounds (Feregrino-Pérez *et al.*, 2008; Cruz-Bravo *et al.*, 2011; Vergara-Castañeda *et al.*, 2012).

The content and composition of NDF are highly variable, depending mainly on variety, crop year, and environmental factors, as shown in Table 5.1. Polysaccharides are the most abundant fraction, followed by resistant protein and peptides.

5.3.2 Polysaccharides

In common beans, polysaccharide content varies from 36.5 to 58.57%, with predominance of insoluble fiber (31–61.8% of NDF) and resistant starch (25.5–39.3% of NDF). Some authors attribute the higher content of insoluble against soluble fiber to the fact that the insoluble cellulose, hemicellulose, lignins, resistant starch, resistant protein, and polyphenols are contained in this fraction (Saura-Calixto *et al.*, 2000).

There is evidence of a wide range of physiological effects associated with insoluble fiber. Insoluble fiber exerts a mechanical action by increasing stool bulk in gastrointestinal tract, improving transit time (Cummings, 2001) and laxation (Tosh and Yada 2010), thus reducing dietary lipid absorption. Specifically, resistant starch from common beans have proven to be beneficial in the management of hyperlipidemia by reducing fat absorption (Han *et al.*, 2003, 2004), and regulating appetite and satiety (Tapsell, 2004; Darzi *et al.*, 2011). It is noteworthy that the traditional cooking and storage methods used for common beans in Latin America (repeated cooling–heating cycles) promote retrogradation of starch, increasing the resistant starch content in this legume (Pujolà *et al.*, 2007).

Table 5.1 NDF composition of different *Phaseolus vulgaris* varieties.

Variety	Processing/ crop year	Polysac-charides (%)	IDF (%)	SDF (%)	RS (%)	Oligosac-charides (mg/g)	Protein (%)	Phenolic compounds (mg/g)	Antioxidant capacity (TEAC/g)	Reference
Negro 8025	Cooked	48.10 ± 2.50	37.50 ± 2.50	11.00 ± 0.00	32.00 ± 2.20	Rf: 9.80 ± 0.15 Sc: 0.90 ± 0.03 Vb: 0.10 ± 0.01		CT: 2.2 ± 0.09		Campos-Vega, *et al.*, 2009
Negro 8025	Cooked	58.57 ± 0.46	57.84 ± 0.46*	0.73 ± 0.01*	26.82 ± 0.10	Rf: 0.23 ± 0.01 Sc: LDL Vb: 0.09 ± 0.00		CT: 20.71 ± 0.44 TF: 0.61 ± 0.30		Cruz-Bravo *et al.*, 2011
Negro 8025	Cooked	57.05 ± 0.05	61.80 ± 0.50	8.70 ± 0.04	39.30 ± 0.15	10.00 ± 4.80	- -	CT: 9.11 ± 0.27		Feregrino-Pérez, *et al.* 2014
Negro 8025	Cooked	42.71 ± 0.66					20.16 ± 0.98			Luna-Vital *et al.*, 2014a
Bayo Madero	Cooked	55.00 ± 2.00	41.00 ± 0.00	14.00 ± 0.50	37.00 ± 3.50	Rf: 9.60 ± 0.00 Sc: 0.10 ± 0.02 Vb: LDL		CT: 0.8 ± 0.03		Campos-Vega *et al.*, 2009
Bayo Madero	Cooked	43.8 ± 0.6	51.1 ± 1.3	0.6 ± 0.1	25.5 ± 0.2	Rf: 1.50 ± 0.10 Sc: 13.80 ± 0.10 Vb: 0.50 ± 0.10	17.1 ± 0.1	TP: 13.80 ± 0.70 CT: 14.0 ± 0.10		Vergara-Castañeda *et al.*, 2010
Bayo Madero	Cooked	46.6 ± 1.53					18.23 ± 0.35			Luna-Vital *et al.*, 2014a
Pinto Durango	Cooked	36.50 ± 0.50	31.10 ± 0.50	5.50 ± 0.00	28.00 ± 0.00	Rf: 15.60 ± 0.00 Sc: 0.60 ± 0.00 Vb: 0.20 ± 0.01		CT : 1.3 ± 0.03		Campos-Vega *et al.*, 2009
Pinto Durango	Cooked	45.63 ± 1.75					16.33 ± 1.10			Luna-Vital *et al.*, 2014a
Azufrado Higuera	Cooked	42.20 ± 1.50	31.00 ± 1.50	11.00 ± 0.00	34.00 ± 1.50	Rf: 1.30 ± 0.09 Sc: 0.20 ± 0.00 Vb: 0.20 ± 0.00		LDL		Campos-Vega *et al.*, 2009
Azufrado Higuera	Cooked	41.3 ± 30.45[a]					19.86 ± 0.25[a]			Luna-Vital *et al.*, 2014a
Black Cotaxtla beans	Cooked	48.93	38.7 ± 0.81	10.22 ± 0.32				TP: 0.30 ± 0.04 CT: 8.30 ± 0.40	4.9 ± 0.10	Hernández-Salazar *et al.*, 2010

IDF, insoluble dietary fiber; SDF, soluble dietary fiber; RS, resistant starch; Rf, Sc and Vb represent farrinose, stachyose and verbascose, respectively; CT, condensed tannins; TP, total phenolics.

Resistant starch and soluble fiber have an important feature in common: fermentability. These fractions are fermented in the proximal colon by the microbiota to produce short-chain fatty acids (SCFAs), which have been shown to be involved in colon cancer prevention by inhibiting survival of colon adenocarcinoma (HT29 cells) (Campos-Vega *et al.*, 2009; Cruz-Bravo *et al.*, 2011), promoting cell cycle arrest and apoptosis (Feregrino-Pérez *et al.*, 2014). On the other hand, soluble fiber is related to reduction of low density lipoproteins (LDL) and cholesterol levels in blood (Jenkins *et al.*, 2006), as well as insulin resistance (Rizkalla *et al.*, 2002; Tungland and Meyer, 2002).

Oligosaccharides consist of monosaccharide residues (3–10 units) linked by glycosidic bonds. In common beans raffinose, stachyose, and verbascose are the main oligosaccharides present in the raw seed and in the cooked and dehydrated product (Ramírez-Jiménez *et al.*, 2014). These compounds are resistant to digestion due to the lack of α-galactosidase in the small intestine of humans, allowing them to pass into the large intestine for fermentation, leading to flatus formation and digestive discomfort (Martín-Cabrejas *et al.*, 2006). Despite this disadvantage, oligosaccharides also exhibit bifidogenic potential, and are considered to be prebiotic agents (Gibson *et al.*, 2004). Moreover, oligosaccharides can be fermented to produce SCFAs, which are associated with hypocholesterolemic and antiproliferative effects (Tungland and Meyer, 2002).

5.3.3 Polyphenols

Although the phenolic compounds are minor components, they confer significant antioxidant capacity; in particular, flavonoids and condensed tannins are considered the most potent antioxidant agents (Cardador-Martínez *et al.*, 2002; Aparicio-Fernández *et al.*, 2005). Unfortunately, only one study assesses the antioxidant value of NDF from *Phaseolus vulgaris* (Hernández-Salazar *et al.*, 2010). According to these authors, polymeric units of condensed tannins are bound to the NDF fraction, whereas some low molecular weight flavonoids, lignins, and hydroxycinnamic acids are found esterified to the cell wall polysaccharides (Shiga *et al.*, 2003). These compounds are retained in the insoluble fraction (Saura-Calixto *et al.*, 2000), which allows polyphenols to reach the colon to exert a biological effect. Phenolic compounds are fermented by local microbiota, producing SCFAs such as acetic, propionic, and butyric acids (Delzenne *et al.*, 2003). In the colonic environment, the release of polyphenols increases the antioxidant capacity *in situ* and in plasma after absorption. Pérez-Jiménez *et al.* (2009) reported that acute intake of dietary fiber rich in polyphenols increased antioxidant capacity in plasma in healthy subjects after 8 hours of intake, suggesting that these associated compounds are partially bioavailable in humans. In another study, a group of rats fed a high fat diet containing 0.5% polyphenols, reduced the amount of fecal bile acids, compounds involved in fat absorption and colon cancer (Han *et al.*, 2009).

5.3.4 Peptides

The second major group of compounds found in the NDF from beans is protein, with values in the range of 16.33–20.16% as shown in Table 5.1. Although significant amounts of proteins are reported in different varieties of beans, its preventive role in health and disease is still unclear. To our knowledge, only one study (Luna-Vital *et al.*, 2014a) has assessed the effect of some peptides extracted from NDF of four Mexican varieties (Azufrado Higuera, Bayo Madero, Negro 8025, and Pinto Durango) on proliferation and protein expression using human colorectal cancer cells. In that study, the peptides extracts were characterized by mass spectrometry (MALDI TOF/TOF) and sequenced. Five major peptides were found in this fraction with molecular mass ranging from 505.48 to 671.68 Da. Pinto Durango was the variety with the higher proportion of peptides. After sequencing, diverse biological potential were predicted for these molecules, including inhibition of angiotensin-converting enzyme, a protein involved in hypertension risk (Rasyid *et al.*, 2012). In subsequent publications, our research group found that peptide extracts were able to downregulate expression of genes related to oxidative processes and to upregulate antioxidant enzymes, suggesting a protective role against proliferation in HCT116 and RKO colorectal cancer cells (Luna-Vital *et al.*, 2014b). Furthermore, synthesized peptides with the same sequence as that originally found in the NDF of common beans showed significant antioxidant capacity measured by four different methods: 421.58 µmol $FeSO_4$/mg by the ferric reducing ability of plasma (FRAP) assay, 2.01 µmol Na_2EDTA/mg using Fe^{2+} chelation assay, 748.39 µmol Trolox/mg of dry peptide by the DPPH method, and 561.42 µmol Trolox/mg by ABTS (Luna-Vital *et al.*, 2015).

5.4 Biological Potential of Antioxidant Fiber of Common Bean

5.4.1 Antioxidant Capacity

Free radicals are generated in the body during respiration in aerobic organisms; imbalance in free radicals can lead to cellular damage. Other oxidative stress promotors are oxidized food constituents and metals in high concentrations in the body (Luna-Vital *et al.*, 2015).

The antioxidant potential of the NDF of common beans is attributed to three main components: (i) polyphenols, (ii) non-digestible carbohydrates (such as soluble and insoluble fiber, resistant starch, oligosaccharides), and (iii) proteins and bioactive peptides. The antioxidant potentials of these components differ and are increased considerably by the microbiota fermentation process (Figure 5.1).

5.4.1.1 Non-Digestible Carbohydrates

NDF is made up of fiber (soluble and insoluble), resistant starch, and oligosaccharides (raffinose, stachyose, and verbascose, mullein) (Escudero and González, 2006). These carbohydrates can be converted to SCFAs such as acetate, propionate, and butyrate by colonic bacteria fermentation (Vergara-Castañeda *et al.*, 2010; Cruz-Bravo *et al.*, 2011; Campos-Vega *et al.*, 2009; Feregrino-Pérez *et al.*, 2008).

The antioxidant potential of SCFAs is related to their ability to modulate enzymes associated with the oxidative stress response. Antioxidant enzymes are

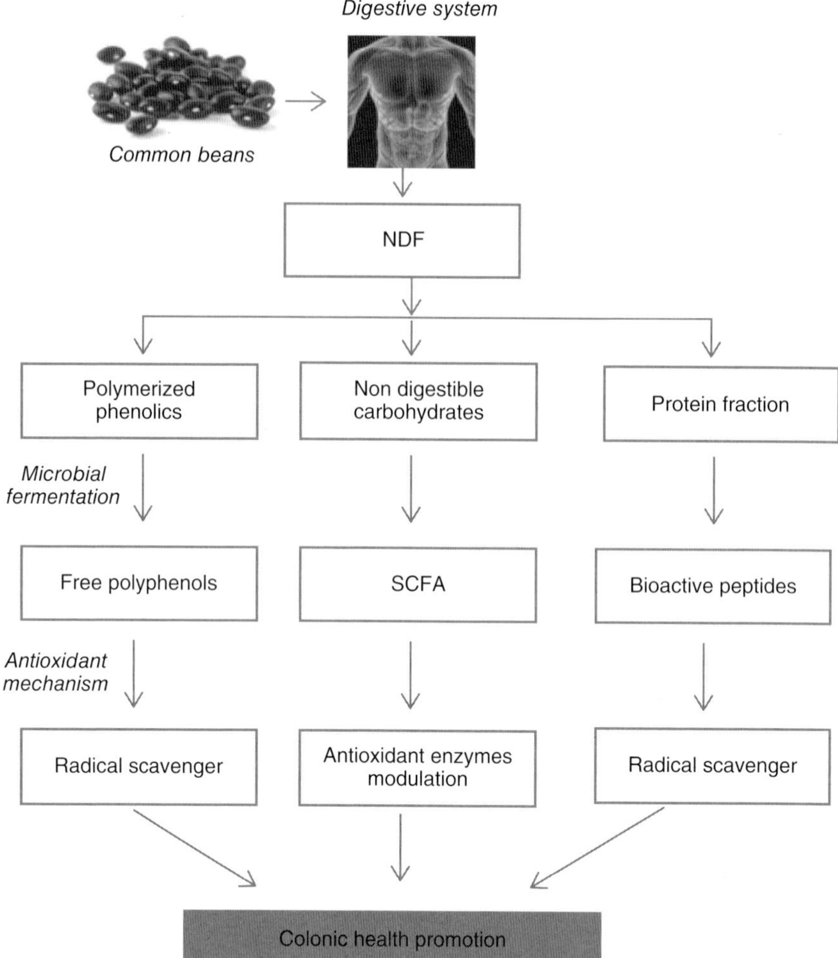

Figure 5.1 Biological potential of common bean antioxidant fiber.

part of a series of defense mechanisms that have evolved by organisms in response to free radicals exposure. The superoxide dismutase (SOD) enzyme family plays a key role in this context by providing a first line of defense against superoxide radicals. In addition, catalase (CAT) enzymes convert hydrogen peroxide to water and molecular oxygen. Butyrate enhances expression of glutathione *S*-transferases (GST) and other enzymes related to detoxification processes (Stein *et al.*, 2010). Upregulation of antioxidant mechanisms is thought to be a protective mechanism in the chemoprevention of colon cancer (Jahns *et al.*, 2015).

Vergara-Castañeda *et al.* (2010) reported the polysaccharide and resistant starch content in the Bayo Madero cultivar to be 55% and 37%, respectively. In this work they found that total and individual oligosaccharide content in beans decreased with cooking (from 59.6 to 55.8 mg/g). Furthermore, the total oligosaccharide content in the NDF was significantly lower compared to that in whole uncooked and cooked beans, representing a loss of 71.7%. This decrease is attributed to solubility processes. Campos-Vega *et al.* (2009) reported polysaccharide content in cooked beans for the cultivars Negro 8025, Bayo Madero, Pinto Durango, and Azufrado Higuera and found it ranged from 36.5% to 55%. Moreover, insoluble fiber from cooked bean seeds ranged from 31% to 41% and was higher than that of soluble fiber (5.5–14%). Fiber content (insoluble and soluble) was higher in cooked beans than in raw, indicating that thermal processes increase non-starch polysaccharide content and modified starch structure, providing resistance to enzymatic action and increasing NDF and their fractions.

5.4.1.2 Phenolic Compounds

Some phenolic compounds such as flavonoids and condensed tannins in beans are complexed with carbohydrates and proteins and can be release during thermal hydrolysis (Vergara-Castañeda *et al.*, 2010). However, most of those phenolic compounds remain in NDF and are finally released during bacterial fermentation in the colon where they exert their beneficial antioxidant activity. Vergara-Castañeda *et al.* (2010) reported total phenols (13.8 mg eq gallic acid/g bean) and condensed tannins (14.0 mg eq chatechin/g bean) in NDF of Bayo Madero cultivar. Condensed tannin and flavonoid contents tend to increase in the cooked beans, suggesting the hydrolysis of complexes with proteins and starch. Condensed tannin content increases in NDF due to concentration effects, however after fermentation the phenolic concentration is small, suggesting their release from the food matrix during fermentation action of colonic bacterial enzymes. This probably reflects increased bioavailability in the large intestine (Cruz-Bravo *et al.*, 2011)

Many researchers have reported that polyphenols from dry beans may act as antioxidants to inhibit the formation of free radicals. Furthermore, flavonoids such as condensed tannins and anthocyanins have been reported as antioxidant and antimutagenic agents. The presence of these bioactive compounds in common beans is related to the decreased incidence of chronic degenerative diseases in people who consume beans (Feregrino-Pérez *et al.*, 2008). Feregrino-Pérez *et al.* (2008) reported differences in condensed tannins in raw beans, cooked beans, and polysaccharide extract (21.04, 15.15, and 9.11 mg of (+)-catechin, respectively). Total phenolic compounds are dependent on the growing and storage conditions as well as thermal treatment. Those differences can be attributed to the climatic conditions during the growing season, or the type of soil in which the beans were grown, as well as the bean genotype and the storage conditions. Total flavonoids were similar in raw and cooked beans and polysaccharide samples (1.9, 1.8, and 1.6 mg rutin eq, respectively).

5.4.1.3 Peptides

Common bean NDF contains a significant amount of protein (17%), which could release amino acids and bioactive peptides with potential health benefits during colon fermentation. Proteins, peptides, and amino acids with potential antioxidant functional groups from foods exert antioxidant properties by inhibiting free radicals and chelating transition metals. Luna-Vital *et al.* (2015) characterized five peptides in NDF that represented 70% of the total protein in NDF of common beans (GLTSK, LSGNK, GEGSGA, MPACGSS, and MTEEY) and evaluated their antioxidant capacity. MPACGSS, for example, showed the highest antioxidant capacity, followed by MTEEY and LSGNK; the lowest values were shown by GLTSK and GEGSGA.

When the FRAP assay was used, the values ranged from 73.8 to 421.58 µmol $FeSO_4$/mg. The FRAP assay measures the ability of antioxidants to reduce the ferric 2,4,6-tripyridyl-s-triazine complex $[Fe^{3+}-(TPTZ)_2]^{3+}$ to the intensely blue-colored ferrous complex $[Fe^{2+}-(TPTZ)_2]^{2+}$ in an acidic medium. The values obtained for the ABTS scavenging activity ranged from 18.14 to 561.42 µmol Trolox/mg, and for the DPPH scavenging activity from 49.98 to 748.39 µmol Trolox/mg. Moreover, the chelating activity of the peptides ranged from 1.01 to 2.01 µmol Na_2EDTA/mg. The antioxidant activity of the peptides was measured using different methods based on different mechanisms to decrease free radicals. The reducing capacity of the peptides may serve as a significant indicator of their potential antioxidant activities as electron-donating reducing agents, which can donate an electron to a free radical. As a result, the radical is neutralized, and the reduced species subsequently acquires a proton from the compound. Previous reports indicated that hydrophobic and sulfur amino acids of peptides contribute to the reducing power. This is in agreement with our results since those types of amino acids are present in the peptide MPACGSS, which was the most potent peptide to reduce $[Fe^{3+}-(TPTZ)_2]^{3+}$. Another antioxidant mechanism is scavenging of free radicals. In this study, we used assays based on $DPPH^{\bullet+}$ and $ABTS^{\bullet}$ radicals.

Peptides are believed to intercept the free radical chain of oxidation and donate a hydrogen from the phenolic, imidazole, and indole groups present in some amino acids, thereby forming stable end-products that do not initiate or propagate further oxidation. Additionally, transition metal ions, such as Fe^{2+} are able to promote the generation of reactive oxygen species. Fe^{2+} can also catalyze the Haber–Weiss reaction and induce superoxide anions to form more hazardous hydroxyl radicals, which can react with neighboring molecules to cause severe tissue damage. Therefore, the chelation of transition metal ions by antioxidative peptides could slow down the oxidation reaction. As in FRAP and the free radical scavenging assays, MPACGSS had the highest ($p < 0.05$) antioxidant activity, but in this case, it was statistically similar to both GLTSK and GEGSGA. The carboxyl and amino groups in the side-chains of the acidic and basic amino acids present in these peptides are thought to play an important role in chelating metal ions, in turn providing them with metal chelating activity.

5.4.2 Anticancer Activity

5.4.2.1 *In Vivo* Studies

According to the World Health Organization (2015) colorectal cancer is the third most common cancer in men (746 000 cases, 10.0% of the total) and the second in women (614 000 cases, 9.2% of the total) worldwide. Almost 55% of the cases occur in more developed regions. Mortality is lower (694 000 deaths, 8.5% of the total) with more deaths (52%) in the less developed regions of the world, reflecting a poorer survival in these regions. There is less variability in mortality rates worldwide (six-fold in men, four-fold in women), with the highest estimated mortality rates in both sexes in Central and Eastern Europe (20.3 per 100 000 for men, 11.7 per 100 000 for women), and the lowest in Western Africa (3.5 and 3.0, respectively).

Common bean NDF has been shown to decrease colorectal cancer *in vitro* and *in vivo*. As can be observed in Table 5.2, the *in vivo* evaluations of antioxidant fiber of common bean have been focused on the early stages of colorectal carcinogenesis using azoxymethane (AOM)-induced rats. One of the known effects caused by common bean fiber is the production of SCFAs, mainly acetate, propionate, and butyrate. Among SCFAs, butyrate represents the most important end-product of colonic bacterial fermentation of fiber and starch (Yang and Rose, 2014). In addition to having a nutrient effect on the mucosa, butyrate is the main energy source for normal colonocytes (Donohoe *et al.*, 2012). Butyrate has been studied due to the proven effect on gene expression, cell growth regulation, and differentiation in several animal cells (Zhou *et al.*, 2011; Yoo *et al.*, 2015; Leonel and Alvarez-Leite, 2012). It has been found to suppress c-*myc* levels and increase c-*jun* transcription, leading to transcriptional activation of specific genes involved in differentiating pathways (Huang and Liu, 2008; Tong *et al.*, 2006). Furthermore, treatment of cultured cells with butyrate promotes reversible hyperacetylated histones that play crucial roles in modulating chromatin structure and its transcriptional activity (Chang *et al.*, 2014; Tan *et al.*, 2015).

Butyrate is also recognized as an anticancer agent in different types of transformed cells (Wang *et al.*, 2013; Foglietta *et al.*, 2014; Yamamura *et al.*, 2014). Feregrino-Pérez *et al.* (2008) studied AOM-induced Wistar rats given 1.84 g of polysaccharide extract (PE) from the antioxidant fiber of common bean Negro 8025 per kg of body weight. Overall, acetate, propionate, and butyrate production was higher in cecal content, followed by colon content and feces except for in the PE + AOM group, for which a higher concentration of these SCFAs was found in feces, colonic content, and cecal content. The increase in butyrate has been reported previously in several studies to be a consequence of fiber administration in clinical studies (Fung *et al.*, 2012). In contrast, other research performed in AOM-induced Wistar rats using 2.5 g/kg body weight of PE extracted from the Bayo Madero cultivar showed that SCFA production was not significantly different among groups in cecal, colonic, and fecal contents (Vergara-Castañeda *et al.*, 2010). However, the fecal content of the PE + AOM group showed a slight increase in propionic (3.71 mM/g) and butyric acid concentrations (3.34 mM/g) compared with that of the AOM group (3.48 and 3.21 mM/g of propionic and butyric acids, respectively). The highest SCFA concentration was present in fecal content. The differences between these results and those reported by Feregrino-Pérez *et al.* (2008) was attributed to the different variety of bean used and the composition of its antioxidant fiber or its fermentation capacity, suggesting that the Bayo Madero bean and its antioxidant fiber could increase SCFAs in fecal content. Butyric acid concentration in the NDF + AOM group was 2.86, 2.63, and 3.34 mM in cecal, colonic, and fecal content, respectively, which is high enough to produce a protective effect in the colon according to the literature.

Table 5.2 Biological effects of antioxidant fiber of *Phaseolus vulgaris* L. on colon cancer models.

Component	Cultivar	Model	Dose	Main effect	Reference
Fermented polysaccharides with human gut flora	Bayo Madero	HT-29 cells	LC_{50} (17% of the extract)	*p53*-mediated pathway affected, mainly in apoptosis, cell cycle and cell proliferation genes	Campos-Vega *et al.*, 2010
Fermented polysaccharides with human gut flora	Bayo Madero	HT-29 cells	LC_{50} (17% of the extract)	Cell growth inhibition, modulation of proteins related to apoptosis, cell cycle arrest and proliferation. Morphological changes associated with apoptosis	Campos-Vega *et al.*, 2012
Human gut microbiota fermented NDF	Negro 8025	HT-29 cells	LC_{50} (7.36, 0.33, and 3.31 mM eq to acetic propionic and butyrate)	Cell growth inhibition, regulation of genes related to apoptosis	Cruz-Bravo *et al.*, 2014
Human gut microbiota fermented NDF	Negro 8025	HT-29	LC_{50} (7.36, 0.33, and 3.31 mM eq to acetic propionic and butyrate)	Cell growth inhibition and DNA fragmentation	Cruz-Bravo *et al.*, 2011
Polysaccharide extract	Negro 8025	AOM-induced wistar rats	1.84 g/kg	Reduction in the number of ACF, differential gene expression related to apoptosis	Feregrino-Pérez *et al.*, 2008
Peptide fraction extracted from the NDF	Azufrado Higuera, Bayo Madero, Negro 8025	HCT116 and RKO cells	IC_{50} (0.44 − 0.79 mg/mL)	Cell growth inhibition, modification of protein expression levels associated to apoptosis and cell cycle arrest	Luna Vital *et al.*, 2014a

Peptide fraction extracted from the NDF	Bayo Madero and Azufrado Higuera	HCT116 and RKO cells	0.5 mg/mL	Differential gene expression corresponding to activation of oxidative stress response pathways	Luna Vital *et al.*, 2014b
Polysaccharide extract	Bayo Madero	AOM-induced Wistar rats	2.5 g/kg	Reduction in the number of ACF. Reduction in β-glucoronidase activity in colonic tissue	Vergara-Castañeda *et al.*, 2010
Polysaccharide extract	Bayo Madero	AOM-induced Wistar rats	2.5 g/kg	Differential gene expression corresponding to p53 pathway activation associated with apoptosis	Vergara-Castañeda *et al.*, 2012

NDF, non-digestible fraction; AOM, azoxymethane; ACF, aberrant crypt foci.

β-Glucuronidase enzymatic activity is also relevant in colon carcinogenesis due to its ability to hydrolyze several glucuronide conjugates and thus release active carcinogenic metabolites in the intestinal lumen (Guo *et al.*, 2013). Diets supplemented with different types of fiber have been suggested to contribute to colon cancer inhibition by increasing non-pathogenic bacteria, fiber fermentation, and reduction of bacterial β-glucuronidase activity (Raman *et al.*, 2016). Vergara-Castañeda *et al.* (2010) reported that feeding antioxidant fiber to AOM-induced rats significantly decreased the β-glucuronidase activity with respect to AOM. This decrease was accompanied by protection against precancerous lesions induced by the chemical carcinogen (AOM), suggesting that reduction of aberrant crypt foci development may be associated with a decrease in cecal, colonic, and fecal activity of this enzyme, because insufficient enzyme prevents carcinogen release in the colon and thus cannot induce the damage produced in the AOM group. According to that finding, the authors suggested that the suppression of aberrant crypt foci formation is strongly influenced by the decrease in the β-glucuronidase activity in the colon, probably by modifying metabolic activities of the intestinal microbiota that prevents AOM release in the colon. These results also indicate that an early stage of colon carcinogenesis, evaluated by aberrant crypt foci formation, *in vivo* is modulated by different mechanisms depending on the cultivar and composition of the common bean and its antioxidant fiber.

5.4.2.2 *In Vitro* Studies

The effects of common bean antioxidant fiber have also been tested in cells in order to determine potential mechanisms of action. Colorectal cancer cells such as HT29, HCT116, RKO, and KM12L4 were used to test the efficacy of common bean fiber. In previous works carried out by Campos-Vega *et al.* (2012), the carbohydrate fermentation products (CFP) of the antioxidant fiber of Negro 8025 beans inhibited the growth of HT29 cells in a concentration-dependent manner. The log-LC$_{50}$ value after 24 hours of treatment was 17%, whereas the untreated cells showed no significant inhibition of cell growth. In order to compare the effect of pure compounds, synthetic SCFAs were also assessed for anticancer potential. The synthetic SCFA mixtures equivalent in the LC$_{50}$ of the CFP (5.1, 0.68, and 1.19 mmol/mL of acetate, propionate, and butyrate, respectively) were less effective in growth inhibition of cells; it was suggested that SCFAs in the CFP are key components responsible for inhibiting HT29 cell survival (35%). Testing the pure compounds as a SCFAs mixture, they induced considerable morphological characteristics (hematoxylin and eosin staining) of apoptosis relative to control cells. These included cellular shrinkage, nuclear condensation, and cytoplasmic vacuoles. A synthetic SCFA mixture induced morphologic signs of apoptosis in more cells than the extracts. The TUNEL assay showed that the CFP and synthetic SCFAs mixture on HT29 cells induced DNA damage; 28% and 51% of HT29 cells were TUNEL-positive after treatment with the LC$_{50}$ of PE and a synthetic SCFAs mixture, respectively, suggesting the occurrence of apoptosis. Interestingly, the fermentation sample was more effective in mediating growth inhibition than the corresponding SCFA mixture. In agreement with *in vivo* studies, this could mean that the activity of fiber derived from beans is mainly based on the SCFAs produced during fermentation.

Although the main mechanism of action of common bean antioxidant fiber was attributed to the CFP, the characterization studies have reported a protein content of approximately 20% (Luna-Vital *et al.*, 2014a), for which role in the chemoprotection remained unknown. Studies performed by our group reported the characterization of the protein fraction from the antioxidant fiber of common bean. In order to simulate the proteolytic effect of the ileal and pancreatic effluents reaching the colon, Luna-Vital *et al.* (2014a) used pepsin–pancreatin hydrolysis in the protein extracted from the antioxidant fiber, observing an increase in the concentration of molecules below 10 kDa, which confirmed the conversion of proteins into peptides. The resulting peptides in the antioxidant fiber extracts had small molecular masses, suggesting that they can cross cell membranes and get internalized into the cells (Koren and Torchilin, 2012). The variability of the responses on proliferation of human colon cancer cells to different cultivar treatments was attributed to the difference in the peptides fraction composition. Even though the molecular masses of the peptides were similar and the sequenced peptides represented around 70% of the protein, small differences in their characteristics and abundance among cultivars were observed. There were 17 peptides with a molecular mass ranging from 505 to 1019 Da; some of these were not present in all of the cultivars. According to the BIOPEP database, the peptides present in the non-digestible fraction of common bean had a predicted inhibitory potential on angiotensin-converting enzyme (ACE), an important member of the renin–angiotensin–aldosterone system. Although this effect is mostly related to cardiovascular processes, it has recently been considered as a possible target for colorectal cancer treatment due to its relation to angiogenesis and cell proliferation through the activation of STAT3 transcription factor (Rodrigues-Ferreira and Nahmias, 2015). The ACE inhibitory potential was later confirmed using the pure peptides originally identified in the antioxidant fiber of common bean, and biochemical assays and detection of substrate–product transformation with HPLC (Luna-Vital *et al.*, 2015). The peak area of the product of the ACE reaction (HHL) decreased as the peptide concentration increased. It is suggested that the peptides inhibited ACE as a function of concentration. The lowest IC_{50} value was for GLTSK (65.4 μM) and the highest for MPACGSS (191.5 μM). The results were significantly higher than those obtained for captopril (17.5 μM), and the five peptides tested had higher (less potent) ACE inhibitory activities than those of previous reports on common bean protein hydrolyzates (de Jesús Ariza-Ortega *et al.*, 2014).

Looking for potential interactions, it was found that the combination of the GLTSK and MTEEY peptides showed a synergistic interaction, reducing the concentration needed to inhibit 50% of the enzymatic activity by approximately 30%. As expected, digestive enzymes did not show an impact on the peptides LSGNK, GEGSGA, and MPACGSS inhibiting ACE, and only a modest significant reduction of the ACE inhibitory activity for the GLTSK and MTEEY peptides was observed.

With regard to the inhibitory potential of the peptides on cancer cells, the peptides extracted from the Bayo Madero (BM), Negro 8025 (N8), and Azufrado

Higuera (AH) cultivars inhibited proliferation of HCT116 and RKO human colorectal cancer cells in a dose–response manner (Luna-Vital *et al.*, 2014a). The most potent results were for HCT116 (AH peptide fraction $IC_{50} = 0.53$ mg/mL; N8 peptide fraction $IC_{50} = 0.80$ mg/mL) and for RKO (BM peptide fraction $IC_{50} = 0.51$ mg/mL, AH peptide fraction $IC_{50} = 0.59$ mg/mL, and N8 peptide fraction $IC_{50} = 0.79$ mg/mL). The effectiveness to reduce cell proliferation varied depending on the cultivar. In KM12L4 cells, whose main characteristic is to be highly metastatic, none of the peptide extracts were effective at inhibiting cell proliferation. Pinto Durango was, in general, less effective at inhibiting cancer cells. Proliferation of HCT116, RKO, and KM12L4 has been reported to be regulated by peptides from food sources such as lunasin, a 43-amino-acid peptide isolated from soybean, which presented an antiproliferative effect on the cell lines mentioned above in a dose-dependent manner (Dia and de Mejía, 2011). The difference in the concentration of the peptides per cultivar could be inducing different responses. However, an interaction between dietary compounds may also occur, including polyphenol–protein bindings, which may be irreversibly enhanced by thermal treatments (Ozdal *et al.*, 2013).

5.4.2.3 Protein Modulation

In the search for potential mechanisms of action, the different components of the antioxidant fiber of common beans have been tested for differential protein expression in human colorectal cancer cells. Table 5.3 summarizes the studies performed using primarily the CFP and the peptide fraction from the antioxidant fiber of common bean on the protein expression of HT29 and HCT116 human colorectal cancer cells. Both fractions targeted the induction of apoptosis caused by proteins transcriptionally activated potentially by the tumor suppressor p53 pathway. Mutations and deletions of the tumor suppressor gene *p53* have been identified in about 50% of colorectal carcinomas and are associated with poor prognosis due to its weaker ability to inhibit cell proliferation (Fearon, 2011). However, in studies performed using the components of the antioxidant fiber of common beans, cells with mutated *p53* (HT29) and wild–type *p53* (HCT116) have been used. As reported by Campos-Vega *et al.* (2012), the levels of the apoptotic proteins SIAH1 and caspase-3 (cleaved) were significantly higher in HT29 cells treated with the CFP and SCFA mixtures than in the untreated cells. Bax was suppressed in both treatments compared to the control. The resultant low expression of Bax observed in this study suggests that the CFP of common bean and SCFAs do not stimulate adenocarcinoma colon cancer cell apoptosis via the intrinsic or mitochondrial Bcl-2/Bax pathway. The authors pointed to a potential role of CFP and SCFAs mixture involvement in an alternative apoptosis-mediated pathway by SIAH1 and caspase-3 activation because those proteins have been associated with tumor suppression and apoptosis (Benhar and Stamler, 2005). Proteins related to cell cycle progression were also affected, such as cyclins and cyclin-dependent kinases. The CFP also caused an increase in the cyclin-dependent kinases inhibitor p21, which corresponds with the potential mechanism of action.

Table 5.3 Protein levels summary of colon cancer models in response to the antioxidant fiber of *Phaseolus vulgaris* L.

Component	Cultivar	Model	Top regulated proteins	Reference
Fermented polysaccharides with human gut flora	Bayo Madero	HT-29 colon adenocarcinoma cells	↑SIAH1 ↑Caspase-3 ↑p21 ↑Rb ↑pRb ↓Bax ↓p53 ↓Cyclin D1 ↓PCNA ↓HDAC1	Campos-Vega *et al.*, 2012
Peptide fraction extracted from the NDF	Bayo Madero and Azufrado Higuera	HCT116 cells	↑p21 ↑p-p53 ↑Bax ↑CytC ↑c-Caspase-3 ↓Livin ↓Survivin ↓XIAP ↓TNRF1 ↓NFκB p65	Luna-Vital *et al.*, 2014a

NDF, non-digestible fraction.

As for peptide fractions from the antioxidant fiber of common bean, treatment with the peptide fraction from the antioxidant fiber of common bean cultivar Azufrado Higuera activated the tumor suppressor p-p53 Ser392 (76% with respect to the control) in HCT116 colon cancer cells. The expression of p21 increased after treatment with AH peptide fraction (64%), whereas cyclin-B1 expression was lower (45%); this could regulate cyclin–CDK complex formation. The regulatory protein cyclin-B1 is expressed predominantly during the G_2/M transition phase of the cell cycle (Lindqvist *et al.*, 2009); therefore, it suggests that the inhibition of cyclin-B1 and overexpression of p21 could be a potential mechanism of action in the antiproliferative effect of AH peptide fraction. Moreover, for cultivar Bayo Madero, p-p53 Ser46 was overexpressed (68%) and potentially triggered the activation of mitochondrial apoptosis pathway. Thus, p-p53 Ser46 led to the activation of pro-apoptotic proteins such as cyt C (106%), Bcl-2-associated with death promoter (BAD) (22%), Bax (50%), and cleaved caspase-3 (115%), an effector caspase which plays an important role in the execution phase of apoptosis.

In a parallel effect contributing to the apoptosis process, TNFR1 (56%) was decreased. TNFR1 is a transmembrane receptor that is able to induce the activation of anti-apoptotic proteins through subunit NFκB p65 signaling (Yu *et al.* 2015). Depending on the stimuli and stress conditions, p53 can be modified at some amino acid residue; for example, by phosphorylation or acetylation among others. Depending on the posttranslational modification, p53 is able to induce either cell cycle arrest or apoptosis (Meek, 2015). This could partially explain the increased expression of p53 in HCT116 cells exposed to peptides of common bean antioxidant fiber of both cultivars but phosphorylated in different residues, leading to modifications of markers associated with cell cycle arrest or apoptosis.

5.4.2.4 Gene Expression

The mechanisms of action of different constituents of common bean has been further studied using gene expression analysis both *in vivo* and *in vitro* in response to the treatment either of the CFP or the peptide fraction from the common bean NDF. In Table 5.4 the different studies analyzing gene expression are listed. In the *in vivo* experiments with the PE of common bean, a PE + AOM group did not show β-catenin and p53 expression compared with the AOM group (Feregrino-Pérez *et al.*, 2008). The increase in β-catenin expression in neoplasic tissue has been related to the acquired aggressiveness of transformed cells, and in advanced stages of carcinogenesis it can trigger metastatic signals (Keerthivasan *et al.*, 2014). Interestingly, a higher p21 expression independent of p53 and an increased expression of Bax and caspase-3, as well as a decreased expression of Rb and Bcl-2 was found in the colon of animals treated with PE + AOM. It was demonstrated that PE + AOM treatment decreased the expression of Bcl-2 and increased the expression of Bax and caspase-3 compared to AOM treatment, suggesting apoptotic induction by butyrate via mitochondria mechanisms.

Another study supporting the hypothesis that the antioxidant fiber from common bean inhibits cancer cell growth through p53-dependent apoptosis induction (Vergara-Castañeda *et al.*, 2012) reported that *Tp53* gene expression pathway analysis modulated 72 genes at least 1.1-fold (induction or inhibition) in the AOM-induced PE group (NDF-AOM) compared with the AOM group. These genes belong to different pathways involved in apoptosis, cell cycle, cell proliferation and differentiation, DNA repair, and inflammatory response. *Tp53* was overexpressed (9.3-fold) in the PE-AOM group compared with the AOM group. In addition, *p21*, participating in the cell cycle G_1/S phase, was also upregulated (5.5-fold), whereas *Ccne2* (cyclin E) and *Cdkn2A* were inhibited (22.6- and 22.4-fold, respectively). Once *Tp53* induces *p21* transcription, it inhibits the cyclin–Cdk complex necessary for the G_1-to-S phase and G_2-to-M phase transitions in colon cancer cells (Zhang *et al.*, 2012). The *FOXO3* gene, which mediates cell proliferation, survival, differentiation, DNA repair, and defense against oxidative stress, was increased by the PE (Bullock *et al.*, 2013).

Differential gene expression has been also studied in cancer cells to evaluate the effect of different constituents of antioxidant fiber from common bean in isolated environments. As reported by Campos-Vega *et al.* (2010), 72 genes were differentially expressed in HT29 cells treated with FCP using a gene array. It was observed that p21 was overexpressed (1.75-fold). Several genes related to apoptosis induction, proliferation, and DNA repair, such as *SIAH1*, *PRKCA*, and *MSH2*, were

Table 5.4 Differential gene expression summary of colon cancer models in response to the antioxidant fiber of *Phaseolus vulgaris* L.

Component	Cultivar	Model	Top 10 regulated genes		Reference
			Genes	**Fold change**	
Fermented polysaccharides with human gut flora	Bayo Madero	HT-29 cells	*SIAH1*	30.5	Campos-Vega *et al.*, 2010
			PRKCA	18.4	
			MSH2	9.8	
			PTEN	6.6	
			CDKN1A	5.9	
			CHEK1	−21.1	
			GADD45A	−9.1	
			NFKB1	−7.9	
			PRC1	−7.0	
			CASP2	−5.7	
Human gut microbiota fermented NDF	Negro 8025	HT-29	*APAF1*	108.3	Cruz-Bravo *et al.*, 2014
			BID	32.0	
			SIRT1	29.8	
			CASP9	12.7	
			SESN1	12.3	
			TP53	−84.4	
			NFKB1	−25.1	
			MDM2	−24.4	
			BIRC5	−24.4	
			BRCA1	−20.1	
Peptide fraction extracted from the NDF	Bayo Madero and Azufrado Higuera	HCT116 and RKO cells	*OSGIN1*	5.5	Luna Vital *et al.*, 2014b
			JUN	3.8	
			FOSL1	3.1	
			AKR1B10	2.5	
			TXNRD1	2.2	
			KRT19	−21.4	
			EEF1A2	−7.5	
			MAGEA2B	−3.8	
			PDE4B	−2.6	
			DHRS2	−2.3	
Polysaccharide extract	Bayo Madero	Azoxy-methane-induced Wistar rats	*CCNG1*	31.1	Vergara-Castañeda *et al.*, 2012
			GADD45A	18.3	
			BAG1	13.7	
			DNMT1	9.3	
			TP53	9.3	
			E2F1	−18.4	
			JUN	−13.7	
			TP73	−12.0	
			MYOD1	−11.8	
			CDC25C	−9.2	

NDF, non-digestible fraction.

the highest upregulated genes (30.5-, 18.4-, and 9.8-fold, respectively), whereas genes related to cell cycle progression, such as *CHEK1* and *GADD45A*, were potently downregulated (21.4- and 9.1-fold, respectively). *SIAH1* was upregulated (30.5-fold), whereas *p53* and *RB* were downregulated (4.8- and 1.1-fold, respectively). *MSH2* gene was upregulated (9.8-fold) by PE extract, supporting its involvement with DNA repair in accordance with earlier observations (Pereira *et al.*, 2013).

With regard to the effect of the peptide fractions on the differential gene expression of HCT116 and RKO cells, Luna-Vital *et al.* (2014b) reported that within the full list of the represented genes on a human genome microarray, 511 and 964 differentially expressed genes (DEGs) were found for AH peptide fraction and BM peptide fraction, respectively, sharing 405 common DEGs among the cultivars. In contrast, 45 and 32 DEGs were found for the AH peptide fraction and the BM peptide fraction, respectively, in RKO cells, sharing 19 common DEGs in both cultivars. It was also found that among these DEGs, the differential expression of only eight genes in both cell lines was commonly triggered by both bean cultivars, namely *C11orf31*, *C9orf169*, *EMP1*, *GEM*, *PLIN2*, *SUN3*, *TRIM16L*, and *TXNRD1*. The oxidation–reduction cluster contained one of the highest numbers of genes, with 34 genes out of a list of 473 genes. Only 32 genes in RKO human colon cancer cells were significantly affected by the BM peptide fraction treatment at 0.5 mg/mL. Moreover, the RKO cell line was affected in the same biological processes by both AH peptide fraction and BM peptide fraction treatments, even for the common DEGs among cultivars. Results showed that the biological functions of the affected gene sets presenting high enrichment scores were cell redox homeostasis, homeostatic process, glutathione metabolic process, peptide metabolic process, and coenzyme metabolic process. The analysis of genes significantly affected by AH peptide fraction and BM peptide fraction in HCT116 and RKO colon cancer cells demonstrated the potential activation of oxidative stress-related pathways, of which the highest scores were in RKO cells glutathione redox reactions I. Examination of downstream targets of NRF2 evidenced transcriptional NRF2-mediated induction of several enzymes in detoxifying metabolism, such as heme oxygenase 1 (HMOX), cytoplasmic pyridine nucleotide oxidoreductase (TRXR1), glutathione reductase (GSR), and superoxide dismutase (SOD). On the other hand, analysis of genes affected by AH polysaccharide extract and BM polysaccharide extract in RKO cell line showed that the highest scored canonical pathway was glutathione redox reactions I, which overlapped with DEGs, showing strong downregulation of glutathione peroxidase 8 (GPX8), glutathione peroxidase 1 (GPX1), and GSR antioxidant enzymes.

The downstream effect analysis for HCT116 cell line treated with AH peptide fraction and BM peptide fraction differential gene expression resulted in a large increase of cell death, apoptosis, and cell death of tumor cell lines. On the other hand, the highest scored decrease was found in the interphase of tumor cell lines, hypertrophy, and hyperplasia of leukocytes, whereas for a RKO cell line treated with AH peptide fraction and BM peptide fraction a significant decrease in proliferation of tumor cell lines and G_1/S phase in cell cycle was predicted.

The RKO highest scored canonical pathway was glutathione redox reactions I. It is widely known that the downregulation of antioxidant enzymes, such as GPX8, GPX1, and GSR, can lead to an increase of reactive oxygen species (ROS) inside the cells, leading to apoptosis induction. Interestingly, the expression of the oxidative stress-induced growth inhibitor 1 (*OSGIN1*) was induced in the colorectal cancer cells in response to the treatment of the peptide fractions. Although Ingenuity Pathway Analysis® (IPA) did not include this gene in NRF2-mediated response to oxidative stress, the expression of *OSGIN1* is known to follow an expression pattern similar to that of *HMOX1* in response to oxidative signals (Valdés *et al.*, 2013). The encoded protein for *OSGIN1* regulates apoptosis intrinsically by inducing cytochrome *c* release from mitochondria. It also appears to be a key regulator of anti-inflammatory molecules and the loss of this protein correlates with uncontrolled cell growth and tumor formation (Yao *et al.*, 2008).

Taking these studies as a whole, the anticancer potential of antioxidant fiber from common bean is the result of the contribution of different food constituents present. The carbohydrate fermentation products play an important role due to the presence of SCFAs. The molecular assessments point to a p53-dependent apoptosis induction and cell cycle arrest. The results were also influenced by the cultivar used, referring to the diversity of nutrients and nutraceutical compounds depending on the bean genotype. The peptides present in the antioxidant fiber of common bean contribute mainly to the induction of apoptosis; however, even though they induced important posttranslational modifications of p53, this may be independent of this transcription factor and instead caused by other apoptosis inductors activated in response to oxidative stress. Further analysis evaluating the pure compounds identified in the antioxidant fiber of common bean are needed in order to elucidate the specific contribution of each one. The evidence presented, however, strongly suggests that consumption of common bean and its antioxidant fiber can give beneficial effects for human health.

References

Anderson, J.W., Baird, P., Davis, R.H., Ferreri, S., Knutson, M., Koraym, A., *et al.* (2009). Health benefits of dietary fiber. *Nutrition Reviews*, 67(4), 188–205.

Aparicio-Fernández, X., Yousef, G.G., Loarca-Pina, G., Mejia, E., and Lila, M.A. (2005). Characterization of polyphenolics in the seed coat of black Jamapa bean (L.). *Journal of Agricultural and Food Chemistry*, 53(11), 4615–4622.

Aune, D., Chan, D.M., Greenwood, D.C., Vieira, A.R., Navarro Rosenblatt, D.A., Vieira, R., *et al.* (2012). Dietary fiber and breast cancer risk: a sytematic review and meta-analysis of prospective studies. *Annals of Oncology*, 23(6), 1394–1402.

Benhar, M. and Stamler, J. S. (2005). A central role for S-nitrosylation in apoptosis. *Nature Cell Biology*, 7(7), 645–646.

Bullock, M.D., Bruce, A., Sreekumar, R., Curtis, N., Cheung, T., Reading, I., *et al.* (2013). FOX03 expression during colorectal cancer progression: biomarker potential reflects a tumour suppressor role. *British Journal of Cancer*, 109(2), 387–394.

Campos-Vega, R., Reynoso-Camacho, R., Pedraza-Aboytes, G., Acosta-Gallegos, J.A., Guzman-Maldonado, S.H., Paredes-Lopez, O., *et al.* (2009). Chemical composition and in vitro polysaccharide fermentation of different beans (*Phaseolus vulgaris* L.). *Journal of Food Science*, 74, T59–T65.

Campos-Vega, R., Guevara-Gonzalez, R.G., Guevara-Olvera, B.L., Oomah, B.D., Loarca-Piña, G. (2010). Bean (*Phaseolus vulgaris* L.) polysaccharides modulate gene expression in human colon cancer cells (HT-29). *Food Research International*, 43, 1057–1064.

Campos-Vega, R., García-Gasca, T., Guevara-Gonzalez, R., Ramos-Gomez, M., Oomah, B.D., and Loarca-Piña, G. (2012). Human gut flora-fermented nondigestible fraction from cooked bean (*Phaseolus vulgaris* L.) modifies protein expression associated with apoptosis, cell cycle arrest, and proliferation in human adenocarcinoma colon cancer cells. *Journal of Agricultural and Food Chemistry*, 60(51), 12443–12450.

Campos-Vega, R., Oomah, B.D., Loarca-Piña, G., and Vergara-Castañeda, H. A. (2013). Common beans and their non-digestible fraction: Cancer inhibitory activity – An overview. *Foods*, 2, 374–392.

Cardador-Martínez, A., Loarca-Piña, G., and Oomah, B. D. (2002). Antioxidant activity in common beans (*Phaseolus vulgaris* L.). *Journal of Agricultural and Food Chemistry*, 50, 6975–6980.

Champ, M., Langkilde, A. M., Brouns, F., Kettlitz, B., and Collet, Y. B. (2003). Advances in dietary fibre characterisation. 2. Consumption, chemistry, physiology and measurement of resistant starch; implications for health and food labeling. *Nutrition Research Reviews*, 16, 143–161.

Chang, P. V., Hao, L., Offermanns, S., and Medzhitov, R. (2014). The microbial metabolite butyrate regulates intestinal macrophage function via histone deacetylase inhibition. *Proceedings of the National Academy of Sciences, U.S.A.*, 111(6). 2247–2252.

Codex (2015). *Codex Alimentarius*. International Food Standards. http://www.fao .org/fao-who-codexalimentarius/en/ (accessed December 8, 2015).

Cruz-Bravo, R. K., Guevara-González, R., Ramos-Gómez, M., García-Gasca, T., Campos-Vega, R., Oomah, B. D., *et al.* (2011). Fermented nondigestible fraction from common bean (*Phaseolus vulgaris* L.) cultivar Negro 8025 modulates HT-29 cell behavior. *Journal of Food Science*, 76, T41–T47.

Cummings, J. H. (2001). The effect of dietary fiber on fecal weight and composition. In *Dietary Fiber in Human Nutrition* (eds. G. Spiller and G. Spiller). CRC Press, Boca Raton, FL, pp. 183–252.

Darzi, J., Frost, G.S., and Robertson, M.D. (2011). Do SCFA hava a role in appetite regulation? *Proceedings of the Nutrition Society*, 70, 119–128.

De Jesús Ariza-Ortega, T., Zenón-Briones, E.Y., Castrejón-Flores, J.L., Yáñez-Fernández, J., de las Mercedes Gómez-Gómez, Y., and del Carmen Oliver-Salvador, M. (2014). Angiotensin-I-converting enzyme inhibitory, antimicrobial, and antioxidant effect of bioactive peptides obtained from different varieties of common beans (*Phaseolus vulgaris* L.) with *in vivo* antihypertensive activity in spontaneously hypertensive rats. *European Food Research and Technology*, 239(5), 785–794.

Del Rio, D., Rodriguez-Mateos, A., Spencer, J.P.E., Tognolini, M., Borges, G., and Crozier, A. (2013). Dietary polyphenolics in human health: Structures, bioavailability, and evidence of protective effects against chronic diseases. *Antioxidants and Redox Signaling*, 18, 1818–1892.

Delzenne, N., Cherbut, C., and Neyrinck, A. (2003). Prebiotics: Actual and potential effects in inflammatory and malignant colonic diseases. *Current Opinion in Clinical Nutrition and Metabolic Care*, 6, 581–586.

Dia, V.P. and de Mejia, E.G. (2011). Lunasin induces apoptosis and modifies the expression of genes associated with extracellular matrix and cell adhesion in human metastatic colon cancer cells. *Molecular Nutrition and Food Research*, 55(4), 623–634.

Díaz, A.M., Caldas, G.V., and Blair, M.W. (2010). Concentrations of condensed tannins and anthocyanins in common bean seed coats. *Food Research International*, 43(2), 595–601.

Díaz-Batalla, L., Widholm, J.M., Fahey, G.C., Castaño-Tostado, E., and Paredes-López, O. (2006). Chemical components with health implications in wild and cultivated Mexican common bean seeds (*Phaseolus vulgaris* L.). *Journal of Agricultural and Food Chemistry*, 54(6), 2045–2052.

Donohoe, D.R., Collins, L.B., Wali, A., Bigler, R., Sun, W., and Bultman, S.J. (2012). The Warburg effect dictates the mechanism of butyrate-mediated histone acetylation and cell proliferation. *Molecular Cell*, 48(4), 612–626.

Doria, E., Campion, B., Sparvoli, F., Tava, A., and Nielsen, E. (2010). Anti-nutrient components and metabolites with health implications in seeds of 10 common bean (*Phaseolus vulgaris* L. and *Phaseolus lunatus* L.) landraces cultivated in southern Italy. *Journal of Food Composition and Analysis*, 26, 72–80.

Escudero, A.E. and González, S.P. (2006). La fibra dietética. *Nutricion Hospitalaria*, 21, 61–72.

FAO (Food and Agriculture Organization of the United Nations) (2014). *The statistics division of the FAO*. http://faostat.fao.org/ (accessed June 1, 2014).

Fearon, E.R. (2011). Molecular genetics of colorectal cancer. *Annual Review of Pathology: Mechanisms of Disease*, 6, 479–507.

Feliciano L.P., Augusto C.C., Chiorato A.F., Fumiko Y. L., Kato M.J., and Morais C. A. F. (2014). Occurrence of isoflavonoids in Brazilia common bean germplasm (*Phaseolus vulgaris* L.). *Journal of Agricultural and Food Chemistry*, 62, 9699–9704.

Feregrino-Pérez, A.A., Berumen, L.C., Garcia-Alcocer, G., Guevara-Gonzalez, R.G., Ramos-Gomez, M., Reynoso-Camacho, R., *et al.* (2008). Composition and chemopreventive effect of polysaccharides from common beans (*Phaseolus vulgaris* L.) on azoxymethane-induced colon cancer. *Journal of Agricultural and Food Chemistry*, 56, 8737–8744.

Feregrino-Perez, A.A., Piñol-Felis, C., Gomez-Arbones, X., Guevara-González, R. G., Campos-Vega, R., Acosta-Gallegos, J., *et al.* (2014). A non-digestible fraction of the common bean (*Phaseolus vulgaris* L.) induces cell cycle arrest and apoptosis during early carcinogénesis. *Plant Foods for Human Nutrition*, 69(3), 248–254.

Foglietta, F., Serpe, L., Canaparo, R., Vivenza, N., Riccio, G., Imbalzano, E., *et al.* (2014). Modulation of butyrate anticancer activity by solid lipid nanoparticle delivery: an in vitro investigation on human breast cancer and leukemia cell lines. *Journal of Pharmacy and Pharmaceutical Sciences*, 17(2), 231–247.

Fung, K. Y., Cosgrove, L., Lockett, T., Head, R., and Topping, D. L. (2012). A review of the potential mechanisms for the lowering of colorectal oncogenesis by butyrate. *British Journal of Nutrition*, 108(05), 820–831.

Gibson, G., Probert, H., Van Loo, J., Rastall, R., and Robertfroid, M. (2004). Dietary modulation of the human colonic microbiota: updating the concept of prebiotics. *Nutrition Research Reviews*, 17, 259–275.

González de Mejía, E., Valadez-Vega, M., Reynoso-Camacho, R., and Loarca-Piña, G. (2005). Tannins, trypsin inhibitors and lectin cytotoxicity in tepary (*Phaseolus acutifolius*) and common (*Phaseolus vulgaris*) beans. *Plant Foods for Human Nutrition*, 60, 137–145.

Guo, Y.W., Chen, Y.H., Chiu, W.C., Liao, H., and Lin, S.H. (2013). Soy saponins meditate the progression of colon cancer in rats by inhibiting the activity of β-glucuronidase and the number of aberrant crypt foci but not cyclooxygenase-2 activity. *ISRN Oncology*, 2013.

Hacisalihoglu G., Larbi B., Settles M. (2010). Near-Infrared reflectance spectroscopy predicts protein, starch and seed weight in intact seed of common bean (*Phaseolus vulgaris* L.). *Journal of Agricultural and Food Chemistry*, 58(2), 702–706.

Han, K., Fukushima, M., Shimizu, K., Kojima, M., Ohba, K., Tanaka, A., *et al.* (2003). Resistant starches of beans reduce the serum cholesterol concentration in rats. *Journal of Nutrition Science and Vitaminology*, 49, 281–286.

Han, K., Sekikawa, M., Shimada, K.-i., Sasaki, K., Ohba, K., and Fukushima, M. (2004). Resitant starch fraction prepared from kintoki bean affects gene expression of genes associated with cholesterol metabolism in rats. *Experimental Biology and Medicine*, 229, 787–792.

Han, Y., Haraguchi, T., Iwanaga, S., Tomotake, H., Okazaki, Y., Mineo, S., *et al.* (2009). Consumption of some polyphenols reduces fecal deoxycholic acid and lithocholic acid, the secondary bile acids of risk factors of colon cancer. *Journal of Agricultural and Food Chemistry*, 57, 8587–8590.

Hansen, L., Skeie, G., Landberg, R., Lund, E., Palmqvist, R., Johansson, I., *et al.* (2012). Intake of dietary fiber, especially from cereal foods, is associated with lower incidence of colon cancer in the HELGA cohort. *International Journal of Cancer*, 131, 469–478.

Hernández-Salazar, M., Osorio-Diaz, P., Loarca-Piña, G., Reynoso-Camacho, R., Tovar, J., and Bello-Perez, L.A. (2010). In vitro fermentability and antioxidant capacity of the indigestible fraction of cooked black beans (*Phaseolus vulgaris*), lentils (*Lens culinaris* L.) and chickpeas (*Cicer arietinum* L.). *Journal of Science of Food and Agriculture*, 90, 1417–1422.

Hoover, R. and Zhou, Y. (2003). In vitro and in vivo hydrolysis of starches by α-amylase and resistant starch formation in legumes – a review. *Carbohydrate Polymers*, 54(4), 401–417.

Huang, H.M. and Liu, J.C. (2008). C-Jun blocks cell differentiation but not growth inhibition or apoptosis of chronic myelogenous leukemia cells induced by STI571 and by histone deacetylase inhibitors. *Journal of Cellular Physiology*, 218, 568–574.

Jahns, F., Wilhelm, A., Jablonowski, N., Mothes, H., Greulich, K.O., and Glei, M. (2015). Butyrate modulates antioxidant enzyme expression in malignant and non-malignant human colon tissues. *Molecular Carcinogenesis*, 54(4), 249–260.

Jenkins, J.A., Kendall, C.C., Faulkner, D.A., Nguyn, T., Kemp, T., Marchie, A., *et al.* (2006). Assessment of the longer-term effects of a dietary portfolio of cholesterol-lowering foods in hypercholesterolemia. *American Journal of Clinical Nutrition*, 83, 582–591.

Jiménez-Escrig, A., Rincón, M., Pulido, R., and Saura-Calixto, F. (2001). Guava fruit (Psidium guajava L.) as a new source of antioxidant. *Journal of Agricultural and Food Chemistry*, 49, 5489–5493.

Keerthivasan, S., Aghajani, K., Dose, M., Molinero, L., Khan, M.W., Venkateswaran, V., *et al.* (2014). β-Catenin promotes colitis and colon cancer through imprinting of proinflammatory properties in T cells. *Science Translational Medicine*, 6(225), 225ra28–225ra28.

Koren, E. and Torchilin, P.T. (2012). Cell-penetrating peptides: breaking through to the other side. *Trends in Molecular Medicine*, 18(7), 385–393.

Kutos, T., Golob, T., Kac, M., and Plestenjak, A. (2003). Dietary fibre content of dry and processed beans. *Food Chemistry*, 80, 231–235.

Leonel, A.J. and Alvarez-Leite, J.I. (2012). Butyrate: implications for intestinal function. *Current Opinion in Clinical Nutrition and Metabolic Care*, 15(5), 474–479.

Lindqvist, A., Rodríguez-Bravo, V., and Medema, R. (2009). The decision to enter mitosis: Feedback and redundancy in the mitotic entry network. *Journal of Cell Biology*, 185, 193–202.

Mojica, L., Meyer, A., Berhow, M.A., and González de Mejía, E. (2015). Bean cultivars (*Phaseolus vulgaris* L.) have similar high antioxidant capacity, *in vitro* inhibition of α-amylase and α-glucosidasewhile diverse phenolic composition and concentration. *Food Research International*, 69, 38–48.

Luna-Vital, D.A., González de Mejía, E., Dia, V.P., and Loarca-Piña, G. (2014a). Peptides in common bean fractions inhibit human colorectal cancer cell. *Food Chemistry*, 157, 347–355.

Luna-Vital, D., Loarca-Piña, G., Vermont, P.D., and González de Mejía, E. (2014b). Peptides extracted from common bean (*Phaseolus vulgaris* L.) non-digestible fraction caused differential gene expression of HCT116 and RKO human colorectal cancer cells. *Food Research International*, 62, 193–204.

Luna-Vital, D., González de Mejía, E., Mendoza, S., and Loarca-Piña, G. (2015). Peptides present in the non-digestible fraction of common beans (*Phaseolus vulgaris* L.) inhibit angiotensin-I converting enzyme by interacting with its catalytic cavity independently of their antioxidant capacity. *Food and Function*, 6(5), 1470–1479.

Luthria, D.L. and Pastor-Corrales, M.A. (2006). Phenolic acids content of fifteen dry edible bean (*Phaseolus vulgaris* L.). *Journal of Food Composition and Analysis*, 19, 205–211.

Martín-Cabrejas, M., Aguilera, Y., Benítez, V., Mollá, E., López-Andréu, F., and Esteban, R. (2006). Effect of industrial dehydration on the soluble carbohydrates and dietary fiber fractions in legumes. *Journal of Agricultural and Food Chemistry*, 54, 7652–7657.

Martinez-Tome, M., Murcia, M.A., Frega, L., Ruggirei, S., Jimenez, A.M., Roses, F., *et al.* (2004). Evaluation of antioxidant capacity of cereal brans. *Journal of Agricultural and Food Chemistry*, 4690–4699.

Meek, D.W. (2015). Regulation of the p53 response and its relationship to cancer. *Biochemical Journal*, 469(3), 325–346.

Miller Jones, J. (2014). CODEX-aligned dietary fiber definitions help to bridge the 'fiber gap'. *Nutrition Journal*, 13, 34.

Oomah, B.D., Tiger, N., Olson, M., and Balasubramanian, P. (2006). Phenolics and antioxidatives activities in narrow-leafed lupins (Lupinus angustifolius L.). *Plant Foods in Human Nutrition*, 61, 91–97.

Oomah, B.D., Corbé, A., and Balasubramanian, P. (2010). Antioxidant and anti-inflammatory activities of bean (*Phaseolus vulgaris* L.) hulls. *Journal of Agricultural and Food Chemistry*, 58, 8225–8230.

Ozdal, T., Capanoglu, E., and Altay, F. (2013). A review on protein-phenolic interactions and associated changes. *Food Research International*, 51, 954–970.

Paredes-López, O. and Valverde, M. (2006). Los recursos nutraceuticos y medicinales que Mesoamerica le ha dado al mundo. *CINVESTAV* 65–73.

Paredes-López, O., Guevara-Lara, F., and Bello-Pérez, L.A. (2006). Frijol. In *Los Alimentos Mágicos de las Culturas Indígenas Mesoamericanas*. Fondo de Cultura Económica-Serie Ciencia para Todos, México, DF, pp. 59–81.

Pereira, C.S., Oliveira, M.V.M.D., Barros, L.O., Bandeira, G.A., Santos, S.H.S., Basile, J.R., *et al.* (2013). Low expression of MSH2 DNA repair protein is associated with poor prognosis in head and neck squamous cell carcinoma. *Journal of Applied Oral Science*, 21(5), 416–421.

Pereira, M., O'Reilly, E., and Augustsson, K. (2004). Dietary fiber and risk of coronary heart disease: a pooled analysisi of cohort studies. *Archives of Internal Medicine*, 164, 370–376.

Pérez-Jiménez, J., Serrano, J., Tabernero, M., Arranz, S., Díaz-Rubio, M.E., García-Diz, L., *et al.* (2009). Bioavailability of phenolic antioxidants associated with dietary fiber: plasma antioxidant capacity after acute and long-term intake in humans. *Plant Foods for Human Nutrition*, 64(2), 102–107.

Prosky, L., Asp, N.G., Schweizer, T.F., DeVries, J.W., and Furda, I. (1988). Determination of insoluble, soluble, and total dietary fiber in foods and food products: interlaboratory study. *Journal of the Association of Official Analytical Chemists*, 71(5), 1017–1023.

Pujolà, M., Farreras, A., and Casañas, F. (2007). Protein and starch content of raw, soaked and cooked beans (*Phaseolus vulgaris* L.). *Food Chemistry*, 102, 1034–1041.

Raman, M., Ambalam, P., and Doble, M. (2016). Bioactive carbohydrate: prebiotics and colorectal cancer. In *Probiotics and Bioactive Carbohydrates in Colon Cancer Management*. Springer, India, pp. 57–82.

Ramírez-Jiménez, A.K., Reynoso-Camacho, R., Mendoza-Díaz, S., and Loarca-Piña, G. (2014). Functional and technological potential of dehydrated *Phaseolus vulgaris* L. flours. *Food Chemistry*, 161, 254–260.

Rasyid, H., Bakri, S., and Yusuf, I. (2012). Angiotensin-converting enzyme gene polymorphisms, blood pressure and pulse pressure in subjects with essential hypertension in a South Sulawesi Indonesian population. *Indonesian Journal of Internal Medicine*, 44(4), 280–283.

Reyes-Moreno, C. and Paredes-López, O. (1993). Hard-to-cook phenomenon in common beans. A review. *Critical Revuews in Food Science and Nutrition*, 33, 227–286.

Rizkalla, S. W., Bellisle, F., and Slama, G. (2002). Health benefits of low glycaemic index foods, such as pulses, in diabetic patients and healthy individuals. *British Journal of Nutrition*, 88, 255–262.

Rocha-Guzmán, N.E., Herzog, A., González-Laredo, R.F., Ibarra-Pérez, F.J., Zambrano Galván, G., and Gallegos-Infante, J.A. (2007). Antioxidant and antimutagenic activity of phenolic compounds in three different colour groups of common bean cultivars (*Phaseolus vulgaris*). *Food Chemistry*, 103, 521–527.

Rodrigues-Ferreira, S. and Nahmias, C. (2015). G-protein coupled receptors of the renin-angiotensin system: new targets against breast cancer? *Frontiers in Pharmacology*, 6.

Rodríguez-Licea, G., García-Salazar, J.A., Rebollar-Rebollar, S., and Cruz-Contreras, A.C. (2010). Preferencias del consumidor de frijol (*Phaseolus vulgaris* L.) en México: factores y características que influyen en la decisión de compra diferenciada por tipo y variedad. *Paradigma Económico*, 1, 121–145.

Saura-Calixto, F. (1998). Antioxidant dietary fiber product: a new concept and a potential food ingredient. *Journal of Agricultural and Food Chemistry*, 46, 4303–4306.

Saura-Calixto, F., García-Alonso, A., Goñi, I., and Bravo, L. (2000). In vitro determination of the indigestible fraction in foods: an alternative to dietary fibre analysis. *Journal of Agricultural and Food Chemistry*, 48, 3342–3347.

Shiga, M., Lajolo, M., and Filisetti, M. (2003). Cell wall polysaccharides of common beans (*Phaseolus vulgaris* L.). *Ciencia e Tecnologia de Alimentos Campinas*, 23(2), 141–148.

Stein, K., Borowicki, A., Scharlau, D., and Glei, M. (2010). Fermented wheat aleurone induces enzymes involved in detoxification of carcinogens and in antioxidative defence in human colon cells. *British Journal of Nutrition*, 104(08), 1101–1111.

Tan, W., Chen, Y., An, P., Wang, A., Chu, M., Shi, L., *et al.* (2015). Sodium butyrate-induced histone hyperacetylation up-regulating WT1 expression in porcine kidney fibroblasts. *Biotechnology Letters*, 37(6), 1195–1202.

Tapsell, L.C. (2004). Diet and metabolic syndrome: where does resistant starch fit in? *Journal AOAC*, 87, 756–760.

Tong, C., Song, Z., Dockendorff, A., Mariadason, J., Nasser, S., Bancroft, L., *et al.* (2006). Butyrate-induced apoptosis is JNK1-dependent in murine embryonic fibroblasts and human colon cancer cells. *Proceedings of the American Association for Cancer Research*, 47, 2473.

Tosh, S. and Yada, S. (2010). Dietary fibres in pulse seeds and fractions: Characterization, functional attributes, and applications. *Food Research International*, 43, 450–460.

Tungland, B. and Meyer, D. (2002). Non-digestible oligo-and polysaccharides (dietary fiber): Their physiology and role in human health and food. *Comprehensive Reviews in Food Science and Food Safety*, 1(3), 90–109.

Valdés A., García-Cañas V., Rocamora-Reverte L., Gómez-Martínez A., Ferragut J.A., and Cifuentes A. (2013). Effect of rosemary polyphenols on human colon cancer cells: Transcriptomic profiling and functional enrichment analysis. *Genes and Nutrition*, 8, 43–60.

Valls, J., Millan, S., Marti, M.P., Borras, E., and Arola, L. (2009). Advanced separation methods for food anthocyanins, isoflavones and flavonols. *Journal of Chromatography A*, 1216, 7143–7172.

Vergara-Castañeda, H.A., Guevara-González, R.G., Ramos-Gómez, M., Reynoso-Camacho, R., Guzmán-Maldonado, H., Feregrino-Pérez, A.A., *et al.* (2010). Non-digestible fraction of cooked bean (*Phaseolus vulgaris* L.) cultivar Bayo Madero suppresses colonic aberrant crypt foci in azoxymethane-induced rats. *Food and Function*, 1(3), 294–300.

Vergara-Castañeda, H.A., Guevara-González, R.G., Guevara-Olvera, B.L., Oomah, B.D., and Loarca-Piña, G.F. (2012). Non-digestible fraction of beans (*Phaseolus vulgaris* L) modulates signaling pathway genes at an early stage of colon cancer in Sprague Dawley rats. *British Journal of Nutrition*, 108, S145–S154.

Wang, H.G., Huang, X.D., Shen, P., Li, L.R., Xue, H.T., and Ji, G.Z. (2013). Anticancer effects of sodium butyrate on hepatocellular carcinoma cells in vitro. *International Journal of Molecular Medicine*, 31(4), 967–974.

World Health Organization (2015). *GLOBOCAN 2012*. International Agency for Research on Cancer. www.globocan.iarc.fr (accessed November 2015).

Yamamura, T., Matsumoto, N., Matsue, Y., Okudera, M., Nishikawa, Y., Abiko, Y., *et al.* (2014). Sodium butyrate, a histone deacetylase inhibitor, regulates lymphangiogenic factors in oral cancer cell line HSC-3. *Anticancer Research*, 34(4), 1701–1708.

Yang, J. and Rose, D.J. (2014). Long-term dietary pattern of fecal donor correlates with butyrate production and markers of protein fermentation during in vitro fecal fermentation. *Nutrition Research*, 34(9), 749–759.

Yao, H., Li, P., Venters, B.J., Zheng, S., Thompson, P.R., Pugh, B.F., *et al.* (2008). Histone Arg modifications and p53 regulate the expression of OKL38, a mediator of apoptosis. *Journal of Biological Chemistry*, 283(29), 20060–20068.

Yoo, D.Y., Kim, D.W., Kim, M.J., Choi, J.H., Jung, H.Y., *et al.* (2015). Sodium butyrate, a histone deacetylase inhibitor, ameliorates SIRT2-induced memory impairment, reduction of cell proliferation, and neuroblast differentiation in the dentate gyrus. *Neurological Research*, 37(1), 69–76.

Yu, S., Hou, D., Chen, P., Zhang, Q., Lv, B., Ma, Y., *et al.* (2015). Adenosine induces apoptosis through TNFR1/RIPK1/P38 axis in colon cancer cells. *Biochemical and Biophysical Research Communications*, 460(3), 759–765.

Zhang, X., Min, K.W., Wimalasena, J., and Baek, S.J. (2012). Cyclin D1 degradation and p21 induction contribute to growth inhibition of colorectal cancer cells induced by epigallocatechin-3-gallate. *Journal of Cancer Research and Clinical Oncology*, 138(12), 2051–2060.

Zhou, Q., Dalgard, C.L., Wynder, C., and Doughty, M.L. (2011). Histone deacetylase inhibitors SAHA and sodium butyrate block G1-to-S cell cycle progression in neurosphere formation by adult subventricular cells. *BMC Neuroscience*, 12(1), 50.

6

In Vivo and *In Vitro* Studies on Dietary Fiber and Gut Health

Rocio Campos-Vega[1], B. Dave Oomah[2] and Haydé A. Vergara-Castañeda[3]

[1] *Programa de Posgrado en Alimentos del Centro de la República (PROPAC), Universidad Autónoma de Querétaro, Querétaro, Mexico*
[2] *Retired, Formerly with Pacific Agri-Food Research Centre, Agriculture and Agri-Food Canada, Summerland, British Columbia, Canada*
[3] *Nucitec, S.A. de C.V., Querétaro, Mexico*

6.1   Introduction

The digestion and absorption of macronutrients (fat, protein, and carbohydrate) is a major factor in health and metabolic disease. In 2015, 2.3 billion adults were overweight and 700 million obese worldwide (Le Magueresse-Battistoni *et al.*, 2015). Dietary fiber intake provides many health benefits, including reduced risk for developing coronary heart disease, stroke, hypertension, diabetes, obesity, and certain gastrointestinal disorders. Furthermore, increased consumption of dietary fiber improves serum lipid concentrations, lowers blood pressure, improves blood glucose control in diabetes, promotes regularity, aids in weight loss, and appears to improve immune function. Unfortunately, most people in the United States consume less than half of the daily-recommended dietary fiber intake (Anderson *et al.*, 2009).

Cereal fiber may partly account for the protective effects of whole grains on mortality and is more predictive of reduced mortality than other fiber sources (Jacobs, 2015). In fact, cereals are the predominant source of dietary fiber, contributing about 50% of the fiber intake in western countries; 30–40% of dietary fiber usually comes from vegetables, about 16% from fruits, and the remaining 3% from other minor sources (Dhingra *et al.*, 2012).

According to the EU Commission Directive EC/2008/100 (European Commission, 2008), dietary fiber includes a wide variety of non-digestible carbohydrates with a degree of polymerization of 3 or more (plus lignin). The main types of dietary fiber are non-starch polysaccharides (cellulose, hemicellulose, pectins, gums, mucilages, and beta-glucans), resistant oligosaccharides (inulin, oligofructose, fructo-oligosaccharides, galacto-oligosaccharides), resistant starch, and lignin (associated with resistant polysaccharides).

The total amount of fermentable carbohydrates in the western diet delivered from the ileum has been estimated at 30–40 g/day. Cecal and colonic carbohydrate fermentation produces short-chain fatty acids (SCFAs), lactate, gasses (hydrogen, carbon dioxide, and methane), and reduces the luminal pH. The SCFAs are largely (95–99%) absorbed, delivering about 10% of the human energy requirement. Butyrate is used directly by the colonic cells, exerting a trophic effect on these cells. SCFAs stimulate salt and water absorption and epithelial growth. The saccharolytic activities increase biomass, fecal bulk, stool weight, and stool frequency (Schaafsma and Slavin, 2015).

Investigation on dietary fiber and gut health has increased dramatically over the last 4 years, with more than 75% (290 out of 379) of the total number of papers published after 1982. A cursory search of "gut health dietary fiber" on PubMed displays 44, 71, 90, and 85 publications annually from 2011 to 2014, while only 120 papers were published from 1982 to 2010 (almost three decades). A newly developed comprehensive fiber database, comprising human intervention studies, identified 141 relevant publications with two major outcomes: modulation of colonic microbiota and/or colonic fermentation/SCFA production. Descriptive analyses were performed to summarize study design characteristics, fiber exposures, and outcomes. The majority of studies were crossover designs (66%) in adult populations (82%) with healthy baseline status; 17% were acute studies (1 day), most (69%) had 1–4 weeks duration, but there were fewer studies (13%) of longer duration. The most frequently examined dietary fibers were resistant starch (14.4%), wheat (7%), inulin (7%), barley (6.4%), and fructo-oligosaccharides (6.4%). A total of 7% of studies administered an intervention that used a combination of fibers.

In the emerging field of dietary fiber and the microbiome, research gaps exist regarding the effects of different fiber types and their combinations on gut microbiota (Sawicki *et al.*, 2015). For decades the contributions of gut microbiota to human health and disease were widely underappreciated. The gut microbiota, now considered central to human biology, was first described in 1992 as an independent organ with immunostimulatory properties. After that, the suite of gut microbial contributions was identified to the human host, such as providing nourishment, regulating epithelial cell development, and modulating innate immune responses. Most studies have focused on species identification and cataloguing, a process that has been hampered by the inability to culture most gut microbes. Species are recognized solely by their 16S rRNA sequence and identification relies heavily on high-throughput technologies such as second- and third-generation sequencing platforms. Success and advancement of these technologies has demonstrated a link between various microbial species and multiple pathologies such as obesity, Crohn's disease and irritable bowel syndrome (Payne *et al.*, 2012). We unravel some of the research gaps between dietary fiber and the gut microbiome through *in vitro* and *in vivo* studies in this chapter. This dietary link is an important component of the gut–brain axis in the prevention/reduction of several chronic immune and psychological diseases.

6.2 Research into Dietary Fiber and Health

Basic research in animal models has been, for some decades, a great source of knowledge for the development of prevention and treatment optimization of diseases. All studies for prevention with chemopreventive drugs and modified diets have previously been tested in animal models. With regard to colorectal cancer management, laboratory animal experiments have advanced knowledge of the carcinogenic process, of colonic tissue, and of modulation of this process by adding various experimental manipulations on the animal model (Noguera-Aguilar and Gamundí-Gamundí, 2006). Animal studies offer greater control of variables, allow for a broader range of interventions, and are generally less expensive than human studies. However, studies should be carefully developed and the animal properly selected to ensure parallel/similar progress of the disease in humans, in order to translate the results more reliably. Biological models have been widely used in the study of the beneficial dietary fiber effects on human physiology and prevention of gastrointestinal disease and provide us with unique opportunities to unravel the metabolic pathways involved in these effects.

On the other hand, the gut microbiota is a highly specialized organ containing host-specific assemblages of microbes whereby metabolic activity directly impacts human health and disease. *In vitro* gut fermentation models present an unmatched opportunity to perform studies that are frequently challenging in humans and animals owing to ethical concerns (Payne *et al.*, 2012). Also, batch *in vitro* systems allow fermentation modeling without absorption and may help to estimate potential health benefits and gastrointestinal tolerances of fibers *in vivo* (Wisker *et al.*, 1998). Despite this, the use of the *in vitro* systems evaluating dietary fiber on gut health *in vitro* remains limited. Only 131 published papers from 1983 to 2014 are displayed when "*in vitro* colonic fermentation dietary fiber" is searched on PubMed; of these, 79 papers have been published in the last decade.

The main topics studied include dietary fiber effect on microbiota metabolism (SCFAs production and prebiotic effect) as well as its relationship with some major diseases. Even though numerous studies have been published on these issues, we will mainly address those using human colonic microbiota and whole dietary fiber, their nutritional and health implications, including some of their fraction according to available information. We also considered studies evaluating the fecal fermentation profile of various fiber substrates usually pool fecal donations, implying that SCFAs accumulation would not vary by donor, but only by substrate.

6.3 *In Vivo* Studies on Intestinal Function

6.3.1 SCFA Production and Intestinal Epithelium Protection

Dietary fiber is the fermentation substrate that produces SCFAs, primarily acetate, propionate, and butyrate, as end-products. The most important factors influencing dietary fiber fermentability include the source of dietary fiber, solubility, degree of lignification, processing, the level of inclusion in the diet, intestinal transit time, the age and weight of the animal and the microbial composition (Montagne *et al.*, 2003). Thus, quantitatively, studies have demonstrated that pectins, hemicelluloses, and gums are fermented, whereas dietary fiber components such as cellulose or wheat bran are not (Wong *et al.*, 2006). Pectin exerts various effects on the gastrointestinal tract such as: (i) maintaining the morphology and structure of the intestinal villi, (ii) increasing lipase activity, (iii) delaying gastric emptying time, (iv) increasing intestinal transit time, and (v) increasing SCFA generation (Andoh *et al.*, 2003). Fermentability (g/g dry weight) of non-starch polysaccharides of five dietary fibers were: pectin, 0.95; soybean, 0.88; sugar beet, 0.68; maize bran, 0.15; and Solka-floc cellulose, 0.06 according to a European inter-laboratory *in vivo* study (Livesey *et al.*, 1995).

Barley (*Hordeum vulgare* L.) grains are relatively rich in dietary fiber such as β-glucan, arabinoxylans, and cellulose. The consumption of β-glucan–rich diets results in several beneficial physiological effects due to a relatively high concentration, soluble state, and high molecular weight of this polysaccharide; β-glucans are fermented by the intestinal microbiota *in vivo*, resulting in the formation of SCFAs. Dongowski *et al.* (2002), investigating the effects of barley-rich diets in the intestinal tract of rats, showed that the greatest fermentation of the dietary fiber components occurred in the cecum with the highest concentrations of SCFAs. Acetic acid was the major SCFA, followed by propionic and butyric acids and small amounts of valeric and iso-valeric acids in the cecum.

Fermentation of different polysaccharides gives rise to distinct patterns of SCFA production. For example, acetate was the main product of pectin and xylan breakdown, whereas large amounts of acetate and propionate were produced from arabinogalactan. Butyrate was only formed in substantial amounts from starch (Macfarlane and Macfarlane, 2003).

The concentration and differential production of SCFAs according to the type of fiber provide significant physiological implications for the specific protection of the colonic epithelium. Such is the case in increased intestinal mucosa permeability. A fructo-oligosaccharide (FOS) diet fed to rats was rapidly fermented, resulting in high SCFA production that increased intestinal permeability and was associated with increased translocation of *Salmonella* (Hamer *et al.*, 2008). Dietary fiber ingestion leads to increased size and length of the digestive organs, including the small intestine, cecum, and colon of pigs, chickens, and rats, and presumably in other non-ruminant animals. These effects are often associated with modification of the gut epithelium morphology, and consequently with the hydrolytic and absorptive functions of the epithelium (Montagne *et al.*, 2003).

Several studies in rats suggest that inclusion of substantial amounts of both soluble and insoluble fibers in the diet benefits colonic health by increasing the protective properties of the colonic mucus layer (Brownlee *et al.*, 2003). Dietary fiber that increases the release of mucin into the lumen furnishes more substrate for the development and growth of commensal as well as pathogenic bacteria in the large intestine; and the variation in the ratio of mucins classes following dietary fiber ingestion has been reported in rats (Montagne *et al.*, 2003). Dietary fiber increases levels of luminal and total (luminal plus tissue) gastric mucin in rats fed 20% psyllium, and such an increase may protect these organs and alter nutrient absorption (Satchithanandam *et al.*, 1996).

The induction of phase II enzymes has been hypothesized as another mechanism by which SFCAs protect intestinal epithelium. For example, glutathione *S*-transferase catalyzes the biotransformation and detoxification of many carcinogens (Scharlau *et al.*, 2009). Thus, the expression of both glutathione transferase isozymes GST A1 and A2 increased significantly in the colon of male Wistar rats fed a diet containing 20% wheat bran (Helsby *et al.*, 2000).

Lange (2015) explored the mechanisms by which dietary fiber and its degradation products (SCFAs) affect the host transcriptional response. Five different fibers (inulin, FOS, arabinoxylan, guar gum, and resistant starch) and a control diet were fed to C57BL/6 mice for 10 days. The peroxisome proliferator-activated receptor (PPARγ) was identified as the potential upstream regulator for the mucosal gene expression response common to all fermented dietary fibers, transactivated by SCFAs, particularly butyrate and to a lesser extent propionate that also regulated the PPARγ target gene *Angpt14* in colonic cells. Furthermore, all fibers, except resistant starch, induced highly similar gene expression and microbiota composition profiles in the colon, which coincided with increased SCFAs concentrations. Resistant starch induced only a few, but includes specific expression of the histone demethylase *KDM5B* gene. Thus, although PPARγ partially governs the response of dietary fermentation in the colon, microbial gene activity, composition, and mucosal transcriptome responses are specifically and differentially affected by dietary fibers (Lange, 2015).

6.3.2 Mineral Absorption

Some minerals bind/complex with fiber-forming insoluble compounds such as phytates in cereals, tannates in spinach, beans, lentils, and oxalates in bananas or cauliflower and spinach. These minerals may be released by bacterial metabolism of these compounds in the colon where they are absorbed in considerable quantities, although their absorption is slower compared to that in the small intestine. Calcium absorption has been widely studied; entrapped calcium is transported to the colon then released by colonic bacteria hydrolyzing the fiber. The SCFAs produced by fiber fermentation facilitate calcium absorption from the colon walls and even the rectum (Escudero-Álvarez and González-Sánchez, 2006).

In experimental animals (mostly rats), many studies demonstrate that inulin-type fructans significantly increase mineral absorption, essentially Ca and Mg. All inulin-type fructans (native inulin, oligofructose, inulin HP, or Synergy 1) were effective in modulating mineral absorption, although some qualitative differences occur with different types of inulin (Roberfroid, 2007). Guar gum also increases Ca absorption in totally gastrectomized rats. Galibois *et al.*, (1994) studied mineral absorption using pectin, cellulose, and oat and wheat fibers on rats and found that the apparent absorption of Zn, Fe, Mg, and Ca was better with pectin than with wheat or oat bran. The effect of pectin on vitamin absorption has been extensively investigated with no definite conclusive results so far (Chawla and Patil, 2010).

6.3.3 Immunomodulation

There is increasing evidence that the addition of fermentable fiber to the diet alters the function and structure of the gut. Several authors have suggested or demonstrated that dietary fiber might enhance protection against enteric infections with pathogenic bacteria, or alternatively might enhance infection and subsequent diseases in young non-ruminant animals (Montagne *et al.*, 2003). Inflammatory bowel diseases such as Crohn's disease and ulcerative colitis may be protected by fiber via increased SCFA production, thereby immunomodulating the inflamed intestine and increasing the proportions of beneficial rather than pathogenic bacteria that make up the gastrointestinal microbiota (Chawla and Patil, 2010).

Dietary fiber has been related to a decrease in proinflammatory cytokine levels and may acutely reduce inflammatory activity. The proposed mechanisms underlying the immunomodulating effects of dietary fibers that alter the gut microbiota are: direct contact of lactic acid bacteria or bacterial products (cell wall or cytoplasmic components) with immune cells in the intestine, SCFA production from fiber fermentation, and modulation of mucin production (Schley and Field, 2002). SCFAs can induce regulatory T-cells (Tregs) and calibrate immune function in ways that over a lifetime may prevent inflammatory disease. Tregs expressing the transcription factor Foxp3 are critical for regulating intestinal inflammation. Thus, SCFAs, gut microbiota-derived bacterial fermentation products, regulated the size and function of the colonic Treg pool and protected against colitis in mice, thereby promoting colonic homeostasis and health (Smith *et al.*, 2013). SCFAs regulate intestinal adaptive immune response and its production through increased ingestion of dietary fiber may be a critical factor that links the gut microbiome to disease. Thus, in rodents, adding fermentable fiber to a diet otherwise high in fat kept the mucous layer healthy and the gut barrier intact, preventing systemic inflammation (Velasquez-Manoff, 2015).

Oral administration of probiotic bacteria increased the production of immunoglobulins, especially IgA, in gut-associated lymphoid tissue (GALT) and modulated both the number and activity of Peyer's patch immune cells. Studies conducted by Field *et al.* (1999) on adult dogs indicate that adding fermentable fiber to the diet can modulate the type and function of cells from different regions of the GALT. In a randomized crossover design, 16 adult dogs were fed two isoenergetic isonitrogenous diets containing 8.3 g/kg non-fermentable or 8.7 g/kg fermentable fibers for 2 weeks. The fermentable fiber diet was a mixture of plant fibers (beet pulp, oligofructose powder, and gum arabic). The fiber content of the diet significantly altered the proportion of T-cells ($CD4^+$ and $CD8^+$) in GALT and their *in vitro* response to mitogens. GALT is the largest and most complex part of the immune system and is able to discriminate effectively between invasive pathogens from innocuous antigens (Ramiro-Puig *et al.*, 2008). One logical mechanism of dietary fiber might be immune stimulation through direct contact of the colonic microbiota with GALT or microbial substances (e.g. cytoplasmic antigens, cell wall components) that penetrate the intestinal epithelia to activate GALT (Schley and Field, 2002).

Other hypotheses have been advanced with regard to the immunomodulatory effect of dietary fibers on gut health. For instance, interleukin-6 (IL-6) cytokine levels were reduced in the serum of obese mice after consumption of a diet supplemented with 5% fungal chitosan for 10 weeks (Sánchez *et al.*, 2012). Furthermore, natural killer cell activity and mucin production increased in response to pH decrease due to SCFA production in a rat model that supplemented total parenteral nutrition (TPN) with SCFAs (Pratt *et al.*, 1996). For example, a cereal fiber diet reduced the volume density of cells containing neutral and sulfomucins in the jejunum of conventional rats, and staining density of neutral and acidic mucins in germ-free rats compared with a diet containing cellulose (Sharma and Schumacher, 1995). Therefore, dietary fiber that increases the release of mucin into the lumen furnishes more substrate for the development and growth of commensal as well as pathogenic bacteria in the large intestine (Montagne *et al.*, 2003). Dietary fiber intake has an impact on the expression of intestinal heat shock proteins (HSP) which have crucial housekeeping functions in maintaining the mucosal barrier integrity in pig guts (Lindberg, 2014). It is believed that such dietary interventions (dietary fiber supplementation) have the potential to improve gut health and simultaneously avoid the use of antibiotics to control enteric diseases common in animal husbandry.

The commercial product ImmuneEnhancer™ AG (arabinogalactan–acacia gum) reflects the immunomodulatory effects of dietary fiber. It is a highly water-soluble fiber larch arabinogalactan extract enhancing the immune system response by increasing levels of interferon gamma (IFNγ), tumor necrosis factor alpha (TNFα), IL-1β, IL-6, and NK (natural killer) cell activity. It also enhances the mononuclear portion of the immune system by supporting monocyte production to defend against foreign invaders (Fitzpatrick *et al.*, 2004). Similar immunomodulatory effects have been observed with another commercial arabinogalactan–acacia gum (AG–Fibergum™) and FOS in gut wall modulation to protect the leaky gut syndrome (Daguet *et al.*, 2015). Both fibers exerted a positive effect on gut barrier and inflammation (modulation of IL-6, IL-8, IL-10, and NFκB cytokines), although AG and FOS showed different fermentation profiles (more proximal for FOS and distal for AG). AG was posited as a potential treatment for conditions characterized by inflammation and increased permeability in the colon, particularly for those affected with irritable bowel syndrome (IBS) (Daguet *et al.*, 2015).

6.3.4 Prebiotic Effect

Today, we know that some fibers also play an important role in maintaining the intestinal flora and the amount of bacteria and fecal excretion is directly proportional to fiber intake in both animal and humans. The prebiotic effects of some fibers are well established since they can stimulate growth of certain intestinal bacteria during fermentation and can therefore be included/added to foods (García-Peris *et al.*, 2002). For example, strong evidence indicates that consumption of prebiotic fibers (inulin and oligofructose) increases the proportion of beneficial lactic acid bacteria in the human colon (Schley and Field, 2002). The addition of guar gum or cellulose to a standard diet also increases ileal bifidobacterial and enterobacterial populations in growing pigs (Owusu-Asiedu *et al.*, 2006). In acidic environment, SCFAs produced by dietary fiber fermentation, as presented below, are capable of inhibiting the growth of some intestinal pathogens such as *Escherichia coli*, *Salmonella* spp., and *Clostridium* spp. Butyrate, in particular, seems to play a selective antimicrobial role, since studies in pigs indicate that *Lactobacillus* spp. and *Streptococcus bovis* are less sensitive to *n*-butyrate than *E. coli*, *Salmonella* spp., *Clostridium acetobutylicum, Streptococcus cremoris, Lactococcus lactis,* and *Lactococcus cremoris* (Montagne *et al.*, 2003). Dietary fiber such as pectin, guar gum, oat gum, or inulin, resistant starch, and non-digestible oligosaccharides (transoligosaccharides, galacto-oligosaccharides, dextrins) exert putative protective effects against colonization by pathogenic bacteria, and their subsequent proliferation and resultant diarrhea. The beneficial effects of these dietary components have been studied largely in animals (Saavedra *et al.*, 2002).

The bifidogenic effect of legume-containing diets with high dietary fiber and resistant starch contents has been investigated on the intestinal microbiota of male Wistar rats (Da. S. Queiroz-Monici *et al.*, 2005). The pea group, which has the second highest amount of total dietary fiber, presented the highest count of *Bifidobacterium*, although the *Lactobacillus* count was similar for all leguminous groups. Animals fed legume-containing diets showed lower *Enterobacter* and *Bacteroides* counts than the control group and no statistical difference was found between groups with respect to *Clostridium* counts and total anaerobes. The bifidogenic effects of different types of arabinoxylans prepared from wheat bran have also been evaluated in rats (Broekaert *et al.*, 2014, 2015). Preparations included: low molecular weight arabinoxylan-oligosaccharides (AXOS), high molecular weight water-soluble arabinoxylan (WS-AX), and high molecular weight water-unextractable arabinoxylan (WU-AX). The preparations were added either alone or in additive combinations to different diets and a range of gut health-related parameters were assessed after 14 days. WS-AX increased butyrate production in both the cecum and the colon and this was further significantly increased in the combination of WS-AX with AXOS. The highest butyrate levels were found in the cecum and colon of rats fed the diet supplemented with the combination of WU-AX, WS-AX, and AXOS. The increase in butyrate levels was accompanied by a reduction in branched SCFAs, a marker of undesired intestinal protein fermentation. Further enzymatic treatment of AXOS produced arabinoxylo-oligosaccharides with low degree of polymerization (DP ≤ 5) that exerted optimal gatrointestinal health effects (increased acetate and butyrate levels in the colon, reduced markers of intestinal protein fermentation, and increased level of bifidobacteria in the cecum) upon digestion.

However, earlier animal (pig) and human studies showed that fiber extracts from fruits or vegetables exerted greater significant beneficial effects on bowel health through increased SCFAs levels in the colon than wheat bran (Lang *et al.*, 2004). The feeding study in humans (12 M + 11 F; average age 51 years; BMI = 24) consisted of a balanced, two-period crossover trial preceded by a baseline period. Subjects were randomly allocated to either wheat bran cereal or the test cereal (PTI fiber – orange and apple fiber extract) supplemented for 14 days and then assigned to the alternating dietary supplement for the same period. Subjects were provided with 34 or 45 g daily portions of PTI or wheat bran, respectively, equivalent to approximately 15 g of dietary fiber. The higher SCFAs in the large bowel (fecal samples) in subjects fed PTI relative to wheat bran was presumed to be associated with its high pectin content, fermentability, and bifidogenic activity in the large bowel.

Furthermore, the combination of two dietary fibers with different fermentation patterns may exert a synergistic effect on bacterial populations

(Rodríguez-Cabezas *et al.*, 2010). In that study, two fibers (FOS and resistant starch) were administered to healthy rats or trinitrobenzenesulfonic acid (TNBS)-colitic rats with an altered colonic immune response. The result was very promising in both groups: the microbiological analysis revealed that all fiber-treated groups exhibited modified intestinal microbiota. Both FOS and the mixture promoted a significant increase of lactobacilli and bifidiobacteria counts both in cecum and colonic contents, whereas resistant starch significantly enhanced only the bifidiobacteria counts in the colonic contents. This prebiotic effect positively influenced the physiological processes of the gut; the fibers upregulated trefoil factor-3 and MUC-2 expression, thereby improving the intestinal barrier function. The anti-inflammatory effect on the colon tissue was positive with a significantly lower colonic damage score compared to control rats.

Enteral formula fortified (15 g/L) with a fiber blend (50:50 insoluble:soluble mixture of FOS and inulin, pea hull fiber, and gum acacia) increased fecal weight and moderated decreases in total bacteria and bifidobacteria compared with fiber-free formula in healthy adults (10 M + 10 F, 26 years old). The fiber blend fortification did not affect overall gastrointestinal quality-of-life scores for subjects consuming formula diets (Koecher *et al.*, 2015). Prebiotics are also used in conjunction with probiotics, the so-called "synbiotic" approach. The inclusion of an inulin/FOS prebiotic enhanced the survival of a double probiotic mixture of *Bifidobacterium bifidum* and *B. lactis* and increased the numbers of native bifidobacterial populations in elderly patients (Flint *et al.*, 2012).

Currently used prebiotics are mainly low digestible carbohydrates that are found naturally in foods. These include xylo-oligosaccharides (XOS), galacto-oligosaccharides (GOS) and fructans including inulin and FOS. Most of the available information on prebiotics has focused on fructans, which were the first carbohydrates used to increase bifidobacteria abundance in the human colon. The inulin-type fructans are present in foods such as onions, garlic, and bananas and other sources are continuously being discovered and/or developed.

New knowledge on gut microbiota modulation by dietary fiber is critical for the development of effective strategies to improve human health and to treat microbiota-associated diseases. Recent developments in community-wide sequencing and glycomics have debated the definition of prebiotics due to the complex interactions between putative prebiotic substrates and gut microbiota revealed by these technologies (Hutkins *et al.*, 2016). This is particularly important because of the overlap between the definitions of prebiotics and dietary fiber, although most dietary fiber sources do not lead to selective changes in gut microbiota. In this context, the following definition has been proposed: a prebiotic is a non-digestible compound that, through its metabolization by gut microorganisms, modulates composition and/or activity of the gut microbiota, thus conferring a beneficial physiological effect on the host (Bindels *et al.*, 2015).

6.3.5 Enteroendocrine Activities

The gut plays key roles in producing various enteroendocrine-derived peptides that control and modulate miscellaneous metabolic and physiological processes, thereby creating a link between the gut and the brain. Glucagon-like peptide-1 (GLP-1) and ghrelin are two such peptides that have been particularly investigated and demonstrated to participate in appetite regulation, with anorexigenic and orexigneic effects, respectively (Roberfroid, 2007). All these molecular mechanisms regulating body weight provide potential opportunities for therapeutic development and renewed hope for potential dietary intervention. An increase in proglucagon mRNA concentration has already been shown in dogs fed fermentable dietary fiber (100 g/kg diet) for 14 days (Massimino *et al.*, 1998); this was accompanied by a higher GLP-1 (7 – 36) amide incremental area under the curve after a glucose load. Zhou *et al.* (2008) provided strong evidence that dietary resistant starch upregulated total GLP-1 in a sustained daylong manner in rodents. These increases were associated with fiber fermentation in the lower intestine. Schroeder *et al.* (2013) showed the effect on satiety and adiposity-related hormones in male Wistar rats fed different types of fiber (fermentable and non-fermentable fiber) for 6 weeks. The fiber sources were either non-fermentable or highly fermentable, each source producing no viscosity, low viscosity, or high viscosity within the small intestinal contents. The non-fermentable fibers were cellulose (no viscosity), low-viscosity hydroxypropyl methylcellulose (LV-HPMC), or high-viscosity HPMC (HV-HPMC). The fermentable fibers were short-chain FOS (no viscosity) (scFOS), scFOS with resistant starch (low viscosity) (scFOS + resistant starch), or oat β-glucan (high viscosity). In the fasted state, scFOS, the fermentable fiber with no viscosity, had the greatest plasma GLP-1 concentration, whereas the GLP-1 concentrations were lowest in the diets containing fermentable fibers with some viscosity. Thus, response of GLP-1 to fermentation was dependent on viscosity. In the fed state, groups administered the non-fermentable fibers with no (cellulose) or low-viscosity HPMC (LV-HPMC) had the numerically highest GLP-1 concentrations, although these groups did not differ from the scFOS and β-glucan groups. Plasma ghrelin concentrations, on the other hand, showed a strong overall trend towards a difference between the fasted and fed states. In the fasted state, animals fed the cellulose diet had significantly lower ghrelin concentrations than those fed all other diets except β-glucan. In the fed state, animals fed the cellulose and LV-HPMC diets had significantly lower ghrelin concentrations than animals on the scFOS + resistant starch and β-glucan diets. The effect of fermentability was statistically significant, such that groups fed the fermentable fibers had a greater ghrelin concentration than the non-fermentable fibers. Non-fermentable dietary fibers promote satiation and satiety and thereby provide an important tool for improving body weight management.

Oligofructose (OFS) has also been shown to increase total cecal GLP-1 (7 – 36) amide concentration in rats. Cani *et al.* (2004) analyzed the modulation of both portal GLP-1 (7 – 36) amide and peripheral ghrelin concentrations in the serum of rats fed three fructan types, differing in their preferential sites and extent of fermentation. The study performed in male Wistar rats showed that both fructans significantly increase GLP-1 (7 – 36) amide concentrations in the proximal colon and in the portal vein, with a reduction in peripheral ghrelin concentration. Adam *et al.* (2014) also demonstrated that different types of soluble fermentable dietary fiber decrease food intake, body weight gain, and adiposity in young adult male rats, through hormone regulation. Diets containing 10% w/w cellulose (CELL), FOS, oat β-glucan (GLUC), or apple pectin (PECT) were administered for 4 weeks in young adult male rats. After supplementation, the GLUC, FOS, and PECT groups had lower food intake percentages, body weight gain, and total body fat than those on the control diet. The three soluble dietary fibers specifically increased concentrations of total GLP-1 and gut hormone peptide YY (PYY; tyrosine amino acids, amino and carboxy terminals) in plasma samples taken in the early part of the light phase at the end of the trial, indicative of raised tonic secretion of these hormones. These studies, combined with other models in different animals, provide strong evidence that inclusion of different fermentable dietary fiber sources may help modulate the activity of specific hormones from the colon, and could be used as functional foods to combat the worldwide obesity problem.

Recent studies have suggested other mechanisms through which dietary fiber fermentation products may help to control body weight beyond that of energy dilution and gut hormone release. For example, novel insight has been provided into the mechanism through which the SCFA acetate mediates some of the protective effects against obesity of fermentable carbohydrate-rich diets directly in the central nervous system (Frost *et al.*, 2014). Oligofructose-enriched inulin (Synergy HF-1) supplementation studies in mice showed that reduction in body weight was partially mediated by acetate independent of changes in peripheral GLP-1 and PYY concentrations. Furthermore, acetate derived from dietary fiber fermentation in the colon was taken up by the hypothalamus in greater amounts than by other brain tissues, inducing a hypothalamic anorectic signal leading to increased lactate and GABA production (Frost *et al.*, 2014).

Acetate also exerted beneficial effects in protection against colitis and arthritis in a mouse model through its association with free fatty acid receptor 2 (FFAR2), also referred to as GPR43 (Trompette *et al.*, 2014 and references therein). Another study highlighted the importance of dietary fermentable fiber (pectin), its influence on intestinal microbiota, increased circulating SCFAs (particularly propionate) in providing a cellular mechanism for an intestinal–bone marrow–lung axis controlling airway inflammation (Trompette *et al.*, 2014). A high fiber diet fed to mice led to increased circulating SCFAs, promoted the outgrowth of bacteria from the *Bacteroidetes* phylum, and protected against allergic lung inflammation by propionate-mediated regulation of airway inflammation involving G protein-coupled receptor 41 (GPR41, also called free fatty acid receptor 3 (FFAR3)) (Trompette *et al.*, 2014). Propionate also activates FFAR3 in the nerves surrounding the portal vein, which transports the nutrients absorbed in the gut to the liver. Feeding FOS instead of propionate induces similar effects, illustrating the importance of metabolites produced by the gut microbiome (Rezzonico *et al.*, 2015).

Eating flaxseed mucilage (10 g/day) over 6 weeks improved insulin sensitivity and modified gut bacteria in obese postmenopausal women ($n = 53$) (Brahe *et al.*, 2015). The flaxseed mucilage treatment altered the abundance of 39 metagenomic species, including decreased and increased relative abundance of eight *Faecalibacterium* species and members of the *Clostridium* genus, respectively. However, the effect on insulin sensitivity was independent of the flaxseed mucilage-induced changes in abundance of bacterial species. The beneficial metabolic effects of flaxseed mucilage observed in this and earlier studies are probably due to the ability of the soluble viscous fibers to delay gastric emptying and inhibit nutrient absorption rather than their ability to induce specific changes in the gut microbiota.

Bifidobacterium species (*B. longum, B. pseudocatenulatum,* and *B. adolescentis* – the dominant species in adult gut microbiota) increased significantly in obese women ($n = 15$) consuming 16 g/day inulin-type fructans (ITF) for 3 months compared to those receiving maltodextrin ($n = 15$) in a randomized, double-blind, parallel, placebo-controlled trial (Salazar *et al.,* 2015). *Bifidobacterium longum* was negatively correlated with serum LPS endotoxin. Total SCFAs, acetate, and propionate, which positively correlated with BMI, fasting insulinemia, and homeostasis (markers of metabolic syndrome) were significantly lower in the prebiotic than in the placebo group after the treatment period. Thus, ITF consumption selectively modulates *Bifidobacterium* species and decreases fecal SCFAs concentration in obese women. It can therefore lessen metabolic risk factors associated with higher fecal SCFA concentration in obese individuals.

6.3.6 Dietary Fiber and Inflammatory Bowel Disease

Dietary fiber use attenuates colonic inflammation by two mechanisms: through beneficial effects on intestinal microbiota and by elevating the colonic SCFA concentration. Inulin reduces dextran sulfate sodium (DSS)-induced colitis mediated intracolonic milieu modification (Videla *et al.,* 2001). Lactulose also dose-dependently affects DSS-induced colitis beneficially in Wistar rats, including improvements in colonic ulceration areas, body weight changes, diarrhea, bloody stools, and myeloperoxidase activity and microscopic colitis reduction (Rumi *et al.,* 2004). Rodríguez-Cabezas *et al.* (2002) studied the probable mechanisms involved in the beneficial effects of a fiber-supplemented diet (5% *Plantago ovata* seeds) in the TNBS model of rat colitis. Rats were fed the fiber-supplemented diet for 2 weeks before TNBS colitis induction and thereafter until one week after colonic evaluation. Supplementation of *P. ovata* seeds (5%) facilitated recovery from TNBS-induced colonic damage, with significant reduction in the extent and severity of involved tissue, and biochemically, by reduced colonic myeloperoxidase activity, a marker of neutrophil infiltration, and restored colonic glutathione content. Intestinal epithelium was restored and edema and granulocyte infiltration reduced in most samples from colitic treated compared to non-treated colitic rats. The study concluded that beneficial effect of dietary fiber on the TNBS model of rat colitis could be ascribed to the enhanced production of propionate and butyrate, which may act through a combination of different mechanisms.

Moreau *et al.* (2003) confirmed the healing effect of resistant starch by the involvement of some types of dietary fiber in inflammatory bowel disease. Resistant starch exhibited beneficial effects on the chronic inflamed cecal and distal mucosa using macroscopic and histological techniques, while FOS showed no beneficial effect in a DSS-induced colitis model (Moreau *et al.,* 2003). The differences could be due to discrepancies in SCFA measurements between diets, because the amount of cecal SCFA measured at day 7 in the FOS-DSS rats was considerably lower than that in the resistant starch-DSS rats. On the other hand, Cherbut *et al.* (2003) demonstrated that intragastric FOS administration significantly reduced intestinal inflammation, producing less damage to the mucosa and decreasing myeloperoxidase (MPO) activity. They concluded that FOS probably decreased colonic damage by modifying the chemical, physicochemical, and bacterial composition of cecal contents.

Previous studies found that germinated barley foodstuff (GBF) ameliorated DSS-induced experimental colitis in rats (Araki *et al.*, 2000). GBF diets (3%) increased acetic and butyric acid concentrations in DSS-induced rat colitis and effectively prevented bloody diarrhea and mucosa damage compared to control rats. However, 10% flaxseed diet containing soluble fiber exacerbated the severity of DSS-induced colitis, despite enhanced SCFA concentrations, cecum weight, and increased mammalian lignin production, indicative of increased microbial activity (Zarepoor *et al.*, 2014). The same group showed that a bean flour diet (20%) attenuated DSS-induced colitis severity by reducing colonic and circulating inflammatory cytokines (IL-1β, IL-6, IFNγ, and TNFα), and beneficially altering the microbiota with enhanced mucus barrier integrity, defense, function, and overall gut health (Monk *et al.*, 2016).

Recently, dietary fiber material extracted from sugarcane has been formulated to ameliorate the effects of intestinal disorders such as the IBS (Ball and Edwards, 2014). The fiber is claimed to be relatively hypoallergenic, containing both soluble and insoluble fiber in beneficial proportions for dietary intake and intestinal health. Three human case studies have demonstrated gut health benefits: (i) in complete remission of multiple digestive stresses after 1 week sugarcane fiber intake; (ii) improvement in bowel movement of a diabetic patient after 12 months fiber intake; and (iii) abating bacterial infection in a 60-year-old individual with poor digestive health (Ball and Edwards, 2014).

Butyrate has been purported to decrease proinflammatory cytokine expression via inhibition of NFκB activation and IκBα degradation. Song *et al.* (2006) found that treatment of sodium butyrate and 5-aminosalicylic acid (5-ASA) combination improved diarrhea, colonic damage score, and MPO activity, increased TFF3 mRNA expression, and decreased serum IL-1β production and tissue NFκB expression. The combination therapy of sodium butyrate and 5-ASA had better effects than any other single treatment. Tedelind *et al.* (2007), however, demonstrated that acetate and propionate ameliorated an ongoing inflammatory response at the cellular level and thus acetate and propionate may also contribute to the anti-inflammatory properties of SCFAs mixtures *in vivo*.

To date, 163 gene loci are known to confer susceptibility to Crohn's disease and/or ulcerative colitis. Genes with the strongest associations are involved in the immune response to microbes, such as the innate bacteria sensing (*NOD2*), the inflammatory response to microbes (*IL23R*), and autophagy (*ATLG16L1*) (Kaplan, 2015 and references therein). Unfortunately, the prevalence of inflammatory bowel disease, currently at 0.5% of the general population, is expected to climb steadily over the next decade in the western world. The annual direct healthcare costs are estimated to be over 1.2 billion Canadian dollars for the over

200 000 Canadians and 4.6–5.6 billion euros for the 2.5–3 million European patients with inflammatory bowel disease (Kaplan, 2015).

6.3.7 Diabetes

A recent meta-analyses of 35 clinical studies over three decades and across three continents showed that psyllium dosed before meals as a dietary supplement effectively lowers elevated fasting blood glucose concentrations (Gibb *et al.*, 2015). This effect was clinically meaningful in lowering glycated hemoglobin, and is comparable to many drugs used to treat diabetes. Furthermore, the blood glucose-dependent effect was most pronounced in patients being treated for type 2 diabetes mellitus and was minimal in euglycemic patients. The authors surmise that the gel-forming characteristic of psyllium may increase its passage to the distal gut, probably due to changes in gastrointestinal hormone secretion rather than effects on the microbiome (Gibb *et al.*, 2015).

6.3.8 Cardiovascular Disorders

Inulin-type fructans can inhibit triglyceride synthesis due to increased SCFA production by bacterial fermentation. Thus, a meta-analysis of 15 studies concluded that the intake of inulin-type fructans (average inulin 14.2 g/day) was associated with a significant decrease in triglyceride level by 15.05 mg/dL (Brighenti, 2007). Furthermore, consumption of inulin (10 g/day) together with a low fat, high carbohydrate diet improved triglyceride level by inhibiting carbohydrate absorption, resulting in reduced chylomicron remnants in the intestine (Letexier *et al.*, 2003). A recent double-blind randomized controlled study confirmed LDL-cholesterol reduction with 1 g phytosterols and 5 g inulin-enriched soymilk twice daily in statin-naive, mild-to-moderate hypercholesterolemia subjects (204 F + 36 M; mean age 47 years) (Kietsiriroje *et al.*, 2015).

6.3.9 Colon Cancer

Many animal studies have examined the relationship between dietary fiber and colon cancer. For example, Hughes and Rowland (2001) studied chicory derived β (2−1) fructans, which are known to exert cancer protective effects in animal models. The effects of two chicory fructans – oligofructose and long-chain inulin – were evaluated on apoptosis and bacterial metabolism associated with carcinogenesis in rats. Chicory fructans significantly affected the number of apoptotic cell per crypt, increasing the colonic apoptotic index in animals fed oligofructose and inulin compared to those fed the basal diet. However, there were no significant dietary effects on bacterial enzyme activities or ammonia concentration.

Fiber is known to bind bile acids, preventing their conversion into secondary bile acids, some of which are considered procarcinogens. Primary bile acid conversion is also inhibited by pH reduction of the enzyme activity of 7-α-hydroxylase in the colon (Escudero-Álvarez and González-Sánchez, 2006). Moreover, the protection afforded by this dietary fiber is through carcinogen inhibition, mutation prevention, and apoptotic effects (Niba and Niba,

2003). The inhibitory mechanisms of carcinogens act on genotoxic injuries produced, for example, by azoxymethane (AOM) and 1,2-dimethylhydrazine (DMH)-induced dysplasia–carcinoma sequence in rodents. Colonic epithelium was examined to evaluate the acute apoptotic response to the genotoxic carcinogens (AARGC) and its regulation by fibers differing in fermentability (Hu *et al.*, 2002). Male Sprague–Dawley rats received a single subcutaneous injection of AOM (10 mg/kg body weight). Two groups of rats were fed diets containing 10% wheat bran fiber (WB; fermentable) or 10% methylcellulose (MC; poorly fermentable) for 4 weeks. The results showed that apoptotic cells were situated predominantly in the lower half of the crypt. Supplementation of diets with WB altered the luminal environment relative to MC, as a result of active fermentation which was associated with a significantly higher AARGC rate in distal colon. SCFA generation, including butyrate, was higher by WB than MC, but proliferation was not different between the fibers. Interestingly, it was concluded that dietary fibers can regulate AARGC; moreover, luminal generation of butyrate may enhance AARGC because butyrate is proapoptotic *in vivo* (Hu *et al.*, 2002).

Numerous authors have investigated the role of SCFAs, specifically butyrate, on colon cancer development. Butyrate influences cell function because of its ability to modulate oxidative stress and gene expression, which is often attributed to histone deacetylase inhibition. In addition, a multiplicity of effects may underlie butyrate's ability to modulate gene expression and thereby impact key apoptosis and cell cycle regulators. This was demonstrated for the cell cycle inhibitor p21 and proapoptotic protein bak, a tumor-induced angiogenesis inhibitor, by modulating two angiogenesis-related proteins – vascular endothelial growth factor and hypoxia-inducible factor 1α (Blottiere *et al.*, 2003; Hamer *et al.*, 2008).

Thus, Avivi-Green *et al.* (2000) evaluated the effect of high intracolonic butyrate concentrations, either through fermentation of a soluble fiber-enriched diet or via intracolonic butyrate instillation, on colon cancer in a chemically induced (DMH) rat model. They concluded that high butyrate levels, instilled or fermented from soluble dietary fibers, inhibit early and late events in colon tumorigenesis by controlling the transcription expression and activity of key proteins involved in the apoptotic cascade: the cleaved poly(ADP-ribose) polymerase product was overexpressed and the anti-apoptotic protein Bcl-2 was suppressed following pectin feeding as well as butyrate instillation. These results confirm the important role of butyrate production by fiber fermentation in intestinal health.

Moreover, the effect of fiber on colorectal carcinogenesis prevention may also result from synergism with other food constituents, some of which are attached to the fiber matrix and reach the colon. Vergara-Castañeda *et al.* (2010) quantified the soluble and insoluble fiber, as well as oligosaccharide fraction, resistant starch, and phenolic compounds in common bean (cultivar Bayo Madero). They demonstrated that common beans are an important source of dietary fiber, with the soluble fiber increasing significantly during the cooking process. The resistant starch proportion in the non-digestible fraction (NDF) of common beans

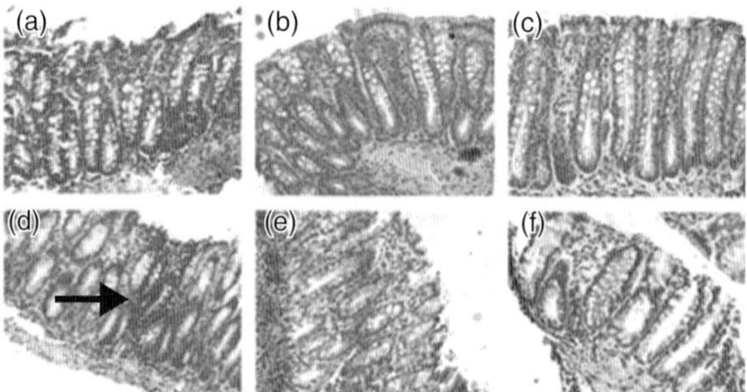

Figure 6.1 Distal colon tissue stained with hematoxylin and eosin. (a) Control; (b) cooked bean; (c) non-digestible fraction; (d) azoxymethane; (e) cooked bean + azoxymethane; (f) non-digestible fraction + azoxymethane. Magnification × 20. The aberrant crypt foci (ACF) (indicated by arrows) increased staining intensity of epithelial cytoplasm and presented irregular elongation of the ducts. Some ACF presented conical shape of the focus. Source: Vergara-Castañeda *et al.* (2010). Reproduced with permission of the Royal Society of Chemistry.

increased with cooking and the oligosaccharide content decreased; similar reductions were observed for the individual oligosaccharides raffinose, stachyose, and verbascose.

All constituents and the NDF of common beans were evaluated in an AOM-induced animal model of colon cancer. Aberrant crypt foci (ACF) development in rats was suppressed by cooked beans and NDF at the end of the experimental period (9 weeks) (Figure 6.1) and β-glucuronidase activity was reduced compared with that in colon cancer-induced rats without treatment. These results indicated that cooked Bayo Madero beans and NDF provide direct chemoprotection against the early stages of colon cancer induced in rats. Feregrino-Pérez *et al.* (2008) found that common beans (cultivar Negro 8025) contain a high proportion of undigested carbohydrates that can be fermented in the large intestine to produce SCFAs. They evaluated the effect of NDF on AOM-induced colon cancer in rats. The number of ACF and the transcriptional expression of Bax and caspase-3 were increased, and Rb expression suppressed. The data suggest that non-digestible compounds decreased ACF and influenced the expression of genes involved in colon cancer because of the action of butyrate.

6.4 *In Vitro* Studies

6.4.1 Prebiotic Effect

The essential role of the gut microbiota in health has generated tremendous interest in modulating its composition and metabolic function. One of these strategies is prebiotics – non-digestible compounds that modulate composition and/or activity of the gut microbiota, thereby conferring a beneficial physiological effect on the host (Bindels *et al.*, 2015). Traditionally, few carbohydrates are considered to be prebiotics (inulin, FOS, GOS, human milk, and oligosaccharides); however, recent research suggests that other compounds that exert their action through gut microbiota modulation (resistant starch, pectin, arabinoxylan, whole grains, and other dietary fibers, as well as non-carbohydrates) should be included (Bindels *et al.*, 2015). The use of *in vitro* models is still limited although many studies have been conducted *in vivo* to evaluate prebiotic effects.

The fermentation properties of prebiotic oligosaccharides were compared *in vitro* (Rycroft *et al.*, 2001). All prebiotics – FOS, inulin, XOS, lactulose, GOS, soybean oligosaccharides, and isomalto-oligosaccharides (IMO) – increased the numbers of bifidobacteria and decreased clostridia. XOS and lactulose produced the highest increases in bifidobacteria numbers; FOS produced the highest lactobacilli population, whereas GOS induced the largest reduction in clostridia numbers. *Bifidobacterium longum, B. bifidum, B. catenulatum, Lactobacillus gasseri,* and *L. salivarius* were the primary members within the complex microbiota directly involved in GOS fermentation (Maathuis *et al.*, 2012). GOS selectively stimulated bifidobacteria, specifically in the presence of β-$(1 \rightarrow 6)$-linkages and FOS lactobacilli (Li *et al.*, 2015). Sugar beet arabino-oligosaccharides also increased *Bifidobacterium* spp. 1.79-fold (high-mass) when fermented with human fecal microbiota, and LC–MS analysis suggested that the bifidobacteria contributed to decomposition of the arabino-oligosaccharide structures, resulting in release of the essential amino acid phenylalanine. During the fermentation process lactobacilli contributed to the release of health-promoting substances such as flavonoids from plant structures (Sulek *et al.*, 2014).

Gut bacteria fermented novel low molecular weight polysaccharides derived from agar and alginate-bearing seaweeds, exhibiting their potential for use as new prebiotic sources. *Gelidium* seaweed CC2253 increased bifidobacterial populations significantly ($p = 0.018$) from $\log_{10}$ 8.06 at the start to $\log_{10}$ 8.55 at 24 hours. Alginate powder CC2238 also increased total bacterial populations significantly ($p = 0.032$) from $\log_{10}$ 9.01 at the start to $\log_{10}$ 9.58 at 24 hours. In this context, pectin increases *Bifidobacterium* almost 25%, while resistant starch increases *Bifidobacterium adolescentis* type 2. Furthermore, inulin utilization was inversely ($r = -0.73$, $p \leq 0.01$) associated with *Subdoligranulum*, while β-glucan utilization was positively ($r = 0.73$, $p \leq 0.01$) correlated with *Firmicutes* and resistant starch utilization with *Blautia wexlerae* ($r = 0.82$, $p < 0.01$) (Yang *et al.*, 2013). Thus, the increased growth of specific microorganisms resulted in increased production of selected SCFAs. The *Firmicutes* families *Lachnospiraceae* and *Ruminococcaceae*, which are representative butyrate-producing anaerobes, are able to grow on short-chain FOS, but their number decreases with increasing chain length of the fructan substrates. Long-chain inulin is utilized by *Roseburia inulinivorans*, with XOS as a more selective growth substrate than FOS (Scott *et al.*, 2014). Thus, *Bacteroides* correlate positively to propionate production ($r = 0.59$, $p < 0.01$), whereas *Ruminococcaceae* and *Faecalibacterium* correlate with butyrate ($r = 0.39$ and 0.54, $p < 0.01$) (Yang *et al.*, 2013).

Wheat dextrin significantly increased total bacteria in vessels simulating the transverse and distal colon according to 16S rRNA-based fluorescence *in situ* hybridization. It also increased the key butyrate-producing bacteria *Clostridium* cluster XIVa and *Roseburia* genus significantly in all segments of a three-stage continuous culture human colonic model (Hobden *et al.*, 2013). *Actinidia chinensis* gold-fleshed kiwifruit cultivar "Zesy002" exerted a bifidogenic effect on *Bacteroides* spp., *Parabacteroides* spp., and *Bifidobacterium* species, reflecting propionate production (Blatchford *et al.*, 2015).

Innovative potential prebiotics are currently being explored. Exopolysaccharides (biopolymers) produced by lactic acid bacteria isolated from a marine environment exhibit strong bifidogenic effect on human fecal microbiota. These biopolymers increase bifidobacteria and lactobacilli as well as acetate and propionate in the transverse and distal colon. In contrast, butyrate decreases in the proximal colon region, but increases in the distal region (Hongpattarakere *et al.*, 2012). Flours from natural sources (whole grain rye, whole grain wheat, chickpeas, and lentils 50:50, and barley milled grains) could be used in the development of a variety of potentially prebiotic food products, since all have shown positive modulations of the microbiota composition and metabolic activity (Maccaferri *et al.*, 2012).

Target organisms other than the *Bifidobacterium* spp., such as *Lactobacillus acidophilus*, have been used to evaluate microbial adhesion of fibers commercially extracted from oat, wheat, rice, potato, pea, carrot, apple, and citrus (Holko and Hrabě, 2012). Wheat and oat fibers had the highest adhesion levels (>60%), whereas apple and citrus fibers had the lowest (≤21%), although all fibers consisted of cellulose ≈ 74%, hemicellulose ≈ 21%, and lignin <0.5%. The study suggests that cereal fibers may be preferably retained and transported to the colon for microbial fermentation (Holko and Hrabě, 2012).

Processing should be taken into account when evaluating prebiotic effect. For example, toasting of whole grain wheat flakes affects lactobacilli growth, whereas fermentation of raw wheat flakes significantly increases these microorganisms. The major bacterial groups and production of SCFAs were compared with those for the prebiotic oligofructose (Connolly *et al.*, 2012).

Age is an important factor that determines microbiota populations when dietary fiber is evaluated on healthy and general microbiota. Likotrafiti *et al.* (2014) reported that elderly gut microbiota can be modulated *in vitro* with the appropriate probiotics (*Bifidobacterium longum* and *Lactobacillus fermentum*), prebiotics (IMO and scFOS), and synbiotics (their mixture). Interestingly, prebiotics such as oligosaccharides and other metabolites are presumably transferred through breastfeeding, modulating their microbiota, thereby influencing their fermentability, reflected in the metabolomic profile of fecal material (Chow *et al.*, 2014). Furthermore, human milk oligosaccharides (HMOS), when fermented by infant microbiota, increase the proportion of *Bifidobacterium* spp. and decrease *Escherichia* and *Clostridium perfringens* proportions. In fact, *B. longum* JCM7007 and *B. longum* ATCC15697 consume oligosaccharides efficiently and produce abundant lactate and SCFAs, whereas *E. coli* K12 and *C. perfringens* do not utilize appreciable fucosylated oligosaccharides, and a typical mixture of organic acid fermentation products inhibits their growth (Yu *et al.*, 2013). Furthermore, microbiota from formula-feed infants ferments specific HMOS, specifically 2′-fucosyl lactose and, lacto-*N*-neotetraose rapidly compared with those from breastfed infants (Vester Boler *et al.*, 2013).

Cereal β-glucans are recognized as functional components of foods with benefits in maintaining digestive health through prebiotic effect. Recently, a groundbreaking study (Beeren *et al.*, 2015) proposed a pathway of enzymatic breakdown on the basis of a time-course experiment, using a fluorescently labeled β-glucan. The initial fast hydrolysis with an endo-1,3 (4)-β-glucanase was followed by slow degradation with an exo-1,4-β-glucanase, and finally slow action of an exo-1,3-β-glucanase.

6.4.2 SCFA Production

The species composition of the gut microbiota responds to dietary change, determined by substrate competition and tolerance of gut conditions. The metabolic outputs of the microbiota, such as SCFAs (the final products of dietary fiber fermentation in the human intestine), are influenced both by the supply of dietary components and via diet-mediated changes in microbiota composition (Flint *et al.*, 2015). These SCFAs also play key role in electrolyte and water transport by the colon, cell differentiation and growth, and can protect against diseases such as colon cancer. Absolute concentrations of individual and total SCFAs vary depending on species, diet, and microbiota diversity and concentration present in the colon (Vinolo *et al.*, 2011). Individual concentrations of SCFAs occur in ratios of 3:2:1 or 3:1:1, with acetate being the most prevalent, followed by propionate and butyrate, respectively, with a total concentration of SCFA around 100 mM. These ratios are location dependent, occurring at highest levels in the proximal colon and decreasing caudally. This pattern correlates with SCFA production by bacteria and absorption by colonic epithelial cells (Tazoe *et al.*, 2008).

Recent studies indicate a role for SCFAs, in particular propionate and butyrate, in metabolic and inflammatory disorders such as obesity, diabetes, and inflammatory bowel diseases, through the activation of specific G-protein-coupled receptors and modification of transcription factors. Established prebiotics, such as FOS and GOS, which support the growth of bifidobacteria, mainly mediate acetate production. Thus, recent identification of prebiotics that are able to stimulate the production of propionate and butyrate by benign saccharolytic populations in the colon is of interest (Puertollano *et al.*, 2014).

Water-insoluble dietary fiber is generally more resistant to colonic fermentation than soluble dietary fiber (Jenkins and Kendall, 2000). The suggested hypothesis that water-insoluble dietary fiber is the major contributor to the protective effects of whole grain type cereal foods emphasizes the importance of dietary fiber structure and the conversions of both carbohydrates and polyphenols in the large intestine (Saura-Calixto, 2010). The type and composition of cereal dietary fiber can consequently be used to modulate the microbial composition and activity as well as the production and molar ratios of SCFAs (Knudsen, 2015). The higher fermentation rate is related to the physical characteristics (higher portion of water-extractable dietary fiber, more degraded cell wall structures, and smaller particle size of bran samples) and, thus, to the better accessibility of microbes to fermentable dietary fiber and associated phenolic compounds. The SCFAs ratios are grain specific and more dependent on the carbohydrate composition than on the physical characteristics of the fiber complex (Nordlund *et al.*, 2012). For example, arabinoxylans (AX) and β-glucan in whole grain cereals and cereal ingredients elevate SCFA production, with the strongest relative effect on butyrate. However, when AX is provided as a concentrate, the effect is only on total SCFA production (Knudsen, 2015).

Wheat is one of the most studied grains, on *in vitro* models, as a dietary fiber source, including the bran and aleurone fractions, which are composed mainly of AX, AXOS, cellulose, lignin, and β-glucans (Rosa-Sibakov *et al.*, 2015). Interestingly, rye bran, especially its aleurone fraction, is fermented much faster and further than wheat bran and its aleurone in 24 hours. Wheat fractions produce, on average, more butyric (21%) and propionic acids (23.5%) than rye fractions (20 and 17.5% propionic and butyric acids, respectively), even higher than oat (bran and cell wall concentrate) (Nordlund *et al.*, 2012).

However, only about 34% of the dietary fiber in wheat is fermentable by gut bacteria (Van Dokkum *et al.*, 1983). Hence, different technological approaches have been used to increase their fermentability. Extrusion of wheat bran improves the fermentability by human fecal microbiota, as reflected in increased SCFA production (40% more) as mediated by higher water-extractability non-starch polysaccharides (Arcila *et al.*, 2015). Repeated cooking and freezing of whole wheat flour increases resistant starch and SCFA production, mainly propionate (Arcila and Rose, 2015). Mechanical (dry grinding) or enzymatic (xylanase with or without feruloyl esterase) modification of aleurone increases the concentration and formation rate of the colonic metabolites of ferulic acids (especially phenylpropionic acids), without significantly altering the formation of SCFAs (Rosa *et al.*, 2013). Other cereals have also been evaluated, especially some of their fractions.

Cereals (and derived products) are not the only source of dietary fiber: potato and legumes, starchy foods (including cereals), and fruits and vegetables (non-starchy foods, including cocoa products) also contribute significantly to the daily intake of dietary fiber, especially from the Mediterranean and Scandinavian diets (Tabernero *et al.*, 2007) and thus to total SCFA production. In the context of the diet, fruit and vegetable dietary fiber generate higher amounts of butyrate than cereal dietary fiber, when an average of 346 and 471.5 g dietary fiber/day are consumed (cereal and fruit/vegetable, respectively). In fact, when equal amount of starchy and non-starchy foods are consumed, more dietary fiber is provided from non-starchy (21.5%) than starchy foods (13.2%) (Tabernero *et al.*, 2011). In contrast, butyrate and propionate yields from polysaccharide extracts of beans (Campos-Vega *et al.*, 2009) are higher (>50%) than those from apple pectin (Waldecker *et al.*, 2008). Nevertheless, phenolic acid contents in fruits, and even in legumes, are one of the factors affecting the conversion of carbohydrates to SCFAs (Bazzocco *et al.*, 2008). Other fruits (and derived products) with interesting SCFA profiles are oranges (Costabile *et al.*, 2015), cranberries, and grape seeds (Sánchez-Patán *et al.*, 2015), as well as blueberries and black raspberries (Goita *et al.*, 2012). Tropical fruits such as mango, papaya, pineapple, and banana are also able to produce those metabolites after gastric and colonic fermentation (Vong and Stewart, 2013).

A range of vegetables have also been evaluated as source of dietary fiber. For example, members of the gourd family (e.g., *Benincasa hispida*, *Lagenaria siceraria*, *Momordica charantia*, *Trichosanthes anguina*, and *Cucurbita maxima*) when fermented by pure cultures or mixed cultures of *E. coli*, *Lactobacillus fermentum*, *Bifidobacterium breve*, and *Clostridium acetobutilicum* species, are able to produce SCFAs, showing, interestingly, higher production than wheat fiber (Sreenivas and Lele, 2013). On the other hand, the production SCFAs from broccoli, carrot, cauliflower, celery, cucumber, lettuce, onion, mushroom sclerotia, and radish is low, at just up to 6.82 mmol/g substrate dry matter (Bourquin *et al.*, 1993; Wong *et al.*, 2005). Mucilage- and pectic-oligosaccharides from nopal (*Opuntia ficus-indica*) increased levels of SCFAs produced in microbial cultures to 71.05 and 62.57 mmol/L, respectively (Guevara-Arauza *et al.*, 2011). Chicory root pulp is also a good substrate for fermentation, close to 8.4 mmol/g fiber are obtained; furthermore, when chicory root pulp is ensiled, the fermentation process is quicker and high levels of SCFAs (10.9 mmol/g fiber) are produced within a short period (6 hours) (Ramasamy *et al.*, 2014). *Agave tequilana* Weber var. *Azul* also yields high SCFA concentrations (up to 39 mmol/L) (Zamora-Gasga *et al.*, 2015), which is even higher than those obtained from fenugreek gum (~20 mmol/L), an ancient grain (Roberts *et al.*, 2015). Surprisingly, polysaccharides from *Cyclocarya paliurus* leaves, a unique plant species in China, can promote SCFA production (~37 mM) (Min *et al.*, 2014).

6.4.3 Dietary Fiber, Microbiota, and Diseases

The gut microbiota makes up the majority of the human bacterial population and exerts systemic effects. Several clinical conditions, including obesity, metabolic and autoimmune diseases, allergy, acute and chronic intestinal inflammation, IBS, allergic gastroenteritis (e.g., eosinophilic gastroenteritis and allergic IBS), and necrotizing enterocolitis, can be impacted by dysbiosis (i.e., when the composition of the gut microbiota is imbalanced) (Ho *et al.*, 2015; Goulet, 2015). The gut microbiota is susceptible to modulation by environmental factors (Kump *et al.*, 2013), such as diet. For instance, children with a high fiber diet (e.g., in some African populations) have high numbers of *Bacteroidetes*, lack *Firmicutes*, but have abundant bacteria from the genera *Prevotella* and *Xylanibacter*; bacteria from these genera are completely absent in children with low fiber, high sugar, starch, and fat diets (e.g., as eaten by many European children) (Vieira *et al.*, 2014). Treatments involving microbiota, including dietary fiber, may be used in attempts to treat illnesses related to gut microbiota imbalances (Ho *et al.*, 2015).

6.4.3.1 Immunity

There is a fascinating relationship between food, immunity, and the microbiota. Many dietary components affect these interactions. We have only limited knowledge on the effects of dietary modification of commensals on the core microbiome and its functional/physiological consequences. Bacterial metabolites such as SCFAs, metabolites generated from food by bacteria, such as trimethylamine-N-oxide (TMAO), and dietary components alone affect the functions of many human systems and tissues. The effects of food on the microbiota and immune system is one of the most exciting areas of science. We now know that microbiota-derived and dietary factors operate together to determine gut health and beyond (Tilg and Moschen, 2015).

Agrarian diets high in fruit/legume fiber are associated with greater microbial diversity and a predominance of *Prevotella* over *Bacteroides*. "Western"-style diets (high fat/sugar, low fiber) lead to lower beneficial *Firmicutes* that metabolize dietary plant-derived polysaccharides to SCFAs and higher levels of mucosa-associated *Proteobacteria* (including enteric pathogens). Short-term diets can also have major effects, particularly those that are exclusively animal-based and the high protein, low fermentable carbohydrate/fiber "weight-loss" diets, which increase the abundance of *Bacteroides* and lower the levels of *Firmicutes*. Long-term adherence to such diets also likely increases the risk of colonic disease. Interventions to prevent intestinal inflammation may be achieved with fermentable prebiotic fibers that enhance beneficial bifidobacteria or with soluble fibers that block bacterial–epithelial adherence (contrabiotics) (Simpson and Campbell, 2015).

Luminal pH is also a major modulator of the intestinal ecosystem, with the natural pH is approximately 7 in the ileum and 5 in the colon. In an *in vitro* fermenter system, low percentage G + C gram-positive *Firmicutes* were dominant when pH was around 5.5, while *Bacteroides* spp. were more competitive at pH 6.7. Dietary fibers whose final product is SCFAs are one of the main determinants of luminal pH, and vegans have a significantly lower stool pH and higher prevalence of *Enterobacteriaceae* compared to omnivores (Shen and Clemente, 2015).

Soluble dietary fiber (complex carbohydrates) is cleaved into SCFAs by bacterial glycoside hydrolases. The SCFAs acetate, propionate, and butyrate have anti-inflammatory effects. In fact, the microbial metabolites that have been mostly studied for their effects on intestinal health and immunity are undoubtedly the SCFAs acetate, propionate, and butyrate (Tilg and Moschen, 2015). A recent review found that SCFAs promoted recruitment of neutrophils while also inhibiting neutrophil production of proinflammatory reactive oxygen species (ROS) and TNFα. SCFAs also promoted a tolerogenic phenotype in dendritic cells and macrophages, and both effector and regulatory T-cells. This newly revealed mechanism of SCFA signaling (e.g., mTOR-mediated pathways (such as glycolysis) shaping T-cell differentiation lineage choice) is intriguing and an important area for further study (Steinmeyer *et al.*, 2015).

SCFAs also bind G protein-coupled receptors, such as GPR41, GPR43, or GPR109A, that activate the transcription factor arrestin-b2 and can lead to NLRP3 inflammasome activation (Macia *et al.*, 2015; Tilg and Moschen, 2015). Butyrate natural inhibitor of the histone deacetylases 6 and 9 can promote peripheral regulatory T-cell development through epigenetic mechanisms (Tilg and Moschen, 2015). Its anti-inflammatory properties in IFN-stimulated macrophages *in vitro* (Park *et al.*, 2007) suggest a likely role for butyrate in modulating host immunity. Acetate can prevent *E. coli* infection by maintaining gut barrier function (Fukuda *et al.*, 2011). Furthermore, depletion of SCFAs correlates with increased incidence of intestinal inflammation. Butyrate and propionate induce the immunosuppressive enzyme Indoleamine 2,3-dioxygenase (IDO) in dendritic cells in an Slc5a8-dependent manner. Furthermore, these dendritic cells are able to suppress conversion of naive T-cells into IFNγ-producing Th1 cells. Therefore, the SCFA transporter Slc5a8 is a key determinant of SCFA-mediated protection against intestinal inflammation (Gurav *et al.*, 2014).

In mouse, SCFAs increase colonic Foxp3$^+$ regulatory T-cell (Treg) function, promote immune tolerance, and ameliorate intestinal inflammation through the G protein-coupled receptor GPR43 (FFAR2). However, despite the compelling literature in mouse, Mamontov *et al.* (2015) revealed for the first time that SCFAs can modulate human Treg function, and that pharmacological GPR43 agonists are sufficient to increase Treg suppressive capacity, with potential therapeutic implications for inflammatory/autoimmune diseases.

The fiber-induced production of cytokines by human peripheral blood mononuclear cells was investigated recently (Breton *et al.*, 2015). A soluble fiber slightly inhibited the production of IL-10 (23% decrease relative to the anti-inflammatory control strain *B. longum* BB3001). More importantly, fiber 1 was associated with much lower levels of IL-12 and IFNα (98% and 89% reduction, respectively, relative to the proinflammatory control strain *L. lactis* MG1363 ($p < 0.001$). This inhibition was dose-dependent and did not occur with any of the other fibers. These results demonstrate that soluble fiber has strong, specific, immunosuppressive effect.

The potential natural immunomodulatory effects of verbascose from mung beans have been explored (Dai *et al.*, 2014). Verbascose can enhance the ability of peritoneal macrophages to devour Neutral Red and promote the release of nitric oxide and immune reactive molecules such as IL-6, IL-1β, IFNα, and IFNγ. A novel water-soluble polysaccharide fraction (SCP-1) from *Sinonovacula constricta*, widely used as a health food and medicine in China, Japan, and Korea, significantly increased macrophage viability and phagocytosis capability, acid phosphatase activity, and promoted nitric oxide production, mouse TNFα, IFNγ, and IL-1β. Thus SCP-1 possesses potent immunomodulating effect and may be explored as a potential biological response modifier (Yuan *et al.*, 2015).

Lactate, acetate, propionate, and butyrate interact on cells relevant to the innate immune response of the gastrointestinal tract (Iraporda *et al.*, 2015). All SCFAs regulated proinflammatory cytokines production by Toll-like receptor (TLR)-4- and TLR-5-activated intestinal epithelial cells in a dose–response manner. Furthermore, SCFAs and lactate dose-dependently modulated cytokine secretion of TLR-activated bone marrow–derived macrophages and also upregulated TLR-dependent CD40 in bone marrow–derived dendritic cells. Butyrate and propionate were effective at 1–5 mM concentrations, whereas acetate and lactate produced modulatory effects at concentrations higher than 20–50 mM in different assays.

Dietary fibers can modulate the host immune system not only by the recognized mechanism of microbiota effects but also by direct interaction with the consumer's mucosa. Non-digestible oligosaccharides exert non-prebiotic effects on intestinal epithelial cells, enhancing the immune response via activation of TLR-4–NFκB (Ortega-González *et al.*, 2014). The interaction of GOS, chicory inulin, wheat AX, and barley β-glucan with epithelial cells and dendritic cells, recognized as an important link between innate and adaptive immunity, altered the production of the Th1 cytokines in autologous T-cells; chicory inulin and barley β-glucan reduced the Th2 cytokine IL-6. The Treg-promoting cytokine IL-10 was induced by GOS, whereas chicory inulin decreased IL-10 production (Bermudez-Brito *et al.*, 2015). An *in vitro* study also showed that GOS could directly enhance intestinal barrier function by modulating goblet cells (Bhatia *et al.*, 2015).

6.4.3.2 Ulcerative Colitis

The imbalances in gut microbiota composition seen in ulcerative colitis indicate a role for the microbiota in propagating the disorder. Interestingly, sulfate-reducing bacteria (SRB) are present in higher numbers in ulcerative colitis than in healthy human inocula. Also, healthy cultures produce two-fold higher growth and SCFA levels with up to 10-fold higher butyrate (Khalil *et al.*, 2014), and increased taurine and cadaverine levels (Le Gall *et al.*, 2011). *In vitro* models revealed a selective increase in *Bifidobacterium* spp. and *Lactobacillus* spp., bacteria that elicit anti-inflammatory responses, and in acetate production after arabino-oligosaccharides (AOS) or FOS fermentation by fecal microbiota derived from patients with ulcerative colitis (Vigsnæs *et al.*, 2011).

6.4.3.3 Irritable Bowel Syndrome

Irritable bowel syndrome is a common functional gastrointestinal disorder defined by the coexistence of abdominal discomfort or pain associated with alterations in bowel habits (Lee and Lee, 2014). A major functional dysbiosis has been observed in constipated–irritable bowel syndrome (C-IBS) gut microbiota, reflecting altered intestinal fermentation. Sulfate-reducing populations increase in the guts of people with C-IBS, accompanied by alterations in other microbial groups. This may be responsible for changes in metabolic output and enhanced toxic sulfide production, which in turn can influence gut physiology and contribute to IBS pathogenesis (Chassard *et al.*, 2012).

There is also evidence that short-chain carbohydrates such as inulin may stimulate or alter the preferential growth of health-promoting species already residing in the colon, leading to potential benefits in IBS. The GOS act as prebiotics in specifically stimulating gut bifidobacteria in IBS patients and are effective in alleviating symptoms (Silk *et al.*, 2009).

6.4.3.4 Crohn's Disease

Crohn's disease is a relapsing inflammatory disease, mainly affecting the gastrointestinal tract, and frequently presents with abdominal pain, fever, and clinical signs of bowel obstruction or diarrhea with passage of blood or mucus, or both. Crohn's disease concerns an increasingly diverse group of clinicians because its incidence and prevalence are rising in all ethnic groups. There are also concerns due to the systemic nature of the illness (Baumgart and Sandborn, 2012). Much has been written about the role of diet and risk for Crohn's disease, however the evidence is contradictory. Recent evidence surmises that fiber plays an important role along with dietary fat and overnutrition (Chan *et al.*, 2015). Brotherton *et al.*, (2012) suggested that, in the absence of contraindications, a dietary pattern featuring daily consumption of concentrated wheat bran cereal and refined carbohydrate restriction can be easily adopted by individuals with moderately active symptoms of Crohn's disease and may improve health-related quality of life and decrease/eliminate gastrointestinal symptoms. This could be related to the fact that patients with Crohn's disease have a compositional and functional dysbiosis in their intestinal microbiota, with high fecal tryptic activity, inversely correlated to *Bacteroides* levels (Midtvedt *et al.*, 2013). This, coupled with functional changes including major shifts in oxidative stress pathways, decreases in butanoate and propanoate metabolism gene expression, lower butyrate levels, and other SCFAs, decreases carbohydrate metabolism and amino acid biosynthesis (Wright *et al.*, 2015). Although *in vitro* colonic fermentation of starch with fecal slurries from ulcerative colitis increases SCFA production (Khalil *et al.*, 2014), no studies are available using feces from patients with Crohn's disease. Dietary fiber intake has recently been associated with increased colonic mucosal GPR43+ polymorphonuclear infiltration using segments of ascending colon and samples of venous blood from patients with Crohn's disease with abnormal neutrophils (Zhao *et al.*, 2015).

6.4.3.5 Weight Management

Obesity is currently a worldwide epidemic that has serious consequences for health. The energy-salvaging capacity of the gut microbiota from dietary ingredients has been proposed as a contributing factor for the development of obesity. This knowledge generated interest in the use of non-digestible dietary ingredients such as prebiotics to manipulate host energy homeostasis (Sarbini *et al.*, 2014). Gut microbiota has been suggested to influence body weight, for example by producing SCFAs, which are substrates for the host, and inducing the release of satiety hormones, such as PYY (de Souza *et al.*, 2014). The gut microbiota is the link in the obesity–adipose tissue axis, and its composition correlates with inflammation, endocannabinoid system, weight control, and diet (Guida and Venema, 2015). Indeed, obesity and associated metabolic dysfunctions often result from disturbed interactions between the intestinal microbiota, dietary changes, and host immune functions (Tilg and Adolph, 2015).

Some studies provide evidence that fermentable carbohydrates are fermented differently by microbiotas from lean and obese people. This contributes to our understanding of the role of diet and the microbiota in tackling obesity. An interesting study suggests that energy harvest (in terms of metabolites) of lean and obese microbiotas is different and may depend on the fermentable substrate (Aguirre *et al.*, 2014); it is therefore necessary to take the dietary components into consideration in future studies. For GOS and lactulose, the cumulative amount of SCFAs plus lactate produced in the TNO dynamic *in vitro* model of the proximal colon (TIM-2) was lower in the fermentation experiments with the lean (L) microbiota (123 and 155 mmol, respectively) compared to the obese (O) (162 and 173 mmol, respectively). This was reversed for pectin and fiber. The absolute amount of SCFAs including lactate was higher after 72 hours in the fermentation experiments with apple fiber–L than with apple fiber–O (108 vs. 92 mmol). Sugar beet–L was also higher than sugar beet–O (130 vs. 103 mmol). GOS and lactulose produced by the microbiota from obese subjects boosted the balance of health-promoting over toxic metabolites. *Firmicutes* were predominant in the inoculum prepared from feces of obese subjects compared to lean subjects. On the other hand, *Bacteroidetes* were dominant in the microbiota prepared with homogenates from lean subjects, with an average abundance of 22% compared with those from obese subjects (3.6%).

De Souza *et al.* (2014) showed, for the first time, the potential prebiotic properties of cassava bagasse, an industrial residue that currently has no or limited commercial value. It induced different effects in microbiota originating from lean and obese individuals, and shifted the obese microbiota composition closer to that of lean individuals. The starch fraction is believed to be responsible for the increase growth of beneficial bacteria, including the bifidogenic effect. Thus, it shows great promise in becoming a future functional food. Dextrans of various molecular weights and degrees of branching were also fermented with the fecal microbiota of healthy obese adults in pH-controlled batch cultures. In contrast, differences were not observed in the profiles between the obese and lean human fecal fermentations of dextrans, although some dextrans altered the composition of the obese human microbiota by increasing the counts of *Bacteroides–Prevotella* and decreasing those of *Faecalibacterium prausnitzii* and *Ruminococcus bromii/R. flavefaciens* (Sarbini *et al.*, 2014). The intake of flaxseed mucilage (10 g/day) over 6 weeks also modified gut bacteria in obese postmenopausal women ($n = 53$) and improved insulin sensitivity (Brahe *et al.*, 2015). The flaxseed mucilage treatment altered the abundance of 39 metagenomic species, including decreased and increased relative abundance of eight *Faecalibacterium* species and the *Clostridium* genus, respectively. The mucilage, similar to flaxseed, can reduce fat absorption resulting in a negative digestive energy value, inducing weight loss (Astrup *et al.*, 2014).

6.4.3.6 Diabetes

Extrinsic factors such as a sedentary lifestyle and excessive caloric intake contribute to the increasing incidence of obesity and type 2 diabetes. It is well established that diet quality can be improved by reducing fat and simple sugars intake while increasing the intake of dietary fiber. Fiber-enriched diets improve insulin sensitivity and glucose tolerance in lean and obese diabetic subjects (De Vadder *et al.*, 2014).

Metagenomic data revealed that type 2 diabetic patients exhibit a moderate degree of gut microbial dysbiosis. Interestingly, the microbiomes of type 2 diabetic patients are characterized by the depletion of several butyrate-producing bacteria, including *Clostridium* spp., *Eubacterium rectale*, *Faecalibacterium prausnitzii*, *Roseburia intestinalis*, and *Roseburia inulinivorans*, and an enrichment of opportunistic pathogens. Bacterial increase in the gut of type 2 diabetic patients also includes the sulfate-reducing bacteria *Desulfovibrio*, as well as *Lactobacillus gasseri*, *L. reuteri*, and *L. plantarum* (Delzenne *et al.*, 2015). *In vitro* studies using human feces from patients with type 2 diabetes have not been conducted to evaluate dietary fiber microbiota modulation.

Viscosity is one of the most studied mechanisms for dietary fiber diabetes modulation since its variation in different dietary fibers impedes glucose diffusion and postpones carbohydrate absorption and digestion. An *in vitro* study evaluating water-soluble and insoluble dietary fibers showed that postprandial serum glucose is lowered by dietary fiber through at least three pathways by: increasing viscosity of the small intestinal content and retarding glucose diffusion; preventing glucose adsorption and diffusion; and α-amylase inhibition and delaying glucose release from starch (Ou *et al.*, 2001). In this regard, our study showed that heat (microwave) treatment increased α-amylase inhibitor concentration, activity, and potency and may be useful in developing novel dietary fibers from beans (*Phaseolus vulgaris* L.) (Oomah *et al.*, 2014). In fact, a proprietary α-amylase inhibitor from white bean (called Phase 2) has been marketed for weight management and glycemic control (www.phase2info.com). Numerous *in vitro* studies confirm these mechanisms of dietary fiber from different sources (Qi *et al.*, 2016; Bae *et al.*, 2016; Chen *et al.*, 2015).

High fiber dietary intervention can regulate glucose metabolism by modulating gut microbiota through colonic fermentation. For example, several studies showed that a barley kernel-based evening meal rich in non-starch polysaccharides and resistant starch improved glucose tolerance in healthy subjects with a normal body mass index (Kovatcheva-Datchary *et al.*, 2015 and references therein). Furthermore, healthy subjects (33 F + 6 M; 50–70 years; BMI 18–28 kg/m^2) exhibiting improved glucose metabolism had increased *Prevotella copri* in their gut microbiota following consumption of barley kernel-based bread (BKB) for 3 days. This crossover randomized study demonstrated that *Prevotella* plays a role in BKB-induced improvement in glucose metabolism in certain individuals by promoting increased glycogen storage. The study also highlights the importance of gut microbiota (abundance and interaction with other microbial species) to host metabolism and responses to changes in the diet to treat metabolic disorders (Kovatcheva-Datchary *et al.*, 2015).

6.4.3.7 Cardiovascular Disorders

The human gut microbiota has been identified as a possible novel cardiovascular disease (CVD) risk factor. Not only are aberrant microbiota profiles associated with metabolic disease, but the flux of metabolites derived from gut microbial metabolism of choline, phosphatidylcholine, and L-carnitine contribute directly to CVD pathology, providing one explanation for the link between increased disease risk and eating too much red meat (Tuohy *et al.*, 2014). TMAO production from dietary phosphatidylcholine depends on metabolism by the intestinal microbiota. Increased TMAO levels are associated with increased risk of major adverse cardiovascular events (Tang *et al.*, 2013).

Diet, especially high intake of fermentable fibers and plant polyphenols, appears to regulate microbial activities within the gut, supporting regulatory guidelines encouraging increased consumption of whole-plant foods (fruit, vegetables, and whole grain cereals), and providing the scientific rationale for the design of efficacious prebiotics. Similarly, recent human studies with carefully selected probiotic strains show that ingestion of viable microorganisms with the ability to hydrolyze bile salts can lower blood cholesterol, a recognized risk factor in CVD (Tuohy *et al.*, 2014).

Microbiota dysbiosis predicted acute cardiovascular events in a large general population (Amar *et al.*, 2013). Bacteria from the class *Erysipelotrichia* (phylum *Firmicutes*) can metabolize choline to trimethylamine (TMA) (Serino *et al.*, 2014). This class of bacteria is increased in obese people with high CVD risk.

Bacteria from the *Collinsella* genus are enriched in patients with symptomatic atherosclerosis, defined as the presence of stenotic atherosclerotic plaques at the carotid artery level, leading to cerebrovascular events. By contrast, the gut microbiotas of healthy individuals contain elevated levels of bacteria belonging to *Roseburia* and *Eubacterium*, which are significant butyrate producers in the colon, compared to those of atherosclerosis patients (Karlsson *et al.*, 2012). Interestingly, wheat dextrin (Nutriose® FB06) mediates significant increases in total bacteria in vessels simulating the transverse and distal colon, and in key butyrate-producing bacteria such as *Clostridium* cluster XIVa and *Roseburia* genus in all vessels of the gut model (Hobden *et al.*, 2013). GOS decreased *Collinsella aerofancies* in a dynamic *in vitro* colon model, using a ^{13}C-labeling technique, demonstrating that carbons are incorporated in their rRNA; it also increased *Eubacterium rectale* (Maathuis *et al.*, 2012).

Other effects related to cardiovascular health, such as cholesterol-lowering effects, have been demonstrated for various dietary fibers, particularly β-glucans from oats and barley. These claims have been substantiated and are used in labeling many food products. Flaxseed fiber added to bread has been shown to lower cholesterol in people with diabetes. This effect was examined in a double-blind randomized crossover study with 16 adults (7 M + 9 F; average age 24.8 years; BMI 23.8 kg/m^2) (Kristensen *et al.*, 2012). Flaxseeds contain ∼30% dietary fibers, of which one-third are water soluble and belong to a group of heterogeneous polysaccharides. The study demonstrated that consumption of 5 g of dietary fiber from flaxseeds daily for one week increased fecal excretion of fat and reduced total and LDL-cholesterols markedly (Kristensen *et al.*, 2012). A follow-up study found that extracted flaxseed fibers reduced weight gain and fat digestibility when fed to growing rats in higher doses (10% w/w) (Kristensen *et al.*, 2013). A recent study reported improved insulin sensitivity and modified gut bacteria in obese postmenopausal women ($n = 53$) following flaxseed mucilage (10 g/day) intake over 6 weeks (Brahe *et al.*, 2015). The flaxseed mucilage treatment altered the abundance of 39 metagenomic species, including reduction in relative abundance of eight *Faecalibacterium* species and increase in the *Clostridium* genus. According to Brahe *et al.* (2015), the beneficial metabolic effects of flaxseed mucilage observed in this and earlier studies are probably due to the ability of the soluble viscous fibers to delay gastric emptying and inhibit nutrient absorption rather than their ability to induce specific changes in the gut microbiota. Prebiotic supplementation also reduced plasma total cholesterol, LDL-cholesterol, and triglycerides, and increased HDL-cholesterol concentrations in diabetic subjects from meta-analysis of 13 trials representing 513 adult participants with ≥25 kg/m^2 body mass index (Beserra *et al.*, 2015).

Markers of cardiovascular risk were not altered by increased whole grain/dietary fiber intake in a randomized, controlled dietary intervention of the UK population (Brownlee *et al.*, 2010). The study consisted of 316 participants (aged 18–65 years; BMI >25 kg/m^2) consuming <30 g whole grain (WG)/day randomly assigned to three groups: (no dietary change), intervention 1 (60 g WG/day for 16 weeks), and intervention 2 (60 g WG/day for 8 weeks followed by 120 g WG/day for 8 weeks). This study demonstrated that increased dietary fiber intake using whole grain food intervention for 4 months may be insufficient to change the lifelong disease trajectory associated with cardiovascular disease in overweight individuals (Brownlee *et al.*, 2010).

6.4.3.8 Colon Cancer

Although cancer treatments have made large strides in recent decades, prevention by diet and other healthy lifestyle factors and habits (e.g., physical exercise) offers a more desirable alternative. Many studies suggest that there is an association between high dietary fiber intake and a low/reduced incidence of colon cancer, and that dietary fiber has anticancer properties. Furthermore, the US Food and Drug Administration have approved health claims supporting the role of dietary fiber in cancer prevention (Zeng *et al.*, 2014). Gut microbiota and fiber fermentation to SCFAs also play critical roles in cancer prevention. In fact, most of the information refers to those compounds with regard to colon cancer prevention in *in vitro* models.

The anti-inflammatory and anti-carcinogenic mechanisms of SCFAs are diverse. They include the ability to inhibit colon cancer cell growth and to suppress LPS-stimulated IL-8 secretion (Asarat *et al.*, 2015). Our research group investigated molecular changes in the p53 pathway in HT29 cells after 24 hours of exposure to an *in vitro* human gut flora (FE-hgf)-fermented extract of NDF from the common bean cultivar Bayo Madero, which is rich in dietary fiber (Campos-Vega *et al.*, 2010). Significant differences were detected in 72 of 84 human p53-mediated signal transduction response genes involved in apoptosis, cell cycle, and cell proliferation. The apoptosis genes *SIAH1* and *PRKCA*, and gene *MSH2*, which is involved in the negative regulation of the cell cycle, were the highest upregulated genes (30.5-, 18.4- and 9.8-fold, respectively), whereas the cell cycle genes *CHEK1* and *GADD45A* were markedly downregulated (21.4- and 9.1-fold, respectively) (Table 6.1). Later, NDF from common beans was demonstrated to elicit beneficial protective effects in colon cancer by modulating protein expression in HT29 cells. NDF inhibited HT29 cell growth and modulated protein expression associated with apoptosis, cell cycle arrest, and proliferation (Figure 6.2) as well as causing morphological changes linked to apoptosis evaluated by TUNEL and hematoxylin and eosin stains, confirming previous results on gene expression (Campos-Vega *et al.*, 2012).

SCFAs can induce autophagy in colon cancer cells by suppressing mTOR activities with rhabdomyosarcoma 2-associated transcript (RMST), a long non-coding RNA, and protein tyrosine phosphatase non-receptor type 7 (PTPN7) as key mediators (Wang and Nie, 2015). Furthermore, butyrate, the primary energy substrate of the colonocyte, regulates gene expression via histone deacetylase (HDAC) inhibition. This mechanism is mediated by carnitine, which is used mainly to shuttle long-chain fatty acids into the mitochondria via CPT1, as required to achieve full butyrate oxidation in the cancerous colonocyte (Han and Donohoe, 2015).

A novel mechanism involving modulation of cancer-associated miRNA profiles that mediate butyrate's anticancer effects has been explored. Among the miRNAs whose expression was suppressed by butyrate, members of the miR-106b family, including miR-17, miR-20a/b, miR-93, and miR-106a/b, regulate p21 translation and cancer cell proliferation (Kim *et al.*, 2009; Hu *et al.*, 2011). Butyrate was found to inhibit pro-proliferative miR-92a by diminishing c-Myc-induced miR-17-92a cluster transcription in human colon cancer cells (Hu *et al.*, 2015).

Table 6.1 Regulated genes in treated (human gut flora-FE-hgf, fermented NDF-cv. Bayo Madero) compared with untreated HT29 cells.

Gene symbol	Biologic gene function	Description	Fold change in response to NDF
Apoptosis			
SIAH1	Apoptosis	Seven in absentia homolog 1	+30.5
GADD45A	Induction of apoptosis	Growth arrest and DNA damage-inducible alpha	−9.1
Cell cycle			
CHEK1	Cell cycle arrest	CHK1 checkpoint homolog	−21.4
CDKN1&2A	Cell cycle arrest	Cyclin-dependent kinase inhibitor A	+5.9; +4.7
Cell proliferation and differentiation			
PTEN	Negative regulation of cell cycle	Phosphatase and tensin homolog	+6.6
PRKCA	Cell proliferation	Protein kinase C alpha	+18.4
DNA repair			
MSH2	DNA repair	MutS homolog 2, colon cancer, non-polyposis type 1 (*E. coli*)	+9.8

Adapted from Campos-Vega *et al.* (2010).

6.5   Current Trends and Perspectives

Several products/innovations are aimed at treating metabolic disorders. For example, a viscous fiber complex consisting (w/w) of glucomannan (70%), xanthan gum (13%), and alginate (17%) in combination with metformin, sitagliptin, or a mixture thereof has been claimed to lower elevated blood glucose, reduce cell damage, increase lean body mass, and prevent, treat, or ameliorate one or more symptoms associated with metabolic disease or disorder in rats (Gahler *et al.*, 2013). Dietary fiber extracted from sugarcane has been formulated to ameliorate the effects of intestinal disorders such as celiac disease and IBS (Ball and Edwards, 2014). The sugarcane fiber is claimed to be relatively hypoallergenic, containing both soluble and insoluble fiber in beneficial proportions for dietary intake, and contains numerous bioactive molecules that affect blood glucose levels and intestinal health. This sugarcane dietary fiber was reported to produce complete remission from multiple digestive disorders after 1 week of fiber intake, to produce marked improvement in bowel movement of a diabetic patient after 12 months fiber intake, and to lead to effective abatement of bacterial infection in a 60-year-old individual with poor digestive health (Ball and Edwards, 2014).

Fiber extracts from apple slices and the albedo of oranges extracted by the countercurrent method altered gut health when supplemented in a human diet.

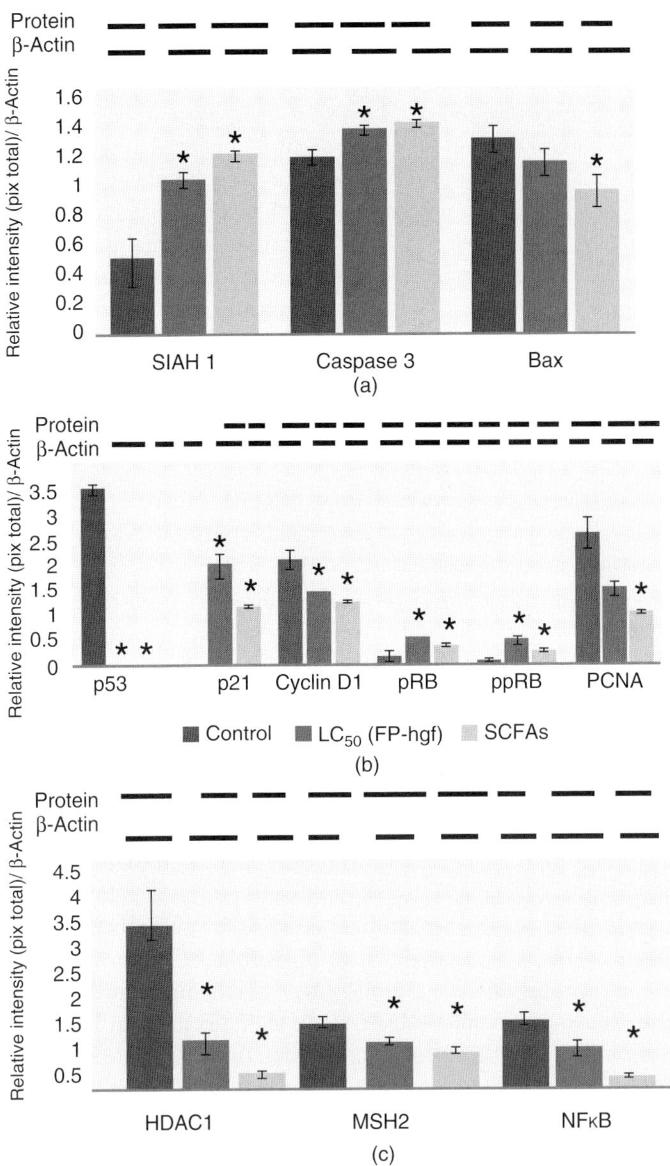

Figure 6.2 Expression of (a) apoptosis-related proteins, (b) cell cycle-related proteins, and (c) expression of MSH2, NFκB, and HDAC1-related proteins in HT29 cells after 24 hours of treatment with LC_{50}/FP (fermented polysaccharide)-hgf and SCFAs mixture found in the LC_{50}/FP-hgf. Expression was analyzed by Western blot using specific antibodies. Control: protein expression in cells without any treatment. The blot was tested with anti-actin antibody to confirm equal protein loading. The protein expression was normalized to β-actin. Data are the mean ± standard errors of three independent experiments ($p < 0.05$ vs. control). Source: Campos-Vega *et al.* (2012). Reproduced with permission of the American Chemical Society.

This beneficial change in indicators of gut health due to increased butyrate production in the distal colon was greater with the fiber mixture compared to the individual fiber extract separately or to wheat bran (Lang *et al.*, 2004). Different types of arabinoxylans prepared from wheat bran also increased butyrate levels in the cecum and colon of rats when supplemented in the diet for 14 days; however, the increased butyrate levels were accompanied with reduced branched SCFA levels, a marker of undesired intestinal protein fermentation (Broekaert *et al.*, 2014). A method has been described for maintaining or restoring a well-balanced flora by administering a liquid or reconstituted powder comprising 4.5–6 g protein/100 mL, a source of digestible carbohydrates, and a source of dietary fiber (2.5 g/100 mL), wherein the source of dietary fiber comprises 20–40% by weight acacia gum, 30–60% by weight of pea outer fiber, and 20–40% by weight of FOS at 30–80 mPas viscosity. This composition is claimed to enhance mucosal function in humans (Ammann *et al.*, 2011).

Many commercial/industrial products have been designed/developed to meet the increasing need for dietary fiber for use in food products. Some examples are: ClearTrac™ AG (arabinogalactan) and Fiber-Aid AG, which are natural prebiotic fibers acting as food sources to stimulate/promote bifidobacteria/lactobacilli growth commonly found in the gastrointestinal tract (colon) and to increase SCFA production. Pea outer fiber (pea hull fiber) is commercially available under the tradenames Exafine® developed by the Belgian company Cosucra or Sofalite® D from the French company Sofalia. Pea outer fiber may be obtained from yellow pea and generally comprises 65–70% cellulose, 22–28% hemicellulose, and about 5–10% lignin. Swelite® from Cosucra is a commercial pea inner fiber, also called pea cellular walls, comprising 10–20% cellulose, 40–50% hemicelluloses, and 35–45% pectin (fiber only). Pea hull fiber has also been used together with a mixture (50:50 soluble:insoluble) of FOS and inulin and gum acacia for enteral nutrition with prebiotic effect to improve gut health in healthy subjects (Koecher *et al.*, 2015). BGOS (Bimuno), a specific non-digestible GOS formulation, also exhibits prebiotic properties by significantly increasing bifidobacteria growth after administration. The anxiolytic effect of this formulation has been associated with cytokine and neurotransmission modulation (cortical IL-1β and 5-HT2A receptor expression), suggesting a potential prebiotic role in anxiety and neuroinflammation-related treatments of neuropsychiatric disorders (Savignac *et al.*, 2015).

Waste reduction and value addition to food-processing by-products has become a major source for developing novel dietary fiber with desirable functional and physiological benefits. For example, a process has been developed to obtain fiber-enriched products from flaxseed hulls (Oomah and Kristensen, 2010). These flaxseed hull fiber products were designed to impart superior physical and potential physiological benefits compared to native dietary fiber when incorporated in processed foods, and to control and optimize the release of essential nutrients and bioactive compounds for absorption in the gut. The dietary fiber extracted from flaxseed hulls reduced apparent energy and fat digestibility, leading to restriction of body weight gain in growing rats (Kristensen *et al.*, 2013). A similar flax dietary fiber extract is now produced commercially in China (Biogin Biochemicals Company Ltd.) and has been proven to suppress appetite and food intake (Ibrügger *et al.*, 2012); and another in Canada (Natunola Health Inc., Ontario). Dietary fiber from fruit processing by-products, such as orange bagasse and passion fruit peel, significantly lowered blood glucose levels in rats when supplemented in their diet for 40 days compared with control animals fed cellulose. These effects were due to the apparent high (7-fold higher than cellulose) digestibility and pH reduction, which contributes to inhibiting pathogenic bacterial growth and prevention of gastrointestinal infections and colon cancer (Macagnan *et al.*, 2015).

Residues or by-products from the vegetable processing and/or other industries, such as sugar beet pulp, tomatoes, or grape skins, have also been used as raw material for producing dietary fibers through intestinal microbial fermentation (Vervoort, 2011). These dietary fiber sources combined with stimulants such as capsiate, caffeine, or epigallocatechin gallate are claimed to accelerate metabolic rate or increase body metabolism designed for weight management. Non-digestible oligosaccharides (manno-oligosaccharides (MOS)) have been derived by hydrolyzing mannan in spent coffee grounds at high temperature and pressure (Campos-Vega *et al.*, 2015 and references therein). MOS promoted bifidobacterial growth in the intestines and daily intake of a 300 mL drink containing MOS (1 or 2 g/100 mL) for 12 weeks reduced abdominal and subcutaneous fat levels in humans. MOS derived from coffee mannan has been developed as an active prebiotic ingredient in Japan (Aginomoto Co. Inc.) and approved as a Food for Specified Health Uses (FOSHU) oligosaccharide functional food ingredient (Fukami, 2010). Other novel dietary fiber sources, such as polysaccharides from water extracts of *Ganoderma lucidum* (2–8% concentration), have been found to reduce obesity and obesity-related features such as fat mass, glucose homeostasis, and liver and adipose tissue inflammation in mice fed a high fat diet. This anti-obesity effect was induced by modulating the gut microbiota (increased abundance of the butyrate-producing *Roseburia* species and immunomodulating species from the *Clostridium* clusters XIVa and XVIII) (Chang *et al.*, 2015).

The dietary fiber market is expected to grow at 13.1% compound annual growth rate from US\$2.27 billion in 2013 to US\$4.21 billion by 2019 (Cantor, 2015). This has led to a surge in demand for whole grains (wheat, oats, brown rice, barley) and seeds (chia, flax, hemp, quinoa, psyllium), resistant starch, and resistant maltodextrin. However, prebiotics dominate the food and beverage industry application probably because of its global market outreach which is estimated at US\$6 billion by 2020 (Cantor, 2015). This may explain the staggering amount of information available on the clinical study of prebiotics, particularly inulin, the largest ingredient segment in the food and beverage category in the digestive health subcategory, accounting for nearly half of the market volume. The *in vitro* and *in vivo* studies demonstrate the benefits of various dietary fibers in modulating gut health through various mechanisms and it has been shown that diets with multiple sources of dietary fiber can benefit overall health and even reduce the risk of chronic metabolic diseases.

Table 6.2 *In vivo and in vitro* dietary fiber effects on gut health.

Compound/metabolite	Effect	Reference
***In vivo* models**		
SCFAs		
Barley grains	↑ Total SCFAs	Dongowski *et al.*, 2002
FOS	↑ Total SCFAs	Hamer *et al.*, 2008
Mineral absorption		
SCFAs	Facilitates the absorption of calcium from the colon walls and even the rectum	Escudero-Álvarez and González-Sánchez, 2006
Inulin-type fructans	Modulate mineral absorption	Roberfroid, 2007
Pectin	Absorption of Zn, Fe, Mg, and Ca	Galibois *et al.*, 1994
Immunomodulation		
Dietary fiber	Protection against enteric infections with pathogenic bacteria	Montagne *et al.*, 2003
SCFAs	↑ Proportions of beneficial rather than pathogenic bacteria	Chawla and Patil, 2010
Dietary fiber	↓ Proinflammatory cytokine levels	Schley and Field, 2002
Fermentable fiber	Modulates GALT	Field *et al.*, 1999
Fungal chitosan	↓ IL-6 level	Sánchez *et al.*, 2012
SCFAs	↑ Natural killer cell activity and mucin production.	Pratt *et al.*, 1996
Cereal fiber	↓ Cells containing neutral and sulfomucins	Sharma and Schumacher, 1995
Prebiotic		
Guar gum and cellulose	↑ Ileal bifidobacterial and enterobacterial populations	Owusu-Asiedu *et al.*, 2006
SCFAs	Inhibition of growth of *Escherichia coli*, *Salmonella* spp., and *Clostridium* spp.	Montagne *et al.*, 2003
Fermentable fibers	Protection effect against colonization by pathogenic bacteria	Saavedra *et al.*, 2002

Dietary fiber and RS	↑*Bifidobacterium* and the *Lactobacillus*, and decrease of *Enterobacter* and *Bacteroides*	Da. S. Queiroz-Monici *et al.*, 2005
FOS and RS	↑ Lactobacilli and bifidobacteria counts, regulated the expression of the trefoil factor-3 and MUC-2	Rodríguez-Cabezas *et al.*, 2010
Enteroendocrine activities		
Fermentable dietary fiber	↑ Proglucagon mRNA concentration and GLP-1 concentration	Massimino *et al.*, 1998
Fermentable dietary fiber	Upregulation of total GLP-1	Zhou *et al.* 2008
Dietary fiber	↑ GLP-1 concentration and decrease of ghrelin concentration. Promote satiation and satiety	Schroeder *et al.*, 2013
Fructans	↑ GLP-1 and decrease of ghrelin concentration	Cani *et al.*, 2004
Soluble fermentable dietary fiber	↓ Food intake, body weight gain, and adiposity ↑ GLP-1 and PYY	Adam *et al.*, 2014
Inulin-type fructans	↑ *Bifidobacterium* species (*B. longum*, *B. pseudocatenulatum*, and *B. adolescentis*)	Salazar *et al.*, 2015
Flaxseed mucilage	Abundance modulation of 39 metagenomic species	Brahe, *et al.*, 2015
Inflammatory bowel disease		
Inulin	↓ DSS-induced colitis	Videla *et al.*, 2001
Lactulose	Beneficial effect on DSS symptoms	Rumi *et al.*, 2004
Plantago ovata seeds	↓ Colonic myeloperoxidase activity, and restoration of colonic glutathione content	Rodríguez-Cabezas *et al.*, 2002
RS	Beneficial effects on the chronic inflamed cecal and distal mucosa	Moreau *et al.*, 2003

(continued overleaf)

Table 6.2 (Continued)

Compound/metabolite	Effect	Reference
FOS	↓ Intestinal inflammation	Cherbut *et al.*, 2003
Germinated barley foodstuff	Prevent bloody diarrhea and mucosa damage	Araki *et al.*, 2000
Butyrate	↑ TFF3 mRNA expression, ↓ serum IL-1β production and tissue NFκB expression	Song *et al.*, 2006
Acetate and propionate	Anti-inflammatory properties	Tedelind *et al.*, 2007
Colon cancer		
Chicory fructans-oligofructose	↑ Colonic apoptotic index	Hughes and Rowland 2001
Dietary fiber	Acute apoptotic response to genotoxic carcinogens regulation	Hu *et al.*, 2002
Butyrate	↓ Colon tumorigenesis, induction of proapoptotic protein transcription	Avivi-Green *et al.*, 2001
NDF of common beans	↓ Aberrant crypt foci development, ↓ β-glucuronidase activity	Vergara-Castañeda *et al.*, 2010
NDF of common beans	↑ Transcriptional expression of bax and caspase-3, ↓ Rb expression	Feregrino-Pérez *et al.*, 2008
NDF of common beans	Modulation of Tp53-mediated signaling pathway	Vergara-Castañeda *et al.*, 2012
***In vitro* models**		
Prebiotic		
Xylo-oligosaccharides	↑ Bifidobacteria	Rycroft *et al.*, 2001
FOS	↑ Lactobacilli	Li *et al.*, 2015
GOS	↓ Clostridia, ↑*Bifidobacterium longum, B. bifidum, B. catenulatum, Lactobacillus gasseri,* and *L. salivarius*	Maathuis *et al.*, 2012
Gelidium seaweed CC2253	↑ Bifidobacterial	Yang *et al.*, 2013
Pectin	↑ Bifidobacterial	

Resistant starch	↑ *Bifidobacterium adolescentis*	
β-Glucan	↑ *Firmicutes*	
Long-chain inulin	↑ *Roseburia inulinivorans*	Scott *et al.*, 2014
Wheat dextrin	↑ *Clostridium* cluster XIVa and *Roseburia* genus	Hobden *et al.*, 2013
Actinidia chinensis gold-fleshed kiwifruit	↑ *Bacteroides* spp., *Parabacteroides* spp., and *Bifidobacterium* spp	Blatchford *et al.*, 2015
Human milk oligosaccharides	↑ *Bifidobacterium* spp., ↓ *Escherichia* and *Clostridium perfringens*	Yu *et al.*, 2013
SCFAs		
Arabinoxylans	↑ Total SCFAs	Knudsen, 2015
β-Glucan	↑ Total SCFAs and butyric acid	Knudsen, 2015
Wheat bran	↑ Butyric and propionic acids	Nordlund *et al.*, 2012
Fruit and vegetable	↑ Butyric acid	Tabernero *et al.*, 2011
Common beans	↑ Total SCFAs	Campos-Vega *et al.*, 2009
Orange	↑ Total SCFAs	Costabile *et al.*, 2015
Gourd family	↑ Total SCFAs	Sreenivas and Lele, 2013
Nopal	↑ Total SCFAs	Guevara-Arauz *et al.*, 2011
Agave tequilana Weber var. *Azul*	↑ Total SCFAs	Zamora-Gasga *et al.*, 2015
Immunity		
SCFAs	Recruitment of neutrophils (N), inhibiting N production of proinflammatory reactive oxygen species (ROS) and TNFα	Steinmeyer *et al.*, 2015
Butyric acid	IFN-stimulated macrophages	Park *et al.*, 2007

(*continued overleaf*)

Table 6.2 (Continued)

Compound/metabolite	Effect	Reference
Butyric and propionic acids	Suppress immune-suppressive enzyme indoleamine 2,3-dioxygenase in dendritic cells in an Slc5a8-dependent manner	Gurav *et al.*, 2014
SCFAs	Modulate human regulatory T cells function	Mamontov *et al.*, (2015)
Soluble fiber	↓ IL-10, IL-12, and IFNγ	Breton *et al.*, 2015
Non-digestible oligosaccharides	Activation of TLR4-NFκB	Ortega-González *et al.*, 2014
Chicory inulin and barley β-glucan	↓ Th2 cytokine IL-6	Bermudez-Brito *et al.*, 2015
GOS	Goblet cells modulation	Bhatia *et al.*, 2015
Ulcerative colitis		
Arabino-oligosaccharides or FOS	↓ Dysbiosis (↑ *Bifidobacterium* spp. and *Lactobacillus* spp)	Vigsnæs *et al.*, 2011
Irritable bowl syndrome		
GOS	↑ Bifidobacteria	Silk *et al.*, 2009
Crohn's disease		
Starch	↑ SCFAs in fecal slurries from patients with Crohn's disease	Khalil *et al.*, 2014
Dietary fiber	Increased colonic mucosal GPR43[+] polymorphonuclear infiltration	Zhao *et al.*, 2015
Weight management		
GOS and lactulose	↑ SCFAs (obese microbiota) ↓ Dysbiosis (obese microbiota)	Aguirre *et al.*, 2014
Dextrans	↑ *Bacteroides − Prevotella* (obese microbiota) ↓ *Faecalibacterium prausnitzii* and *Ruminococcus bromii/ R. flavefaciens* (obese microbiota)	Sarbini *et al.*, 2014

Diabetes

Water-soluble dietary fibers	↓ Postprandial serum glucose	Ou *et al.*, 2001

Cardiovascular disease

Wheat dextrin	↑ Butyric-producing bacteria *Clostridium* cluster XIVa and *Roseburia*	Hobden *et al.*, 2013
GOS	↓ *Collinsella aerofancies and* ↑ *Eubacterium rectale*	Maathuis *et al.*, 2012

Colon cancer

NDF common bean	Modulates genes related to ↑ apoptosis, cell cycle, and ↓ cell proliferation	Campos-Vega *et al.*, 2010
NDF common bean	Modulates proteins related to ↑ apoptosis, cell cycle, and ↓ cell proliferation	Campos-Vega *et al.*, 2012
Butyrate	↓ miR-106b family, including miR-17, miR-20a/b, miR-93, and miR-106a/b	Kim *et al.*, 2009; Hu *et al.*, 2011
Butyrate	c-Myc-induced miR-17-92a cluster transcription	Hu *et al.*, 2015
SCFAs	↓ mTOR activities	Wang and Nie, 2015

FOS, fructo-oligosaccharide; GOS, galacto-oligosaccharide; RS, resistant starch; DSS, dextran sulfate sodium; NDF, non-digestible fraction; SCFA, short-chain fatty acid.

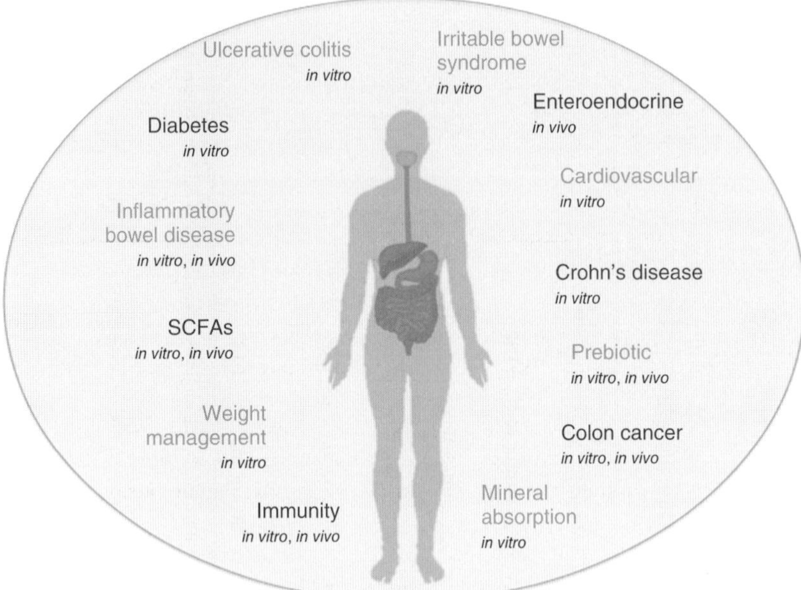

Figure 6.3 Dietary fiber effects on gut health: *in vitro* and *in vivo* evidence. Short-chain fatty acids (SCFAs), metabolic products from dietary fiber (DF), play a role in cell differentiation and growth, have anti-inflammatory effects by promoting recruitment of neutrophils, while butyrate is a natural inhibitor of the histone deacetylases. SCFAs confer protection again chronic diseases such colon cancer. Dietary fiber increases mineral absorption, mainly Ca and Mg. It has also been related to a decrease in proinflammatory cytokine levels and may acutely reduce inflammatory activity. Certain types of fibers stimulate growth of intestinal bacteria during fermentation. Dietary fiber has a key role in the gut in producing a variety of enteroendocrine-derived peptides that control and modulate miscellaneous metabolic and physiological processes and create a link between the gut and the brain. Their health benefits on attenuation of colonic inflammation is mediated through beneficial effects on intestinal microbiota and by increasing the colonic SCFAs concentration. Prevention of intestinal inflammation may be achieved with fermentable prebiotic fibers that enhance beneficial bifidobacteria or with soluble fibers that block bacterial–epithelial adherence (contrabiotics). The dysbiosis (perturbations to the structure of complex commensal communities) observed in inflammatory bowel diseases, such as ulcerative colitis, irritable bowel syndrome, and dietary fiber can modulate Crohn's disease. Weight management effects are linked to SCFAs, which are substrates for the host and induce the release of satiety hormones, and regulate microbiota in obesity. Fiber-enriched diets improve insulin sensitivity and glucose tolerance and increase butyrate-producing bacteria. Postprandial serum glucose is lowered by dietary fiber through at least three pathways: increasing the viscosity of the small intestinal content and slowing the diffusion of glucose; adsorbing glucose and preventing its diffusion; and inhibiting the activity of α-amylase and postponing the release of glucose from starch. Interestingly, dietary fiber improves microbiota dysbiosis, which predicts acute cardiovascular events in a large general population. Finally, *in vitro* and *in vivo* evidence supports health claims about the role of dietary fiber in cancer prevention.

6.6   Conclusion

The *in vivo* and *in vitro* evidence on the effect of dietary fiber on gut health high-lights the relevance of including dietary fiber as a part of a healthy diet (Table 6.2). The mechanisms whereby dietary fiber modulates gut health, as summarized in Figure 6.3, expand our understanding of the related diseases. It is anticipated that further unraveling of the mechanisms underlying dietary fiber beneficial effects will identify new therapeutic strategies to prevent and treat many diseases related to gut health.

References

Adam, C.L., Williams, P.A., Dalby, M.J., Garden, K., Thomson, L.M., Richardson, A.J., *et al.* (2014). Different types of soluble fermentable dietary fibre decrease food intake, body weight gain and adiposity in young adult male rats. *Nutrition and Metabolism*, 11, 36.

Aguirre, M., Jonkers, D.M., Troost, F.J., Roeselers, G., and Venema, K. (2014). *In vitro* characterization of the impact of different substrates on metabolite production, energy extraction and composition of gut microbiota from lean and obese subjects. *PloS One*, 9(11), e113864.

Amar, J., Lange, C., Payros, G., Garret, C., Chabo, C., Lantieri, O., *et al.* (2013). Blood microbiota dysbiosis is associated with the onset of cardiovascular events in a large general population: the DESIR study. *PLoS One*, 8(1), e54461.

Ammann, C., Rochat, F., and Roessle, C. (2011). High fibre high calorie liquid or powdered nutritional composition. US Patent 8067356 B2, issued November 29, 2011.

Anderson, J. W., Baird, P., Davis, R. H., Ferreri, S., Knudtson, M., Koraym, A., *et al.* (2009). Health benefits of dietary fiber. *Nutrition Reviews*, 67(4), 188–205.

Andoh, A., Tsujikawa, T., and Fujiyama, Y. (2003). Role of dietary fiber and short-chain fatty acids in the colon. *Current Pharmaceutical Design*, 9, 347–358.

Araki, Y., Andoh, A., Koyama, S., Fujiama, Y., Kanauchi, O., and Bamba, T. (2000). Effects of germinated barley foodstuff on microflora and short chain fatty acid production in dextran sulfate sodium-induced colitis in rats. *Bioscience, Biotechnology, and Biochemistry*, 64(9), 1794–1800.

Arcila, J.A. and Rose, D.J. (2015). Repeated cooking and freezing of whole-wheat flour increases resistant starch with beneficial impacts on *in vitro* fecal fermentation properties. *Journal of Functional Foods*, 12, 230–236.

Arcila, J.A., Weier, S.A., and Rose, D.J. (2015). Changes in dietary fiber fractions and gut microbial fermentation properties of wheat bran after extrusion and bread making. *Food Research International*, 74, 217–223.

Asarat, M., Vasiljevic, T., Apostolopoulos, V., and Donkor, O. (2015). Short-chain fatty acids regulate secretion of IL-8 from human intestinal epithelial cell lines *in vitro*. *Immunological Investigations*, 44(7), 678–693.

Astrup, A.V., Tetens, I., and Thomsen, A.D. (2014). Flaxseeds for body weight management. US Patent 8877267 B2, issued November 4, 2014.

Avivi-Green, C., Polak-Charcon, S., Madar, Z., and Schwartz, B. (2000). Apoptosis cascade proteins are regulated *in vivo* by high intracolonic butyrate concentration: Correlation with colon cancer inhibition. *Oncology Research*, 12(2), 83–95.

Bae, I.Y., Jun, Y., Lee, S., and Lee, H.G. (2016). Characterization of apple dietary fibers influencing the *in vitro* starch digestibility of wheat flour gel. *LWT-Food Science and Technology*, 65, 158–163.

Ball, M. and Edwards, G. (2014). Use of a dietary fibre supplement in a food formulation. World Patent WO 2014/162303 A1, issued October 9, 2014.

Baumgart, D.C. and Sandborn, W.J. (2012). Crohn's disease. *The Lancet*, 380(9853), 1590–1605.

Bazzocco, S., Mattila, I., Guyot, S., Renard, C.M., and Aura, A.M. (2008). Factors affecting the conversion of apple polyphenols to phenolic acids and fruit matrix to short-chain fatty acids by human faecal microbiota *in vitro. European Journal of Nutrition*, 47(8), 442–452.

Beeren, S.R., Christensen, C.E., Tanaka, H., Jensen, M.G., Donaldson, I., and Hindsgaul, O. (2015). Direct study of fluorescently-labelled barley β-glucan fate in an *in vitro* human colon digestion model. *Carbohydrate Polymers*, 115, 88–92.

Bermudez-Brito, M., Sahasrabudhe, N.M., Rösch, C., Schols, H.A., Faas, M.M., and Vos, P. (2015). The impact of dietary fibers on dendritic cell responses *in vitro* is dependent on the differential effects of the fibers on intestinal epithelial cells. *Molecular Nutrition and Food Research*, 59(4), 698–710.

Beserra, B.T.S., Fernandes, R., Do Rosario, V.A., Mocellin, M.C., Kuntz, M.G.F., and Trindade, E.B.S.M. (2015). A systematic review and meta-analysis of the prebiotics and synbiotics effects on glycemia, insulin concentrations and lipid parameters in adult patients with overweight or obesity. *Clinical Nutrition*, 34, 845–858.

Bhatia, S., Prabhu, P.N., Benefiel, A.C., Miller, M.J., Chow, J., Davis, S.R., *et al.* (2015). Galacto-oligosaccharides may directly enhance intestinal barrier function through the modulation of goblet cells. *Molecular Nutrition and Food Research*, 59(3), 566–573.

Bindels, L.B., Delzenne, N.M., Cani, P.D., and Walter, J. (2015). Towards a more comprehensive concept for prebiotics. *Nature Reviews Gastroenterology and Hepatology*, 12(5), 303–310.

Blatchford, P., Bentley-Hewitt, K.L., Stoklosinski, H., McGhie, T., Gearry, R., Gibson, G., *et al.* (2015). *In vitro* characterisation of the fermentation profile and prebiotic capacity of gold-fleshed kiwifruit. *Beneficial Microbes*, 1–12.

Blottiere, H.M., Buecher, B., Galmiche, J.P., and Cherbut, C. (2003). Molecular analysis of the effect of short-chain fatty acids on intestinal cell proliferation. *Proceedings of the Nutrition Society*, 62(01), 101–106.

Bourquin, L.D., Titgemeyer, E.C., and Fahey JR.C. (1993). Vegetable fiber fermentation by human fecal bacteria: cell wall polysaccharide disappearance and short-chain fatty acid production during *in vitro* fermentation and water-holding capacity of unfermented residues. *Journal of Nutrition*, 123, 860–869.

Brahe, L.K., Le Chatelier, E., Prifti, E., Pons, N., Kennedy, S., Blædel, T., *et al.* (2015). Dietary modulation of the gut microbiota – a randomised controlled trial in obese postmenopausal women. *British Journal of Nutrition*, 114(03), 406–417.

Breton, J., Plé, C., Guerin-Deremaux, L., Pot, B., Lefranc-Millot, C., Wils, D., and Foligné, B. (2015). Intrinsic immunomodulatory effects of low-digestible carbohydrates selectively extend their anti-inflammatory prebiotic potentials. *BioMed Research International*, 2015.

Brighenti, F. (2007). Dietary fructans and serum triacylglycerols: a meta-analysis of randomized controlled trials. *Journal of Nutrition*, 137 (11 Suppl), 2552S–2556S.

Broekaert, W., Courtin, C., Damen, B., and Delcour, J. (2014). Nutriment containing arabinoxylan and oligosaccharides. US Patent 8741376 B2, issued June 3, 2014.

Broekaert, W., Courtin, C., and Delcour, J. (2015). (Arabino) xylan oligosaccharide preparation. US Patent 8927038 B2, issued January 6, 2015.

Brotherton, C.S., Taylor, A.G., and Anderson, J.G. (2012). Can a high fiber diet improve bowel function and health-related quality of life in patients with Crohn's disease?. *The FASEB Journal*, 26(1_MeetingAbstracts), lb338.

Brownlee, I.A., Havler, M.E., Dettmar, P.W., Allen, A., and Pearson, J.P. (2003). Colonic mucus: secretion and turnover in relation to dietary fibre intake. *Proceedings of the Nutrition Society*, 62, 245–249.

Brownlee, I.A., Moore, C., Chatfield, M., Richardson, D.P., Ashby, P., Kuznesof, S.A., *et al.* (2010). Markers of cardiovascular risk are not changed by increased whole-grain intake: the WHOLEheart study, a randomized, controlled dietary intervention. *British Journal of Nutrition*, 104(1), 125–134.

Campos-Vega, R., Reynoso-Camacho, R., Pedraza-Aboytes, G., Acosta-Gallegos, J. A., Guzman-Maldonado, S.H., Paredes-Lopez, O., *et al.* (2009). Chemical composition and *in vitro* polysaccharide fermentation of different beans (*Phaseolus vulgaris* L.). *Journal of Food Science*, 74(7), T59–T65.

Campos-Vega, R., Guevara-Gonzalez, R.G., Guevara-Olvera, B.L., Oomah, B.D., and Loarca-Piña, G. (2010). Bean (*Phaseolus vulgaris* L.) polysaccharides modulate gene expression in human colon cancer cells (HT-29). *Food Research International*, 43(4), 1057–1064.

Campos-Vega, R., García-Gasca, T., Guevara-Gonzalez, R., Ramos-Gomez, M., Oomah, B.D., and Loarca-Piña, G. (2012). Human gut flora-fermented nondigestible fraction from cooked bean (*Phaseolus vulgaris* L.) modifies protein expression associated with apoptosis, cell cycle arrest, and proliferation in human adenocarcinoma colon cancer cells. *Journal of Agricultural and Food Chemistry*, 60(51), 12443–12450.

Campos-Vega, R., Loarca-Piña, G., Vergara-Castañeda, H.A., and Oomah, B.D. (2015). Spent coffee grounds: A review on current research and future prospects. *Trends in Food Science and Technology*, 45, 24–36.

Cani, P.D., Dewever, C., and Delzenne, N.M. (2004). Inulin-type fructans modulate gastrointestinal peptides involved in appetite regulation (glucagon-like peptide-1 and ghrelin) in rats. *British Journal of Nutrition*, 92, 521–526.

Cantor, S. (2015). Digestive dynamos. *Prepared Foods*, 184(11), 28–43.

Chan, D., Kumar, D., and Mendall, M. (2015). What is known about the mechanisms of dietary influences in Crohn's disease? *Nutrition*, 31(10), 1195–1203.

Chang, C.J., Lin, C-S., Lu, C-C., Martel, J., Ko, Y-F., Ojcius, D.M., *et al.* (2015). *Ganoderma lucidum* reduces obesity in mice by modulating the composition of the gut microbiota. *Nature Communications*, 6, 7489.

Chassard, C., Dapoigny, M., Scott, K.P., Crouzet, L., Del'Homme, C., Marquet, P., *et al.* (2012). Functional dysbiosis within the gut microbiota of patients with constipated-irritable bowel syndrome. *Alimentary Pharmacology and Therapeutics*, 35(7), 828–838.

Chawla, R. and Patil, G.R. (2010). Soluble dietary fiber. *Comprehensive Reviews in Food Science and Food Safety*, 9, 178–196.

Chen, C., You, L.J., Abbasi, A.M., Fu, X., and Liu, R.H. (2015). Optimization for ultrasound extraction of polysaccharides from mulberry fruits with antioxidant and hyperglycemic activity *in vitro. Carbohydrate Polymers*, 130, 122–132.

Cherbut, C., Michel, C., and Lecannu, G. (2003). The prebiotic characteristics of fructooligosaccharides are necessary for reduction of TNBS-induced colitis in rats. *Journal of Nutrition*, 133, 21–27.

Chow, J., Panasevich, M.R., Alexander, D., Vester Boler, B.M., Rossoni Serao, M.C., Faber, T.A., *et al.* (2014). Fecal metabolomics of healthy breast-fed versus formula-fed infants before and during *in vitro* batch culture fermentation. *Journal of Proteome Research*, 13(5), 2534–2542.

Connolly, M.L., Lovegrove, J.A., and Tuohy, K.M. (2012). *In vitro* fermentation characteristics of whole grain wheat flakes and the effect of toasting on prebiotic potential. *Journal of Medicinal Food*, 15(1), 33–43.

Costabile, A., Walton, G.E., Tzortzis, G., Vulevic, J., Charalampopoulos, D., and Gibson, G.R. (2015). Effects of orange juice formulation on prebiotic functionality using an *in vitro* colonic model system. *PloS One*, 10(3).

Da S. Queiroz-Monici, K., Costa, G.E., da Silva, N., Reis, S.M., and de Oliveira, A.C. (2005). Bifidogenic effect of dietary fiber and resistant starch from leguminous on the intestinal microbiota of rats. *Nutrition*, 5, 602–608.

Daguet, D., Pinheiro, I., Verhelst, A., Possemiers, S., and Marzorati, M. (2015). Acacia gum improves the gut barrier functionality *in vitro. Agro Food Industry HI Tech*, 26(4), 29–33.

Dai, Z., Su, D., Zhang, Y., Sun, Y., Hu, B., Ye, H., *et al.* (2014). Immunomodulatory activity *in vitro* and *in vivo* of verbascose from mung beans (*Phaseolus aureus*). *Journal of Agricultural and Food Chemistry*, 62(44), 10727–10735.

de Souza, C. B., Roeselers, G., Troost, F., Jonkers, D., Koenen, M. E., and Venema, K. (2014). Prebiotic effects of cassava bagasse in TNO's *in vitro* model of the colon in lean versus obese microbiota. *Journal of Functional Foods*, 11, 210–220.

De Vadder, F., Kovatcheva-Datchary, P., Goncalves, D., Vinera, J., Zitoun, C., Duchampt, A., *et al.* (2014). Microbiota-generated metabolites promote metabolic benefits via gut-brain neural circuits. *Cell*, 156(1), 84–96.

Delzenne, N.M., Cani, P.D., Everard, A., Neyrinck, A.M., and Bindels, L.B. (2015). Gut microorganisms as promising targets for the management of type 2 diabetes. *Diabetologia*, 58(10), 2206–2217.

Dhingra, D., Michael, M., Rajput, H., and Patil, R. T. (2012). Dietary fibre in foods: a review. *Journal of Food Science and Technology*, 49(3), 255–266.

Dongowski, G., Huth, M., Gebhardt, E., and Flamme, W, (2002). Dietary fiber-rich barley products beneficially affect the intestinal tract of rats. *Journal of Nutrition*, 132, 3704–3714.

Escudero-Álvarez, E. and González-Sánchez., P. (2006). La fibra dietética. *Nutrición Hospitalaria*, 21, 61–72.

European Commission (2008). Commission Directive 2008/100/EC of 28 October 2008 amending Council Directive 90/496/EEC on nutrition labeling for foodstuffs as regards recommended daily allowances, energy conversion factors and definitions.

Feregrino-Pérez, A.A., Berumen, L.C., Guadalupe García-Alcocer, Ramón G. Guevara-Gonzalez, Ramos-Gomez, M., Reynoso-Camacho, R., Acosta-Gallegos, J.A., and Loarca-Piña, G. (2008). Composition and chemopreventive effect of polysaccharides from common beans (*Phaseolus vulgaris* L.) on azoxymethane-induced colon cancer. *Journal of Agricultural and Food Chemistry*, 56(18), 8737–8744.

Field, C.J., McBurney, M.I., Massimino, S., Hayek, M.G., and Sunvold, G.D. (1999). The fermentable fiber content of the diet alters the function and composition of canine gut associated lymphoid tissue. *Veterinary Immunology and Immunopathology*, 72, 325–341.

Fitzpatrick, A., Roberts, A., and Witherly, S. (2004). Larch arabinogalactan: a novel and multifunctional natural product. *AgroFood Industry HI-Tech*, 15(1), 30–32.

Flint, H.J., Scott, K.P., Duncan, S.H., Louis, P., and Forano, E. (2012). Microbial degradation of complex carbohydrates in the gut. *Gut Microbes*, 3(4), 289–306.

Flint, H.J., Duncan, S.H., Scott, K.P., and Louis, P. (2015). Links between diet, gut microbiota composition and gut metabolism. *Proceedings of the Nutrition Society*, 74(01), 13–22.

Frost, G., Sleeth, M.L., Shari-Arisoylu, M., Lizarbe, B., Cerdan, S., Brody, L., *et al.* (2014). The short-chain fatty acid acetate reduces appetite via a central homeostatic mechanism. *Nature Communications*, 5, 3611.

Fukami, H. (2010). Functional foods and biotechnology in Japan. In *Biotechnology in Functional Foods and Nutraceuticals* (eds. D. Bagchi, F.C. Lau., and D.K. Ghosh). Taylor and Francis, Boca Raton, FL, pp. 29–49.

Fukuda, S., Toh, H., Hase, K., Oshima, K., Nakanishi, Y., Yoshimura, K., *et al.* (2011). Bifidobacteria can protect from enteropathogenic infection through production of acetate. *Nature*, 469(7331), 543–547.

Gahler, R.J., Lyon, M.R., and Wood, S. (2013). Dietary fiber composition for the treatment of metabolic disease. *Canadian Patent Application 2870813 A1*, 2013/10/31.

Galibois, I., Desrosier, T., Guevin, N., Lavigne, C., and Jacques, H. (1994). Effects of dietary fiber mixtures on glucose and lipid metabolism onmineral absorption in rats. *Annals of Nutrition and Metabolism*, 38, 203–211.

García-Peris, P., Bretón-Lesmes, I., de la Cuerda-Compes, C., and Camblor-Álvarez, M. (2002). Metabolismo colónico de la fibra. *Nutrición Hospitalaria*, 17, 11–16.

Gibb, R.D., McRorie, J.W., Russell, D.A., Hasselblad, V., and D'Alessio, D.A. (2015). Psyllium fiber improves glycemic control proportional to loss of glycemic control: a meta-analysis of data in euglycemic subjects, patients at risk of type 2 diabetes mellitus, and patients being treated for type 2 diabetes mellitus. *American Journal of Clinical Nutrition*, 102(6), 1604–1614.

Goita, M.L., McCutcheon, K.L., Raggio, A.M., and Finley, J.W. (2012). Determining functional fiber properties of berry pomaces via an anaerobic fermentation system. *FASEB Journal*, 26(1_MeetingAbstracts), 646–647.

Goulet, O. (2015). Potential role of the intestinal microbiota in programming health and disease. *Nutrition reviews,* 73(Suppl 1), 32–40.

Guevara-Arauza, J.C., Pimentel-González, D.J., and de J. Órnelas-Paz, J. (2011, November). Preliminary *in vitro* assessment of the bifidogenic properties of mucilage and pectic-derived oligosaccharides from *Opuntia ficus-indica* (nopalitos). In *International Symposium on Medicinal and Aromatic Plants IMAPS2010 and History of Mayan Ethnopharmacology IMAPS2011 964* (pp. 221–228).

Guida, S. and Venema, K. (2015). Gut microbiota and obesity: Involvement of the adipose tissue. *Journal of Functional Foods,* 14, 407–423.

Gurav, A., Singh, N., and Ganapathy, V. (2014). A critical role for Slc5a8 in the suppression of colonic inflammation by commensal bacteria-derived metabolites (MUC9P. 821). *Journal of Immunology,* 192(1 Suppl), 199–198.

Hamer, H.M., Jonkers, D., Venema, K., Vanhoutvin, S., Troost, F.J., and Brummer, R.J. (2008). Review article: the role of butyrate on colonic function. *Alimentary Pharmacology and Therapeutics,* 27, 104–119.

Han, A. and Donohoe, D. (2015). Carnitine is a pivotal contributor for butyrate oxidation in colon cancer cells. *FASEB Journal,* 29(1 Suppl), 394–396.

Helsby, N.A., Zhu, S., Pearson, A.E., Tingle, M.D., and Ferguson, L.R. (2000). Antimutagenic effects of wheat bran diet through modification of xenobiotic metabolising enzymes. *Mutation Research,* 454(1–2), 77–88.

Ho, J.T., Chan, G.C., and Li, J.C. (2015). Systemic effects of gut microbiota and its relationship with disease and modulation. *BMC immunology,* 16(1), 21.

Hobden, M.R., Martin-Morales, A., Guérin-Deremaux, L., Wils, D., Costabile, A., Walton, G.E., *et al.* (2013). *In vitro* fermentation of NUTRIOSE® FB06, a wheat dextrin soluble fibre, in a continuous culture human colonic model system. *PLoS One,* 8(10), e77128.

Holko, I. and Hrabě, J. (2012). The adhesion of *Lactobacillus acidophilus* to dietary fiber. *International Journal of Probiotics and Prebiotics,* 7(3/4), 165–168.

Hongpattarakere, T., Cherntong, N., Wichienchot, S., Kolida, S., and Rastall, R.A. (2012). *In vitro* prebiotic evaluation of exopolysaccharides produced by marine isolated lactic acid bacteria. *Carbohydrate Polymers,* 87(1), 846–852.

Hu, S., Dong, T.S., Dalal, S.R., Wu, F., Bissonnette, M., Kwon, J.H., and Chang, E.B. (2011). The microbe-derived short chain fatty acid butyrate targets miRNA-dependent p21 gene expression in human colon cancer. *PloS One,* 6(1), e16221.

Hu, S., Liu, L., Chang, E.B., Wang, J.Y., and Raufman, J.P. (2015). Butyrate inhibits pro-proliferative miR-92a by diminishing c-Myc-induced miR-17-92a cluster transcription in human colon cancer cells. *Molecular Cancer,* 14(1), 1.

Hu, Y., Martin, J., Le Leu, R., and Young, G.P. (2002). The colonic response to genotoxic carcinogens in the rat: regulation by dietary fibre. *Carcinogenesis,* 23(7), 1131–1137.

Hughes, R. and Rowland, I.R. (2001). Stimulation of apoptosis by two prebiotic chicory fructans in the rat colon. *Carcinogenesis,* 22(2), 43–47.

Hutkins, R.W., Krumbeck, J.A., Bindels, L.B., Cani, P.D., Fahey, G., Goh, Y.J., *et al.* (2016). Prebiotics: why definitions matter. *Current Opinion in Biotechnology,* 37, 1–7.

Ibrügger, S., Kristensen, M., Mikkelsen, M.S., and Astrup, A. (2012). Flaxseed dietary fiber supplements for suppression of appetite and food intake. *Appetite*, 58, 490–495.

Iraporda, C., Errea, A., Romanin, D. E., Cayet, D., Pereyra, E., Pignataro, O., *et al.* (2015). Lactate and short chain fatty acids produced by microbial fermentation downregulate proinflammatory responses in intestinal epithelial cells and myeloid cells. *Immunobiology*, 220(10), 1161–1169.

Jacobs Jr, D.R. (2015). Nutrition: The whole cereal grain is more informative than cereal fibre. *Nature Reviews Endocrinology*, 11, 389–390.

Jenkins, D.J. and Kendall, C.W. (2000). Resistant starches. *Current Opinion in Gastroenterology*, 16(2), 178–183.

Kaplan, G.G. (2015). The global burden of IBD: from 2015 to 2025. *Nature Reviews Gastroenterology and Hepatology*, 12(12), 720–727.

Karlsson, F.H., Fåk, F., Nookaew, I., Tremaroli, V., Fagerberg, B., Petranovic, D., *et al.* (2012). Symptomatic atherosclerosis is associated with an altered gut metagenome. *Nature Communications*, 3, 1245.

Khalil, N.A., Walton, G.E., Gibson, G.R., Tuohy, K.M., and Andrews, S.C. (2014). *In vitro* batch cultures of gut microbiota from healthy and ulcerative colitis (UC) subjects suggest that sulphate-reducing bacteria levels are raised in UC and by a protein-rich diet. *International Journal of Food Sciences and Nutrition*, 65(1), 79–88.

Kietsiriroje, N., Kwankaew, J., Kitpakornsanti, S., and Leelawattana, R. (2015). Effect of phytosterols and inulin-enriched soymilk on LDL-cholesterol in Thai subjects: a double-blinded randomized controlled trial. *Lipids and Health and Disease*, 14, 146.

Kim, Y.K., Yu, J., Han, T.S., Park, S.Y., Namkoong, B., Kim, D.H., *et al.* (2009). Functional links between clustered microRNAs: suppression of cell-cycle inhibitors by microRNA clusters in gastric cancer. *Nucleic Acids Research*, 37(5), 1672–1681.

Knudsen, K.E.B. (2015). Microbial degradation of whole-grain complex carbohydrates and impact on short-chain fatty acids and health. *Advances in Nutrition*, 6(2), 206–213.

Koecher, K.J., Thomas, W., and Slavin, J.L. (2015). Healthy subjects experience bowel changes on enteral diets: addition of a fiber blend attenuates stool weight and gut bacteria decreases without changes in gas. *Journal of Parenteral and Enteral Nutrition*, 39(3), 337–343.

Kovatcheva-Datchary, P., Nilsson, A., Akrami, R., Lee, Y.S., De Vadder, F., Arora, T., *et al.* (2015). Dietary fiber-induced improvement in glucose metabolism is associated with increased abundance of *Prevotella*. *Cell Metabolism*, 22, 1–12.

Kristensen, M., Jensen, M.G., Aarestrup, J., Petersen, K.E., Søndergaard, L., Mikkelsen, M.S., *et al.* (2012). Flaxseed dietary fibers lower cholesterol and increase fecal fat excretion, but magnitude of effect depend on food type. *Nutrition and Metabolism*, 9, 8.

Kristensen, M., Knudsen, K.E.B., Jørgensen, H., Oomah, D., Bügel, S., Toubro, S., *et al.* (2013). Linseed dietary fibers reduce apparent digestibility of energy and fat and weight gain in growing rats. *Nutrients*, 5, 3287–3298.

Kump, P.K., Gröchenig, H.P., Lackner, S., Trajanoski, S., Reicht, G., Hoffmann, K.M., *et al.* (2013). Alteration of intestinal dysbiosis by fecal microbiota transplantation does not induce remission in patients with chronic active ulcerative colitis. *Inflammatory Bowel Diseases*, 19(10), 2155–2165.

Lang, T., Denton, D., Bird, A.R., and Topping, D. (2004). Food supplement. US Patent 6753019 B1, issued June 22, 2004.

Lange, K. (2015). Molecular mechanisms underlying the effects of dietary fiber in the large intestine. PhD Thesis, Wageningen University, Wageningen, NL, 202 pp. ISNB 978-94-6257-270-6.

Le Gall, G., Noor, S.O., Ridgway, K., Scovell, L., Jamieson, C., Johnson, I.T., *et al.* (2011). Metabolomics of fecal extracts detects altered metabolic activity of gut microbiota in ulcerative colitis and irritable bowel syndrome. *Journal of Proteome Research*, 10(9), 4208–4218.

Le Magueresse-Battistoni, B., Vidal, H., and Naville, D. (2015). Lifelong consumption of low-dosed food pollutants and metabolic health. *Journal of Epidemiology and Community Health*, 69(6), 512–515.

Lee, K.N. and Lee, O.Y. (2014). Intestinal microbiota in pathophysiology and management of irritable bowel syndrome. *World Journal of Gastroenterology: WJG*, 20(27), 8886.

Letexier, D., Diraison, F., and Beylot, M. (2003). Addition of inulin to a moderately high carbohydrate diet reduces hepatic lipogenesis and plasma triacylglycerol concentrations in humans. *American Journal of Clinical Nutrition*, 77(3), 559–564.

Li, W., Wang, K., Sun, Y., Ye, H., Hu, B., and Zeng, X. (2015). Influences of structures of galactooligosaccharides and fructooligosaccharides on the fermentation *in vitro* by human intestinal microbiota. *Journal of Functional Foods*, 13, 158–168.

Likotrafiti, E., Tuohy, K.M., Gibson, G.R., and Rastall, R.A. (2014). An in vitro study of the effect of probiotics, prebiotics and synbiotics on the elderly faecal microbiota. *Anaerobe*, 27, 50–55.

Lindberg, J.E. (2014). Fiber effects in nutrition and gut health in pigs. *Journal of Animal Science and Biotechnology*, 5, 15. doi: 10.1186/2049-1891-5-15.

Livesey, G., Smith, T., Eggum, B.O., Tetens, I.H., Nyman, M., Roberfroid, M., *et al.* (1995). Determination of digestible energy values and fermentabilitiesof dietary fibre supplements: a European interlaboratory study *in vivo*. *British Journal of Nutrition*, 74, 289–302.

Maathuis, A.J., van den Heuvel, E.G., Schoterman, M.H., and Venema, K. (2012). Galacto-oligosaccharides have prebiotic activity in a dynamic *in vitro* colon model using a 13C-labeling technique. *Journal of Nutrition*, 142(7), 1205–1212.

Macagnan, F.T., Dos Santos, L.R., Roberto, B.S., De Mura, F.A., Bizzani, M., and Da Silva, L.P. (2015). Biological properties of apple pomace, orange bagasse and passion fruit peel as alternative sources of dietary fibre. *Bioactive Carbohydrates and Dietary Fibre*, 6, 1–6.

Maccaferri, S., Klinder, A., Cacciatore, S., Chitarrari, R., Honda, H., Luchinat, C., *et al.* (2012). *In vitro* fermentation of potential prebiotic flours from natural sources: impact on the human colonic microbiota and metabolome. *Molecular Nutrition and Food Research*, 56(8), 1342–1352.

Macfarlane, S. and Macfarlane, G.T. (2003). Regulation of short-chain fatty acid production. *Proceedings of the Nutrition Society*, 62, 67–72.

Macia, L., Tan, J., Vieira, A.T., Leach, K., Stanley, D., Luong, S., *et al.* (2015). Metabolite-sensing receptors GPR43 and GPR109A facilitate dietary fibre-induced gut homeostasis through regulation of the inflammasome. *Nature Communications*, 6, 6734.

Mamontov, P., Neiman, E., Cao, T., Perrigoue, J., Friedman, J., Das, A., *et al.* (2015). Effects of short chain fatty acids and GPR43 stimulation on human Treg function (IRC5P. 631). *Journal of Immunology*, 194(1), 58–14.

Massimino, S.P., McBurney, M.I., Field, C.J., Thomson, A.B., Keelan, M., Hayek, M.G., *et al.* (1998). Fermentable dietary fiber increases GLP-1 secretion and improves glucose homeostasis despite increased intestinal glucose transport capacity in healthy dogs. *Journal of Nutrition*, 128, 1786–1793.

Midtvedt, T., Zabarovsky, E., Norin, E., Bark, J., Gizatullin, R., Kashuba, V., *et al.* (2013). Increase of faecal tryptic activity relates to changes in the intestinal microbiome: analysis of Crohn's disease with a multidisciplinary platform. *PLoS One*, 8(6), e66074.

Min, F.F., Hu, J.L., Nie, S.P., Xie, J.H., and Xie, M.Y. (2014). *In vitro* fermentation of the polysaccharides from Cyclocarya paliurus leaves by human fecal inoculums. *Carbohydrate Polymers*, 112, 563–568.

Monk, J.M., Lepp, D., Zhang, C.P., Wu, W., Zarepoor, L., Lu, J.T., *et al.* A. (2016). Diets enriched with cranberry beans alter the microbiota and mitigate colitis severity and associated inflammation. *Journal of Nutritional Biochemistry*, 28, 129–139.

Montagne, L., Pluske, J.R., and Hampson, D.J. (2003). A review of interactions between dietary fibre and the intestinal mucosa, and their consequences on digestive health in young non-ruminant animals. *Animal Feed Science and Technology*, 108, 95–117.

Moreau, N.M., Martin, L.J., Toquet, C.S., Laboisse, C.L., Nguyen, P.G., Siliart, B.S., *et al.* (2003). Restoration of the integrity of rat caeco-colonic mucosa by resistant starch, but not by fructo-oligosaccharides, in dextran sulfate sodium-induced experimental colitis. *British Journal of Nutrition*, 90, 75–85.

Niba, L.L. and Niba, S.N. (2003). Role of non-digestible carbohydrates in colon cancer protection. *Nutrition and Food Science*, 33(1), 28–33.

Noguera-Aguilar, J.F. and Gamundí-Gamundí, A. (2006). Carcinogénesis cólica experimental. *Revista Española de Enfermedades Digestivas*, 98(9), 637–643.

Nordlund, E., Aura, A.M., Mattila, I., Kössö, T., Rouau, X., and Poutanen, K. (2012). Formation of phenolic microbial metabolites and short-chain fatty acids from rye, wheat, and oat bran and their fractions in the metabolical *in vitro* colon model. *Journal of Agricultural and Food Chemistry*, 60(33), 8134–8145.

Oomah, B.D. and Kristensen, M. (2010) Fibre-enriched products from flaxseed hulls. http://flintbox.com/public/filedownload/1867/Business%200pportunity%20Document%2015%20April%202010.pdf (accessed August 2016).

Oomah, B.D., Kotzeva, L., Allen, M., and Zaczuk, P. (2014). Microwave and micronization treatments affect dehulling characteristics and bioactive contents of dry beans (Phaseolus vulgaris L.). *Journal of the Science of Food and Agriculture*, 94, 1349–1358.

Ortega-González, M., Ocón, B., Romero-Calvo, I., Anzola, A., Guadix, E., Zarzuelo, A., *et al.* (2014). Nondigestible oligosaccharides exert nonprebiotic effects on intestinal epithelial cells enhancing the immune response via activation of TLR4-NFκB. *Molecular Nutrition and Food Research*, 58(2), 384–393.

Ou, S., Kwok, K.C., Li, Y., and Fu, L. (2001). *In vitro* study of possible role of dietary fiber in lowering postprandial serum glucose. *Journal of Agricultural and Food Chemistry*, 49(2), 1026–1029.

Owusu-Asiedu, A., Patience, J.F., Laarveld, B., Van Kessel, A.G., Simmins, P.H., and Zijlstra, R.T. (2006). Effects of guar gum and cellulose on digesta passage rate, ileal microbial populations, energy and protein digestibility, and performance of grower pigs. *Journal of Animal Science*, 84, 843–852.

Park, J.S., Lee, E.J., Lee, J.C., Kim, W.K., and Kim, H.S. (2007). Anti-inflammatory effects of short chain fatty acids in IFNγ-stimulated RAW 264.7 murine macrophage cells: Involvement of NF-κB and ERK signaling pathways. *International Immunopharmacology*, 7(1), 70–77.

Payne, A.N., Zihler, A., Chassard, C., and Lacroix, C. (2012). Advances and perspectives in *in vitro* human gut fermentation modeling. *Trends in Biotechnology*, 30(1), 17–25.

Pratt, V.C., Tappenden, K.A., McBurney, M.I., and Field, C.J. (1996). Short-chain fatty acid-supplemented total parenteral nutrition improves nonspecific immunity after intestinal resection in rats. *Journal of Parenteral and Enteral Nutrition*, 20, 264–271.

Puertollano, E., Kolida, S., and Yaqoob, P. (2014). Biological significance of short-chain fatty acid metabolism by the intestinal microbiome. *Current Opinion in Clinical Nutrition and Metabolic Care*, 17(2), 139–144.

Qi, J., Li, Y., Masamba, K.G., Shoemaker, C.F., Zhong, F., Majeed, H., and Ma, J. (2016). The effect of chemical treatment on the *In vitro* hypoglycemic properties of rice bran insoluble dietary fiber. *Food Hydrocolloids*, 52, 699–706.

Ramasamy, U.S., Venema, K., Schols, H.A., and Gruppen, H. (2014). Effect of soluble and insoluble fibers within the *in vitro* fermentation of chicory root pulp by human gut bacteria. *Journal of Agricultural and Food Chemistry*, 62(28), 6794–6802.

Ramiro-Puig, E., Pérez-Cano, F.J., Castellote, C., Franch, A., and Castell, M. (2008). El intestino: pieza clave del sistema inmunitario. *Revista Española de Enfermedades Digestivas*, 100(1), 29–34.

Rezzonico, E., Mercenier, A., Baetge, E., Parkinson, S., Beck, T., Le Coutre, J., and Brüssow, H. (2015). Nestlé's research on nutrition and the human gut microbiome. *Scientific American*, 158(3), W1–W6.

Roberfroid, M.B. (2007). Inulin-type fructans: functional food ingredients. *Journal of Nutrition*, 137(11), 2493S–2502S.

Roberts, K.T., Allen-Vercoe, E., Williams, S.A., Graham, T., and Cui, S.W. (2015). Comparative study of the *in vitro* fermentative characteristics of fenugreek gum, white bread and bread with fenugreek gum using human faecal microbes. *Bioactive Carbohydrates and Dietary Fibre*, 5(2), 116–124.

Rodríguez-Cabezas, M.E., Gálvez, J., Lorente, M.D., Concha, A., Camuesco, D., Azzouz, S., *et al.* (2002). Dietary fiber down-regulates colonic tumor necrosis factor α and nitric oxide production in trinitrobenzenesulfonic acid-induced colitic rats. *Journal of Nutrition*, 132, 3263–3271.

Rodríguez-Cabezas, M.E., Camuesco, D., Arribas, B., Garrido-Mesa, N., Comalada, M., Bailón, E., *et al.* (2010). The combination of fructooligosaccharides and resistant starch shows prebiotic additive effects in rats. *Clinical Nutrition*, 29, 832–839.

Rosa, N.N., Aura, A.M., Saulnier, L., Holopainen-Mantila, U., Poutanen, K., and Micard, V. (2013). Effects of disintegration on *in vitro* fermentation and conversion patterns of wheat aleurone in a metabolical colon model. *Journal of Agricultural and Food Chemistry*, 61(24), 5805–5816.

Rosa-Sibakov, N., Poutanen, K., and Micard, V. (2015). How does wheat grain, bran and aleurone structure impact their nutritional and technological properties?. *Trends in Food Science and Technology*, 41(2), 118–134.

Rumi, G., Tsubouchi, R., Okayama, M., Kato, S., Mózsik, G., and Takeuchi, K. (2004). Protective effect of lactulose on dextran sulfate sodium-induced colonic inflammation in rats. *Digestive Diseases and Sciences*, 49(9), 1466–1472.

Rycroft, C.E., Jones, M.R., Gibson, G.R., and Rastall, R.A. (2001). A comparative *in vitro* evaluation of the fermentation properties of prebiotic oligosaccharides. *Journal of Applied Microbiology*, 91(5), 878–887.

Saavedra, J.M., Saavedra, J.M., and Tschernia, A. (2002). Human studies with probiotics and prebiotics: clinical implications. *British Journal of Nutrition*, 2, 241–246.

Salazar, N., Dewulf, E.M., Neyrinck, A.M., Bindels, L.B., Cani, P.D., Mahillon, J., *et al.* (2015). Inulin-type fructans modulate intestinal Bifidobacterium species populations and decrease fecal short-chain fatty acids in obese women. *Clinical Nutrition*, 34(3), 501–507.

Sánchez-Patán, F., Barroso, E., Van de Wiele, T., Jiménez-Girón, A., Martín-Alvarez, P.J., Moreno-Arribas, M.V., *et al.* (2015). Comparative *in vitro* fermentations of cranberry and grape seed polyphenols with colonic microbiota. *Food Chemistry*, 183, 273–282.

Sánchez, D., Miguel, M., and Aleixandre, A. (2012). Dietary fiber, gut peptides, and adipocytokines. *Journal of Medicinal Food*, 15(3), 223–230.

Sarbini, S.R., Kolida, S., Deaville, E.R., Gibson, G.R., and Rastall, R.A. (2014). Potential of novel dextran oligosaccharides as prebiotics for obesity management through *in vitro* experimentation. *British Journal of Nutrition*, 112(08), 1303–1314.

Satchithanandam, S., Klurfeld, D.M., Calvert, R.J., and Cassidy, M.M. (1996). Effects of dietary fibers on gastrointestinal mucin in rats. *Nutrition Research*, 16(7), 1163–1177.

Saura-Calixto, F. (2010). Dietary fiber as a carrier of dietary antioxidants: an essential physiological function. *Journal of Agricultural and Food Chemistry*, 59(1), 43–49.

Savignac, H.M., Couch, Y., Stratford, M., Bannerman, D.M., Tzortzis, G., Anthony, D.C., *et al.* (2015). Prebiotic administration normalizes lipopolysaccharide (LPS)-induced anxiety and cortical 5-HT2A receptor and IL1-β levels in male mice. *Brain, Behavior, and Immunity*, 52, 120–131.

Sawicki, C., Livingston, K., Obin, M., Roberts, S., Chung, M., and McKeown, N. (2015). Dietary fiber and the human gut microbiome: application of evidence mapping methodology. *FASEB Journal*, 29(1 Suppl), 736–727.

Schaafsma, G. and Slavin, J.L. (2015). Significance of inulin fructans in the human diet. *Comprehensive Reviews in Food Science and Food Safety*, 14(1), 37–47.

Scharlau, D., Borowicki, A., Habermann, N., Hofmann, T., Klenow, S., Miene, C., *et al.* (2009). Mechanisms of primary cancer prevention by butyrate and other products formed during gut flora-mediated fermentation of dietary fibre. *Mutation Research*, 682(1), 39–53.

Schley, P.D. and Field, C.J. (2002). The immune-enhancing effects of dietary fibres and prebiotics. *British Journal of Nutrition*, 87, S221–S230.

Schroeder, N., Marquart, L.F., and Gallaher, D.D. (2013). The role of viscosity and fermentability of dietary fibers on satiety-and adiposity-related hormones in rats. *Nutrients*, 5, 2093–2113.

Scott, K.P., Martin, J.C., Duncan, S.H., and Flint, H.J. (2014). Prebiotic stimulation of human colonic butyrate-producing bacteria and bifidobacteria, *in vitro. FEMS Microbiology Ecology*, 87(1), 30–40.

Serino, M., Blasco-Baque, V., Nicolas, S., and Burcelin, R. (2014). Far from the eyes, close to the heart: Dysbiosis of gut microbiota and cardiovascular consequences. *Current Cardiology Reports*, 16, 540.

Sharma, R. and Schumacher, U. (1995). Morphometric analysis of intestinal mucins under different dietary conditions and gut flora in rats. *Digestive Diseases and Sciences*, 40, 2532–2539.

Shen, N. and Clemente, J. C. (2015). Engineering the microbiome: a novel approach to immunotherapy for allergic and immune diseases. *Current Allergy and Asthma Reports*, 15(7), 1–10.

Silk, D.B.A., Davis, A., Vulevic, J., Tzortzis, G., and Gibson, G.R. (2009). Clinical trial: the effects of a trans-galactooligosaccharide prebiotic on faecal microbiota and symptoms in irritable bowel syndrome. *Alimentary Pharmacology and Therapeutics*, 29(5), 508–518.

Simpson, H.L. and Campbell, B.J. (2015). Review article: dietary fibre–microbiota interactions. *Alimentary Pharmacology and Therapeutics*, 42(2), 158–179.

Smith, P.M., Howitt, M.R., Panikov, N., Michaud, M., Gallini, C.A., Bohlooly-Y, M., *et al.* (2013). The microbial metabolites, short-chain fatty acids, regulate colonic T_{reg} cell homeostasis. *Science*, 341, 569–573.

Song, M., Xia, B., and Li, J. (2006). Effects of topical treatment of sodium butyrate and 5-aminosalicylic acid on expression of trefoil factor 3, interleukin 1β, and nuclear factor κB in trinitrobenzene sulphonic acid induced colitis in rats. *Postgraduate Medical Journal*, 82, 130–135.

Sreenivas, K.M. and Lele, S. S. (2013). Prebiotic activity of gourd family vegetable fibres using *in vitro* fermentation. *Food Bioscience*, 1, 26–30.

Steinmeyer, S., Lee, K., Jayaraman, A., and Alaniz, R. C. (2015). Microbiota metabolite regulation of host immune homeostasis: a mechanistic missing link. *Current Allergy and Asthma Reports*, 15(5), 1–10.

Sulek, K., Vigsnaes, L.K., Schmidt, L.R., Holck, J., Frandsen, H.L., Smedsgaard, J., *et al.* (2014). A combined metabolomic and phylogenetic study reveals putatively prebiotic effects of high molecular weight arabino-oligosaccharides when assessed by *in vitro* fermentation in bacterial communities derived from humans. *Anaerobe*, 28, 68–77.

Tabernero, M., Serrano, J., and Saura-Calixto, F. (2007). Dietary fiber intake in two European diets with high (Copenhagen, Denmark) and low (Murcia, Spain) colorectal cancer incidence. *Journal of Agricultural and Food Chemistry*, 55(23), 9443–9449.

Tabernero, M., Venema, K., Maathuis, A.J., and Saura-Calixto, F.D. (2011). Metabolite production during *in vitro* colonic fermentation of dietary fiber: analysis and comparison of two European diets. *Journal of Agricultural and Food Chemistry*, 59(16), 8968–8975.

Tang, W.W., Wang, Z., Levison, B.S., Koeth, R.A., Britt, E.B., Fu, X., *et al.* (2013). Intestinal microbial metabolism of phosphatidylcholine and cardiovascular risk. *New England Journal of Medicine*, 368(17), 1575–1584.

Tazoe, H., Otomo, Y., Kaji, I., Tanaka, R., Karaki, S. I., and Kuwahara, A. (2008). Roles of short-chain fatty acids receptors, GPR41 and GPR43 on colonic functions. *Journal of Physiology and Pharmacology*, 59(Suppl 2), 251–262.

Tedelind, S., Westberg, F., Kjerrulf, M., and Vidal, A. (2007). Anti-inflammatory properties of the short-chain fatty acids acetate and propionate: A study with relevance to inflammatory bowel disease. *World Journal of Gastroenterology*, 13(20), 2826–2832.

Tilg, H. and Adolph, T.E. (2015). Influence of the human intestinal microbiome on obesity and metabolic dysfunction. *Current Opinion in Pediatrics*, 26(4), 496–501.

Tilg, H. and Moschen, A.R. (2015). Food, immunity, and the microbiome. *Gastroenterology*, 148(6), 1107–1119.

Trompette, A., Gollwitzer, E.S., Yadava, K., Sichelstiel, A.K., Sprenger, N., Ngom-Bru, C., *et al.* (2014). Gut microbiota metabolism of dietary fiber influences airway disease and hematopoiesis. *Nature Medicine*, 20(2), 159–166.

Tuohy, K.M., Fava, F., and Viola, R. (2014). 'The way to a man's heart is through his gut microbiota' – dietary pro- and prebiotics for the management of cardiovascular risk. *Proceedings of the Nutrition Society*, 73(02), 172–185.

Van Dokkum, W., Pikaar, N.A., and Thissen, J.T.N.M. (1983). Physiological effects of fibre-rich types of bread. *British Journal of Nutrition*, 50(01), 61–74.

Velasquez-Manoff, M. (2015). The peace-keepers. *Scientific American*, 518(3), S3–S11.

Vergara-Castañeda, H.A., Guevara-González, R.G., Ramos-Gómez, M., Reynoso-Camacho, R., Guzmán-Maldonado, H., Feregrino-Pérez, A.A., *et al.* (2010). Non-digestible fraction of cooked bean (*Phaseolus vulgaris* L.) cultivar Bayo Madero suppresses colonic aberrant crypt foci in azoxymethane-induced rats. *Food and Function*, 1, 294–300.

Vergara-Castañeda, H., Guevara-González, R., Guevara-Olvera, L., Oomah, B.D., Reynoso-Camacho, R., Wiersma, P., *et al.* (2012). Non-digestible fraction of beans (*Phaseolus vulgaris* L.) modulates signalling pathway genes at an early stage of colon cancer in Sprague–Dawley rats. *British Journal of Nutrition*, 108, S145–S154.

Vervoort, M.J. (2011). Process for the manufacture of an edible dietary fibre composition and a dietary fibre composition. World Patent WO 2011/096807 A1, issued August 11, 2011.

Vester Boler, B.M., Rossoni Serao, M.C., Faber, T.A., Bauer, L.L., Chow, J., Murphy, M.R., *et al.* (2013). *In vitro* fermentation characteristics of select nondigestible oligosaccharides by infant fecal inocula. *Journal of Agricultural and Food Chemistry*, 61(9), 2109–2119.

Videla, S., Vilaseca, J., Antolin, M., Garcia-Lafuente, A., Guarner, F., Crespo, E., *et al.* (2001). Dietary inulin improves distal colitis induced by dextran sodium sulfate in the rat. *American Journal of Gastroenterology*, 96, 1486–1493.

Vieira, S.M., Pagovich, O.E., and Kriegel, M.A. (2014). Diet, microbiota and autoimmune diseases. *Lupus*, 23(6), 518–526.

Vigsnæs, L.K., Holck, J., Meyer, A.S., and Licht, T.R. (2011). *In vitro* fermentation of sugar beet arabino-oligosaccharides by fecal microbiota obtained from patients with ulcerative colitis to selectively stimulate the growth of *Bifidobacterium* spp. and *Lactobacillus* spp. *Applied and Environmental Microbiology*, 77(23), 8336–8344.

Vinolo, M.A., Rodrigues, H.G., Nachbar, R.T., and Curi, R. (2011). Regulation of inflammation by short chain fatty acids. *Nutrients*, 3(10), 858–876.

Vong, M.H., and Stewart, M.L. (2013). *In vitro* bacterial fermentation of tropical fruit fibres. *Beneficial Microbes*, 4(3), 291–295.

Waldecker, M., Kautenburger, T., Daumann, H., Veeriah, S., Will, F., Dietrich, H., *et al.* (2008). Histone-deacetylase inhibition and butyrate formation: Fecal slurry incubations with apple pectin and apple juice extracts. *Nutrition*, 24(4), 366–374.

Wang, J. and Nie, D. (2015). Abstract B19: Short chain fatty acids suppress mTOR activation in colon cancer cells via the long noncoding RNA rhabdomyosarcoma 2 associated transcript. *Molecular Cancer Therapeutics*, 14(7 Suppl), B19–B19.

Wisker, E., Daniel, M., Rave, G., and Feldheim, W. (1998). Fermentation of non-starch polysaccharides in mixed diets and single fibre sources: comparative studies in human subjects and *in vitro*. *British Journal of Nutrition*, 80(03), 253–261.

Wong, J.M.W., de Souza, R., Kendall, C.W.C., Emam, A., and Jenkins, D.J.A. (2006). Colonic health: fermentation and short chain fatty acids. *Journal of Clinical Gastroenterology*, 40, 235–243.

Wong, K.H., Wong, K.Y., Kwan, H.S., and Cheung, P.C. (2005). Dietary fibers from mushroom sclerotia: 3. *In vitro* fermentability using human fecal microbiota. *Journal of Agricultural and Food Chemistry*, 53(24), 9407–9412.

Wright, E.K., Kamm, M.A., Teo, S.M., Inouye, M., Wagner, J., and Kirkwood, C.D. (2015). Recent advances in characterizing the gastrointestinal microbiome in Crohn's disease: a systematic review. *Inflammatory Bowel Diseases*, 21(6), 1219–1228.

Yang, J., Martínez, I., Walter, J., Keshavarzian, A., and Rose, D.J. (2013). *In vitro* characterization of the impact of selected dietary fibers on fecal microbiota composition and short chain fatty acid production. *Anaerobe*, 23, 74–81.

Yu, Z.T., Chen, C., Kling, D.E., Liu, B., McCoy, J.M., Merighi, M., *et al.* (2013). The principal fucosylated oligosaccharides of human milk exhibit prebiotic properties on cultured infant microbiota. *Glycobiology*, 23(2), 169–177.

Yuan, Q., Zhao, L., Cha, Q., Sun, Y., Ye, H., and Zeng, X. (2015). Structural characterization and immunostimulatory activity of a homogenous polysaccharide from sinonovacula constricta. *Journal of Agricultural and Food Chemistry*, 63(36), 7986–7994.

Zamora-Gasga, V.M., Loarca-Piña, G., Vázquez-Landaverde, P.A., Ortiz-Basurto, R. I., Tovar, J., and Sáyago-Ayerdi, S.G. (2015). *In vitro* colonic fermentation of food ingredients isolated from *Agave tequilana* Weber var. *azul* applied on granola bars. *LWT-Food Science and Technology*, 60(2), 766–772.

Zarepoor, L., Lu, J.T., Zhang, C., Wu, W., Lepp, D., Robinson, L., *et al.* (2014). Dietary flaxseed intake exacerbates acute colonic mucosal injury and inflammation induced by dextran sodium sulfate. *American Journal of Physiology and Gastrointestinal Liver Physiology*, 306, G1042–G1055.

Zeng, H., Lazarova, D.L., and Bordonaro, M. (2014). Mechanisms linking dietary fiber, gut microbiota and colon cancer prevention. *World Journal of Gastrointestinal Oncology*, 6(2), 41.

Zhao, M., Zhu, W., Gong, J., Zuo, L., Zhao, J., Sun, J., *et al.* (2015). Dietary fiber intake is associated with increased colonic mucosal GPR43[+] polymorphonuclear infiltration in active crohn's disease. *Nutrients*, 7(7), 5327–5346.

Zhou, J., Martin, R.J., Tulley, R.T., Raggio, A.M., McCutcheon, K.L., Shen, L., *et al.* (2008). Dietary resistant starch upregulates total GLP-1 and PYY in a sustained day-long manner through fermentation in rodents. *American Journal of Physiology, Endocrinology and Metabolism*, 295, E1160–E1166.

7

Dietary Fiber and Colon Cancer

Maria Elena Maldonado and Luz Amparo Urango

Escuela de Nutrición y Dietética, Universidad de Antioquia, Medellín, Colombia

7.1 Introduction

According to the International Agency for Research on Cancer (IARC, 2011), colon cancer was the fourth most common cancer worldwide in 2012. It is the third most common cancer for men and the second for women. Approximately 55% of cases occur in developed countries. Dietary habits and lifestyle are crucial factors in the development of colon cancer. For example, the consumption of red meat, saturated fat, refined carbohydrates, alcohol intake are positively associated with increased risk, whereas intake of dietary fiber, vegetable, fruits, antioxidants, vitamins, calcium, and folate are negatively associated (WCR/AIRC, 2007, 2011).

The American Association of Cereal Chemists (2001) defined dietary fiber as the edible part of plants and analogs of carbohydrate that are resistant to digestion and absorption in the human small intestine, with partial or total fermentation in colon. This includes polysaccharides, oligosaccharides, lignin, and associated plant substances. The Codex Alimentarius, on the other hand, defines dietary fiber as carbohydrate polymers with a degree of polymerization not less than 3, which are neither digested nor absorbed in the small intestine. This definition classifies these polymers as: (i) natural carbohydrate polymers; (ii) carbohydrate polymers obtained from raw material by physical, enzymatic, or chemical methods; (iii) synthetic polymers (Food and Agriculture Organization, 1997; Phillips, 2011). From a microbiological point of view, fiber is classified into degradable or non-degradable by colonic flora (Ajila *et al.*, 2008). Fiber can be classified as: (i) associated structural cell wall polysaccharides comprising mainly cellulose, hemicellulose, and pectin; (ii) structural non-polysaccharides such as lignin; and (iii) non-structural polysaccharides such as gums and mucilages based on its functions in the plant.

From a nutritional point of view, dietary fiber classification is based on its ability to generate hydration and gel formation. In this classification there are two types: (i) soluble fiber, comprising gums, pectins, mucilages, and some hemicelluloses, and (ii) insoluble fibers, which are cellulose, hemicellulose, and lignin (López and Suárez, 2002). Partially soluble fiber has beneficial physiological effects on intestinal motility, weight and volume of the bolus, and intestinal transit time.

Dietary Fiber Functionality in Food and Nutraceuticals: From Plant to Gut, First Edition.
Edited by Farah Hosseinian, B. Dave Oomah and Rocio Campos-Vega.
© 2017 John Wiley & Sons Ltd. Published 2017 by John Wiley & Sons Ltd.

It contributes to the removal of bile acids and reduces cholesterol levels in the blood, lowering the risk of cardiovascular diseases and disorders of the colon (Wollowski and Pool-Zobel, 2001).

The evolution of the definitions of dietary fiber can be attributed to numerous studies on the functional, biological, and physiological characteristics, including the protective effect against colon carcinogenesis extensively investigated since the early 1970s. It was realized that African populations, whose diet was characterized by a high intake of fiber and low refined carbohydrates, presented low or no incidence of colon cancer (Kim, 2000).

Numerous epidemiological studies have shown the protective effects of consuming 11.1 g/day dietary fiber 3–3.5 times a day, although cohort studies have shown conflicting results, specifically the Follow-up Nurses Health Study or the Health Professionals (Michels *et al.*, 2000). The discrepancies between studies have been attributed to errors in some definitions, such as dietary fiber in the population, and high fiber consumption below the recommended daily levels (30 g/day) (Ferguson, 2005). Moreover, considering that one of the products of fermented dietary fiber in the colon is butyrate, it has been proposed that resistant cancerous lesions to this short-chain fatty acid (SCFA) exist. For example, *in vitro* studies found that adenocarcinoma colon cells were resistant to 5 mM butyrate after 24 hours of treatment, because of suppression of Wnt/catenin and inhibition of apoptosis (Lazarova *et al.*, 2013). This could explain the existence of tumors resistant or partially resistant to butyrate (Zeng *et al.*, 2014).

On the other hand, the European Prospective Investigation into Cancer and Nutrition (EPIC) analyzed fiber intake and incidence of colorectal cancer in more than 500 000 individuals. They showed that total fiber consumption at twice the recommended level decreases incidence by 40%. In particular, the incidence was 25% lower in individuals with a high intake of fruits and vegetables than in the rest of the population (Bingham *et al.*, 2003; van Duijnhoven *et al.*, 2009). The World Cancer Research Fund/American Institute for Cancer Research (WCR/AICR, 2011) also reported convincing evidence of the protective effect of dietary fiber against colorectal cancer. This expert panel found cohort studies with up to 25% colorectal cancer risk reduction at dietary fiber consumption between 33.1 and 12.6 g/day in a dose–dependent response in men and women. These findings were supported by evidence on mechanisms of action such as blocking conversion of primary to secondary bile acids, antiproliferative, apoptotic, and anti-inflammatory properties of SCFAs (butyrate, acetate, and propionate). Dietary fiber led to a reduction in the amount of time carcinogens were in contact with epithelial cells, dilution of carcinogenic substances by increasing the fecal mass, and a reduction in postprandial hyperinsulinemia because of a delay in the absorption of complex sugars (Baena and Salinas, 2015).

In view of the evidence, it is considered reasonable to recommend a total of 21–38 g/day of dietary fiber distributed in 5 to 7 servings of fruits, vegetables, and whole grain (American College of Gastroenterology, 2000). However, there is uncertainty as to what type or source of fiber is the most effective in preventing colon cancer. Therefore, the American College of Gastroenterology states that the most prudent recommendation is to intake a high fiber diet from all sources (vegetables, fruits, cereals, grains, and legumes). It is also important to include in the colon cancer prevention recommendations a healthy lifestyle (low intakes of saturated animal fat, moderate red meat, avoid obesity, low alcohol consumption, smoking, and regular physical activity) (American College of Gastroenterology, 2000; WCR/AICR, 2011).

The type of dietary fiber affects the composition and physiological properties of the gut microbiota as well as production of SCFAs whose concentration may exceed 100 mmol/L. Acetate comprises 60–70% of total SCFAs (Cummings *et al.*, 1987; Cummings and Macfarlane 1991) produced by the fermentation of pectin (Lupton and Kurtz, 1993). Propionate is produced by *Bacteroides* species from succinate, resulting from gum arabic and cyclodextrin fermentation (Kaewprasert *et al.*, 2001; Ushida *et al.*, 2011). Butyrate is produced by colonic bacteria belonging to the clostridial clusters I, III, IV, VI, XIVa, XV, and XVI. Cluster IV *Faecalibacterium prausnitzii* comprises 7–24% of total intestinal bacteria in healthy individuals, along with *Eubacterium rectale* and *Roseburia* spp. cluster XIVa (Barcenilla *et al.*, 2000). Chen *et al.* (2013) found that decreased dietary fiber intake led to reduced production of SCFAs and prevalence of *Enterococcus* and *Streptococcus* spp. in individuals at risk for colon cancer, while in a group of healthy subjects *Clostridium, Roseburia,* and *Eubacterium* spp. were more prevalent.

Acetate has been reported to stimulate proliferation of normal crypts in the colon mucosa and exert anti-inflammatory effect mediated by the reduction of tumor necrosis factor (TNFα), interleukin-6 (IL-6), IL-1β, IL-4, IL-5, IL-13, and activation of nuclear factor-κB (NFκB). Propionate and butyrate also exhibit this anti-inflammatory ability, particularly butyrate, which increases the expression of IL-8, IL-10, IL-12, induces apoptosis and cell cycle arrest, and inhibits histone deacetylase (Tedelind *et al.*, 2007; Bailón *et al.*, 2010; Comalada *et al.*, 2006; Archer *et al.*, 2005; Chuang *et al.*, 2011).

Moreover, the chemopreventive properties of dietary fiber are attributed to the ability to bind or to contribute to the excretion of carcinogens into the intestinal lumen and decrease in fecal pH colon. Its anticancer potential is also associated with the content of phenolic compounds: carotenoids, lignans, terpenes, β-glucans, and inulin (Surh, 2003; Lattimer and Haub, 2010).

This chapter is a review summarizing current knowledge on the potential preventive effects in the colon of dietary fiber obtained from different sources, based on evidence from *in vitro* and animal models, human intervention studies, and epidemiological findings linking dietary fiber intake and the occurrence of colon cancer in humans.

7.2 Physiological Action and Function of Dietary Fiber in Colon Cancer

Dietary fiber affects the entire gastrointestinal tract from the mouth to the anus, and is responsible for much of its physiological and functional processes (Anderson *et al.*, 2009). It reaches the large intestine where it is fermented by the colonic microflora, leading to the production of SCFAs, hydrogen, carbon dioxide, and biomass. This fermentation is the most important function of the human large intestine and provides a means by which energy is obtained from undigested carbohydrates from the small intestine by SCFAs absorption.

Two types of fermentation – saccharolytic and proteolytic – occur in the colon. Saccharolytic fermentation produces mainly SCFAs (acetate, propionate, and butyrate) in a molar ratio 60:25:15. These fatty acids are generated through the metabolism of pyruvate produced by glucose oxidation via the glycolytic Embden–Meyerhof pathway. Butyrate is the preferred energy substrate of colonocytes. There are two pathways for the use of pyruvate, which is converted to propionate or acetyl-CoA. This is subsequently hydrolyzed to acetate or butyrate (Valenzuela and Maiz, 2006). In contrast, proteolytic fermentation produces nitrogen derivatives such as amines, ammonia, and phenolic compounds, some of which are carcinogens (Guarner and Malagelada, 2003a; McCrea *et al.*, 2009).

Not all types of dietary fiber contribute effectively to colon health. Soluble fiber captures more water and toxic substances, in addition to its fermentable action.

The benefits of soluble fiber and their mechanisms of action in colonic health have been investigated in many studies. These effects may be mediated by factors such as SCFAs production and regulation of energy homeostasis, modulation of signaling pathways that alter histone acetylation, and activation of G protein-coupled receptors (FFAR2 and FFAR3) (Layden *et al.*, 2013; Brown *et al.*, 2003; De Vadder *et al.*, 2014). Once absorbed, the SCFAs (particularly butyrate) are used as an energy source by the colonic epithelium. The SCFAs contribute up to 80% of the energy requirements of colonocytes and 5–10% of the total energy requirements of the individual (Balanzà, 2007).

The gastrointestinal tract has the highest density and variety of bacteria in the human body (about 100 trillion microbes of more than 1000 species), making it the ideal host for microorganisms. In the colon, there are approximately 10^{12} microbes per gram of luminal contents, representing 60% of feces weight (Viladomiua *et al.*, 2013). The resident flora in the gastrointestinal tract protects against pathogen invasion by the so-called "barrier effects." These include resistance to colonization by exogenous bacteria and overgrowth of opportunistic species that reside in the colon, whose growth is controlled by the balance with other species. In order to study trophic functions on the epithelium it is important to know the role of the flora in the pathogenesis of colorectal cancer (Guarner and Malagelada, 2003a, 2003b). When the host relationship is initiated, the colonization of bacteria creates an optimal environment that leads to symbiosis, in which the different bacterial genera and species use the metabolic products for their proliferation (Guarner and Malagelada, 2003a, 2003b).

Instability in the intestine–bacteria relationship can lead to different physiological changes, such as inflammatory bowel disease (IBD), since the epithelial cells of the gut mucosal layer are formed by goblet cells, producing antimicrobial peptides (AMP) and segregating immunoglobulin A (IgA) to maintain homeostasis (Viladomiua *et al.*, 2013).

7.3 Colon Cancer Chemopreventive Bioactivities

7.3.1 *In Vitro* Evidence

In recent years many *in vitro* studies have examined the mechanisms involved in the chemopreventive effect of dietary fiber on colon mucosa. Sporn (1976) first introduced the concept of chemoprevention in a study concerning the preventive properties of natural forms of vitamin A in epithelial carcinogenesis. Today, chemoprevention generally refers to the use of natural, synthetic, biological, or chemical agents to reverse, suppress, or prevent either the initial phase of carcinogenesis or the progression of neoplastic cells to cancer.

There are three strategies for cancer chemoprevention: (i) *Primary chemoprevention* is designed to help healthy individuals prevent the development of a certain cancer type. These individuals may be high risk and/or predisposed to cancer development. (ii) *Secondary chemoprevention* is designed to provide treatment of premalignant lesions (colon adenomas) with the aim of preventing cancer progression. (iii) *Therapy chemoprevention* aims to help patients with a history of cancer treatment to prevent the development of a second primary cancer.

Phytochemicals present in the diet can be classified according to their ability to block the initiation stage of carcinogenesis (cancer-blocking agents for primary chemoprevention) or to suppress (cancer-supressing agents) the proliferative capacity of pre-neoplastic lesions in the stages of tumor promotion and progression (secondary chemoprevention and therapy).

Butyrate has been implicated in the chemoprevention of colon cancer at the secondary level since it inhibits growth and induces apoptosis of HT29, HT1080, LT97, and HCT116 colon cancer cell lines at >1 mM. However, at concentrations equal to or less than 0.5 mM butyrate is mitogenic and an energy metabolite in colon mucosa (Zeng and Briske-Anderson, 2005; Blottière *et al.*, 2003; Emenaker *et al.*, 2001; Richter *et al.*, 2002; Miyanishi *et al.*, 2001; Grubben *et al.*, 2001; Bultman, 2014; Zeng *et al.*, 2015). When these cells are exposed to 1–2 mM butyrate concentrations it may accumulate in the nucleus, favoring the inhibition of histone deacetylase activity and the acetylation of gene promoters that contribute to altered cell cycle and apoptosis (Fung *et al.*, 2012).

Butyrate at concentrations up to 2 mM metabolizes β-oxidation of fatty acids into the mitochondria. The acetyl-CoA produced is condensed by oxaloacetate to form citrate. The citrate is used in the Krebs cycle or transported to the cytoplasm or the nucleus, where the citrate lyase enzyme (nuclear or cytoplasmic) makes it useful for lipid biosynthesis in the cytoplasm or for histone acetylation by inhibiting histone deacetylase enzymes. High dose of butyrate (5 mM) increases gene expression of cell cycle arrest and activation of apoptosis (Donohoe *et al.*, 2012; Bultman, 2014). For example, HCT116 cell growth was inhibited by 80% and 89% after treatment with 0.5–2 mM butyrate for 48 hours and 72 hours, respectively, compared to untreated cells. Apoptotic cells increased by 1.0 and 3.1-fold compared to controls after treatment with 1.0 and 1.5 mM butyrate for 48 hours. In addition, HCT116 cells accumulated in G_2 phase and expression of p21 tumor suppressor protein increased under the same conditions. This suggests that butyrate may exert its antiproliferative activity on the apoptotic pathway through p21/p53 (Zeng *et al.*, 2015). Growth of LT97 colon adenoma cells and HT29 human colon adenocarcinoma cells was inhibited by 50% at 1.9 mM and 4.0 mM butyrate, respectively (Kautenburger *et al.*, 2005).

The anti-inflammatory activity of butyrate has also been reported using human carcinoma cells and wild-type, Fas-deficient (Faslpr), or FasL-deficient (Fasgld) colonic T-cells from BALB/c mice (Zimmerman *et al.*, 2012). The wild-type T-cells of the gut lamina propria (T-LPL) expressed high levels of Fas, but during inflammation Fas is reduced, and consequently cells increase resistance to apoptosis. However, butyrate at 5 mM for 24 hours restores sensitivity via Fas in the wild-type T-cells (Garrett *et al.*, 2010; Zimmerman *et al.*, 2012). Butyrate inhibits the enzyme activity of histone H1 deacetylase (HDAC1), which binds to the Fas promoter of T-cells, resulting in hyperacetylation of Fas promoter and increase of Fas receptor in these cells, which favors sensitivity to Fas-mediated apoptosis (Zimmerman *et al.*, 2012).

DNA hyperacetylation may also be induced with physiological concentrations of SCFAs, specifically facilitating the acetylation of histone H4 in HT29 cells (Kiefer *et al.*, 2006). In this context, treatment of HT29 cells with supernatants obtained from fermented soybeans, inulin, wheat, grains, and leafy vegetables with human feces, as a source of microorganisms, showed greater antiproliferative activity than individual SCFAs or their mix. This suggests that the presence of other phytochemicals are capable of inhibiting HT29 and LT97 cell growth (Beyer-Sehlmeyer *et al.*, 2003; Glei *et al.*, 2006; Scharlau *et al.*, 2009).

Furthermore, butyrate inhibits hyperactivation of STAT1 induced by IFNγ in colonic epithelial cells (Hanada *et al.*, 2006; Klampfer *et al.*, 2003). STAT1 is a transcription factor that regulates the expression of inducible nitric oxide synthase enzyme (iNOS) and cyclooxygenase-2 (COX-2) (Hanada *et al.*, 2006; Klampfer *et al.*, 2003). Activated T-cells accumulated and IFNγ synthesis was sustained in the colon mucosa of patients with ulcerative colitis, thereby favoring STAT1 activation. This situation is transient under normal physiological conditions, but it can promote chronic inflammation in the colon mucosa, which is a risk factor for colorectal cancer (Hanada *et al.*, 2006). Taking these findings together it can be concluded that butyrate is an anti-inflammatory agent that removes activated T-cells and suppresses the HDAC1 – Fas – STAT1 pathway.

A primary chemopreventive mechanism of butyrate is the upregulation at transcriptional level of glutathione *S*-transferases (GSTs) enzymes in colon cancer cells (Hayes *et al.*, 2005). The GSTs transform carcinogens from food or smoking, and protect cells from genotoxicity (Hayes *et al.*, 2005). The activation of GST expression by butyrate may occur by phosphorylation of ERK signaling via the mitogen-activated protein kinase pathway (MAPK). The ERK activates the transcription factor AP-1 that has binding sites in the promoters of GST genes. However, the evidence is inadequate to prove this hypothesis (Tsai *et al.*, 2007; Shah *et al.*, 2006; Ebert *et al.*, 2001).

Evidence of the antigenotoxic role of butyrate is based on its ability to prevent DNA damage of HT29, LT97, and HT29-19A cells exposed to 10–15 µM H_2O_2 or 5 µM 4-hydroxy-2-nonenal (HNE) (Ebert *et al.*, 2001; Rosignoli *et al.*,

2001). When these cells were pre-incubated with physiological (6.25 and 12 mM) butyrate concentrations, H_2O_2-induced DNA damage in HT29 decreased by 45% and 75%, respectively, and by 30% and 80% in HT29-19A, respectively. This protective effect was similar when cells were pre-incubated with 50 mM acetate, 20.8 mM propionate, and 12.5 mM butyrate. These results suggest that propionate and acetate do not affect the antigenotoxic and scavenger ability of butyrate against reactive oxygen species (ROS) such as H_2O_2.

ROS production and accumulation in colonic mucosal cells promotes initiation of pre-neoplastic cells by genotoxic damage. This alters the activation or expression of transcription factors, oncogenes, anti- and pro-apoptotic proteins favoring the transformation of normal epithelium, with the appearance of precancerous lesions (aberrant crypt foci, ACF), leading to the formation of adenomatous polyps, prior to the appearance of adenocarcinoma (Yeum *et al.*, 2010; Renehan *et al.*, 2002).

Ebert *et al.* (2001) also demonstrated that 4 mM butyrate reduced DNA damage induced by HNE, with increased levels of GST mRNA and GSTP1 protein activity, and the maintenance of glutathione (GSH) levels in cells. Yadav *et al.* (2008) supported these findings, demonstrating that HNE genotoxicity is dependent on intracellular GSH content and GST expression in K562 human erythroleukemia cells. GSH depletion in K562 cells exposed to 100 µM L-buthionine-[*S,R*]-sulfoximine (BSO) for 16 hours (pretreatment), followed by 5 µM HNE for 3 hours, significantly increased HNE-induced DNA damage compared to cells treated with HNE alone. In contrast, GSH supplementation decreased genotoxicity. Furthermore, overexpression of the GST isoenzyme GSTA4-4 prevented the HNE-induced genotoxic effect, because respective use of GSTA4-4 siRNAs increased DNA damage produced by HNE (Yadav *et al.*, 2008).

Relative to the stimulation of GST activity, the same effect was observed on HT29 cells treated with fermentation products and SCFAs. However, inulin fermentation did not produce this result on GST (Grubben *et al.*, 2001; Miyanishi *et al.*, 2001; Richter *et al.*, 2002; Scharlau *et al.*, 2009).

The findings presented here indicate the need for *in vitro* studies to understand the mechanisms of action involved in the protective effect of SCFAs and dietary fiber. There is also a need for animal and human studies to define the physiological effects of dietary fiber, dietary fiber types, butyrate, and propionate in colon cancer chemoprevention.

7.3.2 *In Vivo* Studies in Animal Models

The evidence for a chemopreventive role of dietary fiber has been obtained in rodents from preclinical models of colorectal cancer, which are induced by chemical agents such as azoxymethane (AOM) (Reddy *et al.*, 1981; Reddy, 2004), 3,29-dimethyl-4-aminobiphenyl (DMAB) (Reddy and Mori, 1981), or 1,2-dimethylhydrazine (DMH) (Hambly *et al.*, 2002).

AOM is a chemical agent that can induce colorectal cancer by DNA guanine alkylation, which results in increased proliferation as well as mutations in the epithelial cells of the colon due to a mismatch of the nitrogenous bases (Bruce,

2003; Papanikolau *et al.*, 1998). AOM and its derivatives are some of the most studied agents in the specific induction of colorectal carcinogenesis. However, AOM does not correspond to the end carcinogenic metabolite. It requires metabolic activation after intraperitoneal injection. This activation process has not been fully elucidated, although AOM is hydroxylated by P450 isoenzymes in the liver (Sohn *et al.*, 2001). After biliary excretion, another chemical change occurs through the presence of intestinal bacterial flora (Reddy *et al.*, 1974; Fiala, 1977). Initiation takes place at the DNA level by introducing mutations that alter the regulation of expression of genes involved in various cell signaling pathways, including anti-tumor, anti-apoptotic, pro-apoptotic, among others (Reddy, 2000; Surh 2003).

In these studies AOM was injected intraperitoneally into animals in two doses one week apart. The animals were randomly divided into a control group and an experimental group after the last injection, and the number of tumors arising after 40 weeks evaluated (Reddy, 2000, 2004). ACF can be used as a biomarker and can be registered by size from 12 to 14 weeks in rats (Reddy, 2000) and about 30 days in mice (Zamora-Ponce *et al.*, 2009) after the last AOM injection. The results are similar to those observed in humans. Epithelial lesions induced by AOM begin with the appearance of ACF as observed in human colon cancer, which is why this model is useful for experiments on environmental factors to estimate the etiology, treatment, and prevention of colon cancer (Montenegro *et al.*, 2003). The ACF become adenomatous polyps after 5 months and develop into adenocarcinomas 8 months later, as a result of successive accumulation of genetic changes leading to malignant (carcinoma) in the distal region, similar to the distribution of tumors in humans.

Among the advantages of this preclinical model are its potency, reproducibility, simplicity, and similarities with carcinogenesis of human colon. For example, the location of tumors in rodents and humans is concentrated in the distal colon. Tumors that develop in the colon of the rodent exhibit a growth polypoid similar to the histopathological features seen in human colon carcinogenesis, except that AOM-induced tumors rarely show mucosal invasiveness and metastases (Nambiar *et al.*, 2003; Boivin *et al.*, 2003).

Reddy *et al.* (1981) performed one of the first studies evaluating the effectiveness of primary chemopreventive dietary fiber in animals. They used 15% wheat bran or fiber dehydrated from citrus fruit plus 5% of fat in diet 2 weeks before AOM (8 mg/kg) administration in F344 rats. The groups fed wheat bran or citrus fiber for 20 weeks showed a significant decrease in the number of colon tumors compared to the group of animals that received the control diet + AOM. A similar result was observed when wheat bran was fed to rats exposed to DMAB (50 mg/kg), but not with citrus fiber. This difference was attributed to the presence of phytate in wheat fiber. However, in a similar study using rats fed with corn fiber and exposed to DMAB, an increase in the number of colon tumors was observed (Reddy *et al.*, 1983). This suggests that it is not only the amount of fiber that is important in the prevention of colon cancer, but also the type of fiber consumed.

This animal model has also explained why people with a low-risk diet are less susceptible to colon cancer compared to those accustomed to a western or high-risk diet. Hambly *et al.* (2002) showed that Sprague–Dawley rats injected with DMH and fed with a low-risk diet for 3 weeks, were protected against the initial stages of colon carcinogenesis by triggering apoptosis in cells with impaired DNA. The low-risk diet contained casein, corn oil, vitamin E, choline, calcium, and 43.5 g of wheat bran, 43.5 g inulin, and 628 g of starch per kg feed. This protective effect was not observed in animals fed the high-risk diet containing 223 g starch, 223 g sucrose per kg feed, free of inulin, wheat bran, calcium, and vitamin E.

The protective role of dietary fiber in the early stages of colon carcinogenesis has been demonstrated in rats fed diets containing wheat bran or resistant starch. Although the prebiotic inulin has shown pro-apoptotic effect (Le Leu *et al.*, 2007; Clarke *et al.*, 2008; Hughes and Rowland, 2002), this effect is partially attributed to the increase of the relative expression of the G protein-coupled butyrate receptor (93.1%) (GPR43). This protein was increased in colonic mucosa of Wistar rats fed a diet containing 5% dietary fiber (cellulose) from the cactus (*Opuntia ficus-indica*) for 16 days, compared to animals receiving the control diet (Corte Osorio *et al.*, 2011). This result suggests that GRP43 may be induced by dietary factors, an event that can be positively associated with histone acetylation and butyrate concentration (Boffa *et al.*, 1992).

Conlon *et al.* (2012) showed that DNA damage of colonocytes decreased by 70% in Sprague–Dawley rats fed a western-style diet moderate in fat (19%) and protein (20%) containing resistant amylose maize starch (HAMS), butylated HAMS (HAMSB), or whole high amylose wheat (HAW) compared to that in those fed with digestible starches (low amylose or low amylose maize whole wheat). In addition, HAMS, HAMSB, and HAW increased SCFAs levels in the large bowel. These findings were confirmed by Le Leu *et al.* (2007) and Clarke *et al.* (2008) using Sprague–Dawley rats that were protected from AOM-induced colon carcinogenesis by feeding dietary resistant starch (high amylose maize starch), reducing the incidence ($p < 0.01$) and multiplicity ($p < 0.05$) of colon adenocarcinomas compared to control diet (without dietary fiber), involving apoptosis of colonocytes in the distal colon.

Pesarini *et al.* (2013) used DMH at 30 mg/kg body weight (2 doses/week for 2 weeks) as carcinogenic agent in male Swiss mice, fed *ad libitum* with a diet containing wheat bran (*Triticum aestivum* variety CD-104) at 100 g/kg for 12 weeks before DMH, simultaneously with DMH, or after DMH administration. They found that wheat bran was antimutagenic and anticarcinogenic, because DNA damage decreased from 90.3% to 26.4% and ACF from 63.4% to 28.7%, respectively. The best antigenotoxic effect was in the group that received a wheat bran diet 2 weeks after DMH injection (post-treatment) and the lowest value of ACF was observed in the pretreatment group (fed with wheat bran diet 2 weeks before DMH). These findings suggest that wheat bran may be useful as a dietary supplement for preventing colon cancer or for treatment as an adjuvant agent.

Another useful model of colon carcinogenesis is the Apc$^{Min/+}$ mouse. This model develops colon cancer spontaneously because there is a dominant germline mutation at codon 850 of the human gene homolog adenomatous polyposis colon (Apc) (McCart *et al.*, 2008). Adenomatous polyps decreased in total number (by 76%) and size (65% <1 mm diameter, 67% 1–2 mm, and 87% >2 mm) in Apc$^{Min/+}$ mice fed with a diet supplemented with red grape powder containing proanthocyanidins and dietary fiber (GADF) compared to those animals that received control diet for 6 weeks (Sánchez-Tena *et al.*, 2013). These effects were mainly associated with cell cycle arrest in phase G_1 through GADD45 upregulation, as well as downregulation of cyclin D and genes related to the immune response and inflammation such as CXCR4, T-cell receptor and CD28, and nuclear factor of activated T-cells (Sánchez-Tena *et al.*, 2013). These important findings showed that GADF specifically might be a promising chemopreventive agent against colon cancer in high-risk populations.

Other chemopreventive agents against colon cancer include prebiotics, such as inulin, which has been used in preclinical DMH-induced model. Hijová *et al.* (2013) evaluated the effect of inulin (80 g/kg of conventional feed) for 28 weeks on the activities of bacterial glycolytic enzymes, SCFAs levels, coliform and lactobacilli counts, proinflammatory cytokine and cyclooxygenase-2 (COX-2) expression, and NFκB in colon mucosa in Sprague–Dawley rats (DMH dose 21 mg/kg body weight 5 times at weekly intervals subcutaneously). They found that in the DMH group (without inulin) coliform counts diminished significantly ($p < 0.001$) and lactobacilli counts increased ($p < 0.001$), and butyrate and propionate were reduced. Inulin increased concentration of SCFAs ($p < 0.001$), however, and reduced the numbers of COX-2- and NFκB-positive cells in the mucous membrane and submucosa of colon. IL-2, TNFα, and IL-10 expressions in the jejunal mucosa were reduced. Taking these results together, Hijová *et al.* (2013) concluded that consumption of inulin by 28 weeks prevented pre-neoplastic changes and was anti-inflammatory.

Recently, Birt and Phillips (2014) have proposed that resistant starch diets modulate colon microbiota and consequently favor microorganisms that produce butyrate. Fischer 344 rats treated or not with AOM (20 mg/kg body weight for 2 weeks) were fed for 8.5 weeks with a diet supplemented with high amylose starch (HA7) or a more resistant processed starch by complexing steric acid (HA7-SA). They observed that although ACF decreased by 16% and 37% in AOM-treated animals and those fed with HA7 and HA7-SA, respectively, this reduction was not statistically significant compared to that in control groups. However, mucin-depleted foci were significantly reduced ($p < 0.05$) by 50% and 90% in the AOM-HA7 and AOM-HA7-SA groups, respectively. These effects were accompanied with changes in colonic bacterial microbiota. Both diets in AOM-treated animals significantly increased levels of *Bacteriodetes*, while *Firmicutes* and *Proteobacteria* were reduced with respect to animals fed a conventional diet. In particular, the *Actinobacteria* were reduced in the group fed the HA7-SA diet.

These latest results led to an ongoing project trying to answer the following questions: Are levels of butyrate and other SCFAs sufficiently elevated to prevent the development of colorectal cancer? Are other microbial metabolites beneficial to the host in preventing cancerous lesion development? The answers to these questions will be important in understanding the mechanisms involved and the impact of dietary fiber on the intestinal microbiota and its role on colon cancer prevention, control, and treatment (Birt and Phillips, 2014).

7.3.3 Human Intervention Studies

The results obtained from studies *in vitro* and *in vivo* support the evaluation of dietary fiber and prebiotics in early-phase chemoprevention trials. One of the first studies of human intervention with dietary fiber was performed by DeCosse *et al.* (1989) in a group of 58 individuals with familial adenomatous polyposis (FAP) over a 4-year period. The subjects were followed with protosigmoidoscopy every 3 months. Individuals were distributed into three groups: (i) a control group that received a low fiber supplement (2.2 g/day) + placebo, (ii) a group receiving low fiber supplement (2.2 g/day) + vitamin C (4 g/day) + vitamin E (400 mg/day), and (iii) a group receiving a high fiber supplement (22.5 g/day) + vitamin C (4 g/day) + vitamin E (400 mg/day). DeCosse *et al.* (1989) found that the protective effect of fiber supplement was low compared to control group. However, polyp was signficantly reduced when consumption of dietary fiber in addition to supplement was continuous. Vitamins C and E had no significant protective effect. A similar result was obtained in a phase III study in 655 patients with a clinical history of colorectal adenomas. In this study 198 patients received 3.5 g/day ispaghula husk fiber for 3 years. Recurrent adenoma risk increased (67%), and 58 of the patients developed at least one adenoma, showing an adverse effect on the recurrence of colorectal adenoma (Bonithon-Kopp *et al.*, 2000).

Similarly, Mathers *et al.* (2012) conducted a phase III study, the CAPP2 (Concerted Action Polyposis Prevention), which evaluated the efficacy of resistant starch (30 g/day) co-administered with aspirin (600 mg) in patients with hereditary risk for colorectal cancer. They reported that resistant starch had no protective effect in individuals with Lynch syndrome because after 52.7 months of intervention, participants developed 27 primary colorectal cancer, an incidence rate ratio (IRR) of 1.15 (95% confidence interval (CI) 0.66 – 2.00; $p = 0.61$). For those participants who completed 2 years of intervention they reported a hazard ratio of 1.09 (0.55 – 2.19, $p = 0.80$) and IRR of 0.98 (0.51 – 1.88, $p = 0.95$) without adverse effects.

The Toronto Polyp Prevention Study Group from Canada in 1994 assessed the effect of a low fat diet (50 g/day or 20 – 25%) + high fiber calories 50 g/day and fiber supplementation versus placebo (normal western diet, 33% high fat, and low fiber 16 g) in 201 randomized polypectomized patients. After 2 years of intervention, the patients were followed with colonoscopy, and the recurrence of adenomatous polyps between dietary groups was not significantly different. However, women who received the low fat/high fiber diet showed a non-significant 50% reduction (relative risk (RR) 0.5; 95% CI 0.2 – 1.9) in polyp recurrence associated with low fecal bile acid concentration. On the other hand, men in the low fat/higher fiber diet group had an increased recurrence of polyps by 90% (RR 1.9; 95% CI 0.8 – 4.4) with respect to the control group, as well as in fecal bile acid concentration (McKeown-Eyssen *et al.*, 1994). In contrast, the Australian Polyp Prevention Project found that a low fat diet (<25% energy) combined with wheat bran supplementation (25 g) significantly reduced the occurrence of adenomas (>10 mm) after 2 and 4 years of follow-up ($p < 0.035$). However, in the same study neither low fat diet nor wheat bran supplementation alone had a significant effect on adenoma recurrence. The results reported in both studies were attributed to the small sample size, high dropout at the end of study, no compliance with low fat/high fiber diet, and short track. Specifically, in the Australia project the use of large adenomas (>1 cm) as a secondary endpoint led to a small number of subjects (McKeown-Eyssen *et al.*, 1994; MacLennan *et al.*, 1995).

Subsequently, the Polyp Prevention Trial, a multicenter study from United States, tried to show for 8 years the reducing effect of a low fat (20% fat calories), high fiber (18 g/1000 kcal day), high fruit and vegetables (3.5 servings/day 1000) on the recurrence of adenomatous polyps in patients (405) and control group (396 participants). This trial had 90% power to achieve 24% reduction in adenoma recurrence/year (Lanza *et al.*, 2007). This study was performed in two phases. During the first 4 years the recurrence of colon adenomas was not significantly different between these groups compared to the control diet. Thus, the study was extended for 4 years under the hypothesis that the diets used affect early event colon carcinogenesis. However, this research failed to show any effect of a low fat, high fiber, high fruit and vegetable dietary pattern; the RR was 0.98 (0.88−1.09) compared to control group. Moreover, the cumulative recurrence of adenomas until the end of the study was 1.04 (0.98−1.09), and no significant differences were observed between intervention and control groups with respect to the RR for recurrence of an advanced adenoma (1.06; 0.81−1.39) or multiple adenomas (0.92; 0.77−1.10) (Lanza *et al.*, 2007).

In contrast to these studies, two trials have shown promising results: the Arizona Cancer Center single-arm study (Alberts *et al.*, 1990) and the Orafty®Synergy-1 study (Limburg *et al.*, 2011). In the Arizona Cancer Center single-arm study, the effect of wheat bran fiber supplementation (13.5 g/day) for 8 weeks was evaluated in 17 subjects who had undergone colon or rectal cancer resection. Researchers found a significant reduction of cell proliferation based on ^{3}H-thymidine-labeling index. However, this index has not been accepted as an appropriate biomarker for colorectal cancer (Alberts *et al.*, 1990). Later, this research group analyzed fecal bile acid concentrations from 100 patients with previous colorectal adenomas. Patients were supplemented with 2.0 or 13.5 g/day wheat bran fiber and calcium carbonate 250 or 1500 mg/day for 9 months, the overall fiber ranging from 14.4 to 17.5 g/day and 25.7 to 28.7 g/day in the low and high fiber groups, respectively. They observed a 52% reduction ($p < 0.05$) of the total bile acid concentrations in the high fiber supplementation group compared to baseline (Alberts *et al.*, 1996, 1997).

In an intervention study in humans with prebiotic fiber made with Orafty®Synergy-1 (Pool-Zobel *et al.*, 2002) combined with *Lactobacillus rhamnosus* GG (LGG) and *Bifidobacterium lactis* Bb12 (BB12) an association was found between intake of this preparation and decreased risk of cancer in colon polypectomized patients. After 12 weeks of treatment, a reduction in DNA damage in the colonic mucosa and a tendency to decrease the proliferative activity of aberrant crypts was demonstrated. While these changes were observed, *Lactobacillus* and *Bifidobacterium* levels increased and *Clostridium perfringens* decreased (Rafter *et al.*, 2007).

Based on previous findings with Orafty®Synergy-1, Limburg *et al.* (2011) studied its effect (6 g twice daily) on the number of ACF and apoptosis of colon mucosa cells (biomarkers Ki67 and caspase-3), through a study of phase II clinical intervention for 6 months in subjects at risk for developing sporadic colorectal cancer. However, the intervention did not show convincing evidence of reduced risk for this cancer because the change in the percentage of ACF, levels of Ki67 and caspase-3 was not statistically significant compared to the control group (6 g maltodextrin). The measurement of biomarkers in the rectum affected the results of this trial (Limburg *et al.*, 2011).

Although low or no protective effects of dietary fiber (diet or supplements) in intervention studies in humans have been shown, there is no evidence of harmful effects in participants. These results should be interpreted with care, and should not be used to controvert the epidemiological findings, because intervention studies are based on *in vitro* and *in vivo* results to identify the mechanisms of action involved. The weakness of intervention studies affects the quality of results due to the short time tracking, insufficient sample sizes, and low compliance with dietary intervention, high dropout rates and the biomarkers used.

7.3.4 Epidemiological Evidence of Dietary Fiber Consumption and Colon Cancer Incidence

Epidemiological studies are important because they allow us to get conclusions about the effects of consumption of dietary fiber or respective sources on colon cancer prevention. The best evidence may be obtained from large-scale prospective studies on healthy people who are asked regularly about their dietary habits and have their colon cancer incidence followed for a long period. These types of studies lead to obtaining the RR that evaluates a dose–response relationship. RR values can be more than 1, equal to 1 or less than 1. If RR is >1 within CI it means there is increased risk; in contrast <1 indicates protection. Those studies with a CI that does not include the null value (RR = 1) are statistically significant.

Another type of epidemiological study, case–control studies compare a group of colon cancer patients with a healthy group (or patients who do not have disease). These studies are important to obtain information about dietary fiber or respective sources restrospectively and are more susceptible to mistakes. The results are presented as odds ratio (OR) which means the ratio of the odds of an event (eats dietary fiber) occurring in the group of colon cancer patients, to the odds of it occurring in the healthy group (control). OR values can be equal to 1, which indicates that dietary fiber consumption is equal in both groups, or <1, showing that the control group is more likely to intake dietary fiber than the group of patients, which would suggest that regular consumption of dietary fiber or respective sources may be associated with reduced risk of developing colon cancer. Taking into account these important epidemiological concepts, in this section we present some important epidemiological studies and findings about the protective role of dietary fiber against colon and/or colorectal cancer incidence.

Howe *et al.* (1992) published some of the first convincing evidence about the inverse association between dietary fiber intake and colon cancer risk in a meta-analysis of 13 case–control studies. This study compared 5287 subjects with colon cancer with 10 470 healthy control subjects from the United States.

They found 12 studies in which RR diminished significantly by 50% as fiber intake increased ($p < 0.0001$) and estimated that consumption of 13 g/day dietary fiber reduced the risk of colon cancer by 30%, similar to the finding of Trock *et al.* (1990), who reported an OR = 0.6 from a meta-analysis of 16 case–control studies. In contrast, a prospective study (Fuchs *et al.*, 1999) showed that there was no protective effect of total dietary fiber or dietary fiber intake from cereals, fruits, or vegetables against colon cancer or adenoma. However, the amount of dietary fiber ingested by the participants in this study was less than 9.8–24.9 g total dietary fiber, 1.0–4.8 g cereal fiber, 0.8–7.2 g fruit fiber, and vegetable fiber 2.7–10.9 g.

A case–control study was performed in the Swiss Canton of Vaud during 1992–2000 to evaluate the relationship between colorectal cancer risk and consumption of different types of dietary fiber (Levi *et al.*, 2001). This study included 550 controls and 286 colorectal cancer patients (149 colon and 137 rectal cancers) and used a food frequency questionnaire (FFQ). A significant inverse association between total fiber intake (non-starch polysaccharides) and its components with the risk of colorectal cancer was found. The OR values calculated for total fiber, soluble non-cellulose polysaccharides (NCPs), total insoluble fiber, cellulose, insoluble NCPs, and lignin were 0.57, 0.55, 0.58, 0.57, 0.62, and 0.62, respectively. The protection varied according to the source of the fiber: fruit fiber (OR 0.78) has an important protective effect against colorectal cancer compared to vegetables (OR 0.60) and grain fiber (0.74) (Levi *et al.*, 2001).

In agreement with these results, a case–control study was performed by Peters *et al.* (2003) within the Prostate, Lung, Colorectal, and Ovarian (PLCO) Cancer Screening Trial. High consumption of dietary fiber from grains, cereals, and fruits, but not from legumes or vegetables, was strongly and inversely associated with adenoma risk (Peters *et al.*, 2003). This study compared 33 971 people who were sigmoidoscopy-negative for colon adenomatous polyps with 3591 cases with at least one identified adenoma in the distal colon, using an FFQ including 137 items to evaluate the relation between dietary fiber consumption and frequency of colorectal adenoma. People in the highest quintile of dietary fiber intake (36.4 g/day) had 27% lower risk of adenoma than those in the lowest quintile (12.6 g/day) (95% CI = 14–38, $p_{\text{trend}} = 0.002$).

An important prospective study called the EPIC, performed in 10 European countries, analyzed 519 978 participants aged 25–70 years old who completed an FFQ and were followed-up for colorectal cancer incidence during 1992–1998. The aim was to determine the association between dietary fiber consumption and incidence of colorectal cancer. Follow-up consisted of 1939011 person-years and 1065 cases of colorectal cancer were reported. Similar to the previous study, a protective effect of dietary fiber was observed. The EPIC study found that in populations with low average intake of dietary fiber, an approximate doubling of total fiber intake from foods could reduce the risk of colorectal cancer by 40%. The adjusted RR was 0.75, 95% CI 0.59–0.95 to incidence of colon cancer for the highest versus lowest quintile of intake. An important finding from this research was that no food source of fiber was significantly more protective than others. Non-food dietary fiber supplementation was not considered in this research (Bingham *et al.*, 2003).

A new analysis from the EPIC study was performed by Murphy *et al.* (2012) to investigate whether an inverse association between dietary fiber intake and colorectal cancer risk exists after 11 years of follow-up, and whether this association is changed by sex and tumor localization. This new EPIC analysis included 4517 people with colorectal cancer, for whom consumption of fruit, vegetable, cereal, and total fiber was estimated by using FFQ. The study confirmed that total dietary fiber was inversely associated with colorectal cancer risk. The hazard ratio (HR) was 0.87, 95% CI 0.79–0.96 with increased intake of 10 g/day. A similar result was observed for colon and rectal cancers. This association was not affected by sex or other variables (dietary habits, lifestyle, age, anthropometric factors). In relation to the fiber sources, dietary fiber sources from cereals, fruits, and vegetables were similarly associated with colon cancer. For rectal cancer, only cereal fiber was inversely associated with rectal cancer (Murphy *et al.*, 2012). In conclusion, these findings support the protective role against colon cancer shown in previous studies.

Two cohorts from the Adventist Health Study-1 of 1976 and the Adventist Health Study-2 during 2002–2005 were analyzed. This research included 2818 participants with high risk of colon adenomatous polyps. The research concluded that individuals who consume low amounts of fiber from vegetables had a higher risk of developing colon adenomatous polyps (95% CI 0.51–0.99, OR = 0.71 highest vs. lowest quartile). Moreover, this study showed the best dose–response effect with vegetable fiber involving legumes (95% CI 0.47–0.90, OR = 0.65; $p < 0.02$) (Tantamango *et al.*, 2011).

The prospective Scandinavian HELGA study cohort examined the association between consumption of dietary fiber contained in vegetables, fruits, potatoes, and cereals and risk of colon cancer by stratifying distal and proximal colon and rectal cancer. In this study 691 colon and 477 rectal cancer cases were followed for 11.3 years. The IRR estimated was related to the consumption of total or specific fiber source. This study reported for the first time the quantity of specific fiber source that protects against colon cancer. Women who increased their intake of cereal fiber by 2 g/day had a lower risk of colon cancer, with IRR = 0.97 (95% CI 0.93–1.00). Similar results were obtained for men for increased total fiber intake 10 g/day (IRR = 0.74; 95% CI 0.64–0.86) and increased cereal fiber or cereal fiber enriched food intake by 2 g/day (IRR = 0.94; 95% CI 0.91–0.98). Thus, contrary to the Adventist Study this research showed that cereal fiber has a protective effect against colon cancer (Hansen *et al.*, 2012).

As mentioned earlier, high dietary fiber intake on its own is not enough to protect the colon mucosa against carcinogenesis, healthy dietary habits are also important. This hypothesis was evaluated by Fu *et al.* (2014), who looked at whether smoking affects the protective role of dietary fiber. This case–control study included 3184 controls and 2275 cases from the Tennessee Colorectal Polyp Study during 2003–2010, in which dietary fiber consumption was estimated by FFQ. They confirmed that consumption of high dietary fiber was associated with reduced risk of colorectal polyps ($p_{\text{trend}} = 0.003$). This association was stronger among cigarette smokers with high risk of colon adenomatous polyps, who had smoked longer than 23 years. For adenomatous polyps the association between smoking and dietary fiber intake was stronger ($p_{\text{interaction}} = 0.09$)

with a 38% reduction for risk of high-risk adenomatous polyps associated with high intake of dietary fiber compared with smokers with low consumption of dietary fiber. Therefore, this study demonstrates that consumption of dietary fiber may modify the risk for colon cancer and protect the colon mucosa against cigarette carcinogens (Fu *et al.*, 2014).

Recently, Song *et al.* (2015) published the results of a case–control study in 265 cases (105 colon cancer, 144 rectal cancer and 16 colon cancer and rectal cancer) and 252 controls from China to analyze the effect of dietary fiber consumption on the risk of colorectal cancer stratified by tumor site, employing a 121-item FFQ. They found an inverse association between total fiber consumption and colorectal, colon, and rectal cancer (Q4 vs. Q1: OR = 0.44, 95% CI 0.27–0.73; OR = 0.40, 95% CI 0.21–0.76; OR = 0.52, 95% CI 0.29–0.91, respectively). The OR values were similar according to vegetable fiber consumption and tumor site (Q4 vs. Q1: colorectal OR = 0.51, 95% CI 0.31–0.85; colon OR = 0.48, 95% CI 0.25–0.91; rectal OR = 0.53, 95% CI, 0.29–0.97). Moreover, inverse associations were found between soluble fiber and insoluble fiber and colorectal and colon cancers (Song *et al.*, 2015).

7.4 Future Directions: Food Designs New Structures for Colon Cancer Prevention

Dietary fiber is often used in the development or design of new foods to offer alternative ways to achieve compliance with recommendations for dietary fiber consumption. The use of dietary fiber for the treatment of diseases, however, has been challenging because clinical studies to establish doses and support the recommendations are required.

The formulation and development of new food products with added ingredients and innovative nutritional properties such as inulin, polydextrose, carboxymethylcellulose (CMC), pectin, and fructo-oligosaccharides (FOS), considered to be fiber, have shown increased use by the food industry. These ingredients, in addition to providing fiber to the body, improve the organoleptic characteristics of the products containing them and are highly fermentable in the gut by colonic bacteria (New Nutrition Business, 2013).

Of the various dietary fibers with functional properties, prebiotic fiber has been the most studied. Research into the characteristics of the structure, for example, of inulin and FOS, have allowed rheological and sensory characteristics to be modified. These non-digestible carbohydrates are found in natural sources such as bananas (*Musa paradisiaca*), garlic (*Allium sativum*), onion leek (*Allium ampeloprasum* var. *porrum*), chicory (*Cichorium intybus* var. *sativum*) and artichoke (*Cynaras colymus*). These fibers are obtained by β-furanosidase and β-inulinase fructosyl-transferase enzymatic reaction (Sabater, 2008).

The application of FOS functionality in foodstuffs provides design features related to the organoleptic aspects, microstructural, mechanical/physical, and chemical properties of food (Sequeira, 2005). The main functional properties evaluated are the water-holding capacity, viscosity, susceptibility to fermentation, substance absorption capacity, and particle size (Conesa *et al.*, 2004; Martínez-Cervera *et al.*, 2012).

Other food components that have been studied for the development of foods with chemopreventive properties for colon cancer are antioxidants such as the polyphenols (Bembu, 2013; Gaviria *et al.*, 2009). Polyphenols are natural compounds found in fruits, vegetables, cereals, and beverages. Fruits such as grapes, apples, pears, cherries, and berries contain 200–300 mg polyphenols per 100 g fresh weight and products made from these fruits may contain polyphenols in significant quantities.

Thus, the use of dietary fiber in food design has evolved not just because of its physiological effect, but also as a useful strategy for preventing diseases related to low dietary fiber intake. Moreover, the nutritional advantages of FOS with its prebiotic effect enables its effective use for bowel function and colonic bacteria.

7.5 Conclusions

Experts in colon cancer and gastroenterology agree that regular consumption of dietary fiber as a component of the human diet in recommended quantities protects against the development of colon cancer. *In vitro* studies provide evidence of mechanisms mediated primarily by butyrate, propionate, and acetate. These findings, together with the evidence from animal studies, validate its protective efficacy in the initiation and promotion stages of colon carcinogenesis. However, the results obtained from clinical studies in humans with dietary fiber do not correspond to the effects observed in *in vitro*, *in vivo*, and epidemiological studies due to errors in design and the compliance of participants. This has prevented a recommended dose definition for use as a chemopreventive agent for at risk populations. One of the challenges of modern medicine and the food industry is the definition of a dose and design of functional food using dietary fiber as a bioactive ingredient for intervention patients and individuals at risk. The challenge for researchers is to demonstrate the functional difference and effectiveness for each type of dietary fiber in the prevention and treatment of colon cancer.

References

Ajila CM, Leelavathi K, Prasada U. (2008). Improvement of dietary fiber content and antioxidant properties in soft dough biscuits with the incorporation of mango peel powder. *J Cereal Sci* 48:319–326.

Alberts DS, Einspahr J, Rees-McGee S, Ramanujam P, Buller MK, Clark L, *et al.* (1990). Effects of dietary wheat bran fiber on rectal epithelial cell proliferation in patients with resection for colorectal cancer. *J Natl Cancer Inst* 82:1280–1285.

Alberts DS, Ritenbaugh C, Story JA, Aickin M, Rees-McGee S, Buller MK, *et al.* (1996). Randomized, double-blinded placebo controlled study of effect of wheat bran fiber and calcium on fecal bile acids in patients with resected adenomatous colon polyps. *J Natl Cancer Inst* 88:81–92.

Alberts DS, Einspahr J, Ritenbaugh C, Aickin M, Rees-McGee S, Atwood J, *et al.* (1997). The effect of wheat bran fiber and calcium supplementation on rectal mucosal proliferation rates in patients with resected adenomatous colorectal polyps. *Cancer Epidemiol Biomarkers Prevent* 6:161–169.

American Association of Cereal Chemists (AACC). (2001). Dietary Fiber Technical Committee. The definition of dietary fiber. *Cereal Foods World* 46:112.

American College of Gastroenterology (ACG) (2000). American gastroenterological association medical position statement: impact of dietary fiber on colon cancer occurrence. *Gastroenterology* 118:1233–1234.

Anderson JW, Baird P, Davis R, Ferreri S, Knudtson M, Koraym A, *et al.* (2009). Health benefits of dietary fiber. *Nutr Rev* 67:188–205.

Archer SY, Johnson J, Kim HJ, Ma Q, Mou H, Daesety V, *et al.* (2005). The histone deacetylase inhibitor butyrate downregulates cyclin B1 gene expression via a p21/WAF-1-dependent mechanism in human colon cancer cells. *Am J Physiol Gastrointest Liver Physiol* 289:G696–G703.

Baena R, Salinas P (2015). Diet and colorectal cancer. *Maturitas* 80:258–264.

Bailón E, Cueto-Sola M, Utrilla P, Rodríguez-Cabezas ME, Garrido-Mesa N, *et al.* (2010). Butyrate in vitro immune-modulatory effects might be mediated through a proliferation-related induction of apoptosis. *Immunobiology* 215:863–873.

Balanzà R (2007). Efectos metabólico-terapéuticos a corto y largo plazo de la suplementación con fibra dietética. *Doctoral thesis*, Universitat Rovira I Virgili, Tarragona.

Barcenilla A, Pryde SE, Martin JC, Duncan SH, Stewart CS, Henderson C, *et al.* (2000). Phylogenetic relationships of butyrate-producing bacteria from the human gut. *Appl Environ Microbiol* 66:1654–1661.

Bembu (2013). *Fighting foods & drinks.* http://bembu.com/cancer-fighting-foods (accessed August 27, 2015).

Beyer-Sehlmeyer G, Glei M, Hartmann E, Hughes R, Persin C, Bohm V, *et al.* (2003). Butyrate is only one of several growth inhibitors produced during gut flora-mediated fermentation of dietary fibre sources. *Br J Nutr* 90:1057–1070.

Bingham SA, Day NE, Luben R, Ferrari P, Slimani N, Norat T, *et al.*; European Prospective Investigation into Cancer and Nutrition (2003). Dietary fibre in food and protection against colorectal cancer in the European Prospective Investigation into Cancer and Nutrition (EPIC): an observational study. *Lancet* 361:1496–1501.

Birt DF, Phillips GJ (2014). Diet, genes, and microbes: complexities of colon cancer prevention. *Toxicol Pathol* 42:182–188.

Blottière HM, Buecher B, Galmiche JP, Cherbut C (2003). Molecular analysis of the effect of short-chain fatty acids on intestinal cell proliferation. *Proc Nutr Soc* 62:101–106.

Boffa LC, Lupton JR, Mariani MR, Ceppi M, Newmark HL, Scalmati A, *et al.* (1992). Modulation of colonic epithelial cell proliferation, histone acetylation, and luminal short chain fatty acids by variation of dietary fiber (wheat bran) in rats. *Cancer Res* 52:5906–5912.

Boivin GP, Washington K, Yang K, Ward JM, Pretlow TP, Russell R, *et al.* (2003). Pathology of mouse models of intestinal cancer: consensus report and recommendations. *Gastroenterology* 124:762–777.

Bonithon-Kopp C, Kronborg O, Giacosa A, Rath U, Faivre J (2000). Calcium and fibre supplementation in prevention of colorectal adenoma recurrence: a randomised intervention trial. European Cancer Prevention Organisation Study Group. *Lancet* 356:1300–1306.

Brown AJ, Goldsworthy SM, Barnes AA., Eilert MM, Tcheang L, Daniels D, *et al.* (2003). The Orphan G protein-coupled receptors GPR41 and GPR43 are activated by propionate and other short chain carboxylic acids. *J Biol Chem* 278:11312–11319.

Bruce WR (2003). Counterpoint: from animal models to prevention of colon cáncer. Criteria for proceeding from preclinical studies and choice of models for prevention studies. *Cancer Epidemiol Biomarkers Prevent* 12:401–404.

Bultman SJ (2014). Molecular pathways: gene–environment interactions regulating dietary fiber induction of proliferation and apoptosis via butyrate for cancer prevention. *Clin Cancer Res* 20:799–803.

Chen HM, Yu YN, Wang JL, Lin YW, Kong X, Yang CQ, *et al.* (2013). Decreased dietary fiber intake and structural alteration of gut microbiota in patients with advanced colorectal adenoma. *Am J Clin Nutr* 97:1044–1052

Chuang SC, Vermeulen R, Sharabiani MT, Sacerdote C, Fatemeh SH, Berrino F, *et al.* (2011). The intake of grain fibers modulates cytokine levels in blood. *Biomarkers* 16:504–510.

Clarke JM, Topping DL, Bird Ar, Young GP, Cobiac L (2008). Effects of high-amylose maize starch and butyrylated high amylose maize starch on azoxymethane-induced intestinal cancer in rats. *Carcinogenesis* 29:2190–2194.

Comalada M, Bailón E, de Haro O, Lara-Villoslada F, Xaus J, Zarzuelo A, Gálvez J (2006). The effects of short-chain fatty acids on colon epithelial proliferation and survival depend on the cellular phenotype. *J Cancer Res Clin Oncol* 132:487–497.

Conesa DP, Martínez GL, Berruezo GFR (2004). Principales prebióticos y sus efectos en la alimentación humana. *In An Vet Murcia* 20:5–20.

Conlon MA, Kerr CA, McSweeney CS, Dunne RA, Shaw JM, Kang S, *et al.* (2012). Resistant starches protect against colonic DNA damage and alter microbiota and gene expression in rats fed a Western diet. *J Nutr* 142:832–840.

Corte Osorio LY, Martínez Flores HE, Ortiz Alvarado R (2011). Effect of dietary fiber in the quantitative expression of butyrate receptor GPR43 in rats colon. *Nutr Hosp* 26:1052–1058.

Cummings JH, Macfarlane GT (1991). The control and consequences of bacterial fermentation in the human colon. *J Appl Bacteriol* 70:443–459.

Cummings JH, Pomare EW, Branch WJ, Naylor CP, Macfarlane GT (1987). Short chain fatty acids in human large intestine, portal, hepatic and venous blood. *Gut* 28:1221–1227.

DeCosse JJ, Miller HH, Lesser ML (1989). Effect of wheat fiber and vitamins C and E on rectal polyps in patients with familial adenomatous polyposis. *J Natl Cancer Inst* 81:1290–1297.

De Vadder F, Kovatcheva-Datchary P, Goncalves D, Vinera J, Zitoun C, Duchampt A, *et al.* (2014). Microbiota-generated metabolites promote metabolic benefits via gut-brain neural circuits. *Cell* 156:84–96.

Donohoe DR, Collins LB, Wali A, Bigler R, Sun W, Bultman SJ (2012). The Warburg effect dictates the mechanism of butyrate-mediated histone acetylation and cell proliferation. *Mol Cell* 48(4):612–626.

Ebert MN, Beyer-Sehlmeyer G, Liegibel UM, Kautenburger T, Becker TW, Pool-Zobel BL (2001). Butyrate induces glutathione S-transferase in human colon cells and protects from genetic damage by 4-hydroxy-2-nonenal. *Nutr Cancer* 41:156–164.

Emenaker NJ, Calaf GM, Cox D, Basson MD, Qureshi N (2001). Short-chain fatty acids inhibit invasive human colon cancer by modulating uPA, TIMP-1, TIMP-2, mutant p53, Bcl-2, Bax, p21 and PCNA protein expression in an in vitro cell culture model. *J Nutr* 131:3041S–3046S.

Ferguson LR (2005). Does a diet rich in dietary fibre really reduce the risk of colon cancer? *Dig Liver Dis* 37:139–141.

Fiala ES (1977). Investigations into the metabolism and mode of action of the colon carcinogens 1,2-dimethylhydrazine and azoxymethane. *Cancer* 40:2436–2445.

Food and Agriculture Organization (FAO) (1997). *Producción y Manejo de Datos de Composición Química de Alimentos en Nutrición*. Santiago de Chile, Chile.

Fu Z, Shrubsole MJ, Smalley WE, Ness RM, Zheng W (2014). Associations between dietary fiber and colorectal polyp risk differ by polyp type and smoking status. *J Nutr* 144:592–598.

Fuchs CS, Giovannucci EL, Colditz GA, Hunter DJ, Stampfer MJ, Rosner B, *et al.* (1999). Dietary fiber and the risk of colorectal cancer and adenoma in women. *N Engl J Med* 340:169–176.

Fung KY, Cosgrove L, Lockett T, Head R, Topping DL (2012). A review of the potential mechanisms for the lowering of colorectal oncogenesis by butyrate. *Br J Nutr* 108:820–831.

Garrett WS, Gordon JI, Glimcher LH (2010). Homeostasis and inflammation in the intestine. *Cell* 140:859–870.

Gaviria C A, Ochoa CI, Sánchez N, Medina C, Lobo M, Tamayo A, *et al.* (2009). Propiedades antioxidantes de los frutos de agraz o mortiño (*Vaccinium meridionale* Swartz). In *Perspectivas del cultivo de agraz o mortiño en la zona altoandina de Colombia*. Universidad Nacional de Colombia, Bogotá, pp. 95–112.

Glei M, Hofmann T, Kuster K, Hollmann J, Lindhauer MG, Pool-Zobel BL (2006). Both wheat (*Triticum aestivum*) bran arabinoxylans and gut flora-mediated fermentation products protect human colon cells from genotoxic activities of 4-hydroxynonenal and hydrogen peroxide. *J Agric Food Chem* 54:2088–2095.

Grubben MJ, Nagengast FM, Katan MB, Peters WH (2001). The glutathione biotransformation system and colorectal cancer risk in humans. *Scand J Gastroenterol* 68–76.

Guarner F, Malagelada JR (2003a). Gut flora in health and disease. *Lancet* 361:512–519.

Guarner F, Malagelada JR (2003b). Prebióticos y probióticos: mecanismos de acción y sus aplicaciones clínicas. La flora bacteriana del tracto digestivo. *Gastroenterol Hepatol* 26(Suppl 1):1–5.

Guarner F, Malagelada JR (2003c). Role of bacteria in experimental colitis. *Best Pract Res Clin Gastroenterol* 17(5):793–804.

Hambly RJ, Saunders M, Rijken PJ, Rowland IR (2002). Influence of dietary components associated with high or low risk of colon cancer apoptosis in the rat colon. *Food Chem Toxicol* 40:801–808.

Hanada T, Kobayashi T, Chinen T, Saeki K, Takaki H, Koga K, *et al.* (2006). IFNgamma-dependent, spontaneous development of colorectal carcinomas in SOCS1-deficient mice. *J Exp Med* 203:1391–1397.

Hansen L, Skeie G, Landberg R, Lund E, Palmqvist R, Johansson I, *et al.* (2012). Intake of dietary fiber, especially from cereal foods, is associated with lower incidence of colon cáncer in the HELGA cohort. *Int J Cancer* 131:469–478.

Hayes JD, Flanagan JU, Jowsey IR (2005). Glutathione transferases. *Annu Rev Pharmacol Toxicol* 45:51–88.

Hijová E, Szabadosova V, Štofilová J, Hrčková G (2013). Chemopreventive and metabolic effects of inulin on colon cancer development. *J Vet Sci* 14:387–393.

Howe GR, Benito E, Castelleto R, Cornée J, Estève J, Gallagher RP, *et al.* (1992). Dietary intake of fiber and decreased risk of cancers of the colon and rectum: evidence from the combined analysis of 13 case control studies. *J Natl Cancer Inst* 84:1887–1896.

Hughes R, Rowland IR. (2002). Stimulation of apoptosis by two prebiotic chicory fructans in the rat colon. *Carcinogenesis* 22:43–47.

IARC (International Agency for Research on Cancer) (2011). GLOBOCAN 2012: Estimated cancer incidence, mortality and prevalence worldwide in 2012. http://globocan.iarc.fr/Pages/fact_sheets_cancer.aspx (accessed August 2016).

Kaewprasert S, Okada M, Aoyama Y (2001). Nutritional effects of cyclodextrins on liver and serum lipids and cecal organi acids in rats. *J Nutr Sci Vitaminol* 47:335–339.

Kautenburger T, Beyer-Sehlmeyer G, Festag G, Haag N, Kuhler S, Kuchler A, *et al.* (2005). The gut fermentation product butyrate, a chemopreventive agent, suppresses glutathione S-transferase theta (hGSTT1) and cell growth more in human colon adenoma (LT97) than tumor (HT29) cells. *J Cancer Res Clin Oncol* 131:692–700.

Kiefer J, Beyer-Sehlmeyer G, Pool-Zobel BL (2006). Mixtures of SCFA, composed according to physiologically available concentrations in the gut lumen, modulate histone acetylation in human HT29 colon cancer cells. *Br J Nutr* 96:803–810.

Kim YI (2000). AGA technical review: impact of dietary fiber on colon cancer occurrence. *Gastroenterology* 18:1235–1257.

Klampfer L, Huang J, Sasazuki T, Shirasawa S, Augenlicht L (2003). Inhibition of interferon gamma signaling by the short chain fatty acid butyrate. *Mol Cancer Res* 1:855–862.

Lanza E, Yu B, Murphy G, Albert PS, Chan B, Marshall JR, *et al.*; Polyp Prevention Trial Study Group (2007). The polyp prevention trial continued follow-up study: No effect of a low-fat, high-fiber, high-fruit and vegetable diet on adenoma recurrence eight years after randomization. *Cancer Epidemiol Biomarkers Prevent* 16:1745–1752.

Lattimer JM, Haub MD (2010). Effects of dietary fiber and its components on metabolic health. *Nutrients* 2:1266–1289.

Layden BT, Angueira AR, Brodsky M, Durai V, Lowe WL (2013). Short chain fatty acids and their receptors: new metabolic targets. *Transl Res* 161:131–140.

Lazarova DL, Chiaro C, Wong T, Drago E, Rainey A, O'Malley S, *et al.* (2013). CBP activity mediates effects of the histone deacetylase inhibitor butyrate on WNT activity and apoptosis in colon cancer cells. *J Cancer* 4:481–490.

Le Leu RK, Brown IL, Hu Y, Esterman A, Young GP (2007). Suppression of azoxymethane-induced colon cancer development in rats by dietary resistant starch. *Cancer Biol Ther* 6:1621–1626.

Levi F, Pasche C, Lucchini F, La Vecchia C (2001). Dietary fibre and the risk of colorectal cancer. *Eur J Cancer* 37:2091–2096.

Limburg PJ, Mahoney MR, Ziegler KLA, Sontag SJ, Schoen RE, Benya R, *et al.* (2011). Randomized phase II trial of sulindac, atorvastatin, and prebiotic dietary fiber for colorectal cancer chemoprevention. *Cancer Prevent Res* 4(2):259–269.

López L, Suárez M. (2002). *Fundamentos de nutrición normal.* Ateneo, Argentina.

Lupton JR, Kurtz PP (1993). Relationship of colonic luminal shortchain fatty acids and pH to in vivo cell proliferation in rats. *J Nutr* 123:1522–1530.

MacLennan R, Macrae F, Bain C, Battistutta D, Chapuis P, Gratten H, *et al.* (1995). Randomized trial of intake of fat, fiber, and beta carotene to prevent colorectal adenomas. The Australian Polyp Prevention Project. *J Natl Cancer Inst* 87:1760–1766.

Martínez-Cervera S, Sanz T, Salvador A, Fiszman SM (2012). Rheological, textural and sensorial properties of low-sucrose muffins reformulated with sucralose/polydextrose. *LWT-Food Sci Technol* 45:213–220.

Mathers JC, Movahedi M, Macrae F, Mecklin JP, Moeslein G, Olschwang S, *et al.*; CAPP2 Investigators (2012). Long-term effect of resistant starch on cancer risk in carriers of hereditary colorectal cancer: an analysis from the CAPP2 randomised controlled trial. *Lancet Oncol* 13:1242–1249.

McCart AE, Vickaryous NK, Silver A (2008). Apc mice: models, modifiers and mutants. *Pathol Res Pract* 204:479–490.

McCrea GL, Miaskowski C, Stotts NA, Macera L, Paul SM, Varma MG (2009). Gender differences in self-reported constipation characteristics, symptoms, and bowel and dietary habits among patients attending a specialty clinic for constipation. *Gender Med* 6:259–271.

McKeown-Eyssen GE, Bright-See E, Bruce WR, Jazmaji V, the Toronto Polyp Prevention Group (1994). A randomized trial of a low fat high fibre diet in the recurrence of colorectal polyps. *J Clin Epidemiol* 47:525–536.

Michels KB, Edward Giovannucci, Joshipura KJ, Rosner BA, Stampfer MJ, Fuchs CS, *et al.* (2000). Prospective study of fruit and vegetable consumption and incidence of colon and rectal cancers. *J Natl Cancer Inst* 92:1740–1752.

Miyanishi K, Takayama T, Ohi M, Hayashi T, Nobuoka A, Nakajima T, *et al.* (2001). Glutathione S-transferase-pi overexpression is closely associated with K-ras mutation during human colon carcinogenesis. *Gastroenterology* 121:865–874.

Montenegro MA, Sánchez-Negrete M, Lértora WJ, Catuogno MS (2003). Focos de criptas displásicas inducidas con 1,2-dimetilhidrazina en intestine grueso de ratas tratadas con Molibdeno y tungsteno. *Rev Vet* 14:15–19.

Murphy N, Norat T, Ferrari P, Jenab M, Bueno-de-Mesquita B, Skeie G, *et al.* (2012). Dietary fibre intake and risks of cancers of the colon and rectum in the European Prospective Investigation into Cancer and Nutrition (EPIC). *Plos One* 7:1–10.

Nambiar PR, Girnun G, Lillo NA, Guda K, Whiteley HE, Rosenberrg DW (2003). Preliminary analysis of azoxymethane induced colon tumors in inbred mice commonly used as transgenic/knockout progenitors. *Int J Oncol* 22:145–150.

New Nutrition Business (2013). *12 Key Trends in Food*. http://www.new-nutrition.com/

Papanikolau A, Shanka A, Delker DA, Povey A (1998). Initial level of azoxymethane-induced DNA methyl adducts are not predictive of tumor susceptibility in inbred mice Toxicol. *Appl Pharmacol* 150:196–203.

Pesarini JR, Zaninetti PT, Mauro MO, Carreira CM, Dichi JB, Ribeiro LR, *et al.* (2013). Antimutagenic and anticarcinogenic effects of wheat bran in vivo. *Genet Mol Res* 12:1646–1659.

Peters U, Sinha R, Chatterjee N, Subar AF, Ziegler RG, Kulldorff M, *et al.*; Prostate, Lung, Colorectal, and Ovarian Cancer Screening Trial Project Team (2003). Dietary fibre and colorectal adenoma in a colorectal cancer early detection programme. *Lancet* 361:1491–1495.

Phillips GO (2011). An introduction: Evolution and finalisation of the regulatory definition of dietary fibre. *FoodHydrocolloids* 25:139–143.

Pool-Zobel B, van Loo J, Rowland I, Roberfroid MB (2002). Experimental evidences on the potential of prebiotic fructans to reduce the risk of colon cancer. *Br J Nutr* 87:S273–S281.

Rafter J, Bennett M, Caderni G, Clune Y, Hughes R, Karlsson PC, *et al.* (2007). Dietary synbiotics reduce cancer risk factors in polypectomized and colon cancer patients. *Am J Clin Nutr* 85:488–496.

Reddy BS (2000). Novel approaches to the prevention of colon cancer by nutritional manipulation and chemoprevention. *Cancer Epidemiol Biomarkers Prevent* 9:239–247.

Reddy BS (2004). Studies with azoxymethane – rat preclinical model for assessing colon tumor development and chemoprevention. *Environ Mol Mutagen* 44:26–35.

Reddy BS, Mori H (1981). Effect of dietary wheat bran and dehydrated citrus fiber on 3,29-dimethyl-4-aminobiphenyl–induced intestinal carcinogenesis in F344 rats. *Carcinogenesis* 2:21–25.

Reddy BS, Weisburger JH, Narisawa T, Wynder EL (1974). Colon carcinogenesis in germ-free rats with 1,2-dimethyl hydrazine and N-methyl1–n'–nitro-nitrosoguanidine. *Cancer Res* 34:2368–2372.

Reddy BS, Mori H, Nicolais M (1981). Effect of dietary wheat bran and dehydrated citrus fiber on azoxymethane-induced intestinal carcinogenesis in Fischer 344 rats. *J Natl Cancer Inst* 66:553–557.

Reddy BS, Maeura Y, Wayman M (1983). Effect of dietary corn bran and autohydrolyzed lignin on 3,29-dimethyl-4-aminobiphenyl–induced intestinal carcinogenesis in male F344 rats. *J Natl Cancer Inst* 71:419–423.

Renehan AG, O'Dwyer ST, Haboubi NJ, Potten CS (2002). Early cellular events in colorectal carcinogenesis. *Colorectal Dis* 4:76–89.

Richter M, Jurek D, Wrba F, Kaserer K, Wurzer G, Karner-Hanusch J, *et al.* (2002). Cells obtained from colorectal microadenomas mirror early premalignant growth patterns in vitro. *Eur J Cancer* 38:1937–1945.

Rosignoli P, Fabiani R, De BA, Spinozzi F, Agea E, Pelli MA, Morozzi G (2001). Protective activity of butyrate on hydrogen peroxide-induced DNA damage in isolated human colonocytes and HT29 tumour cells. *Carcinogenesis* 22:1675–1680.

Sabater M (2008). Efecto de las poliaminas y los FOS en la dieta sobre la maduración intestinal en cerdos destetatos precozmente. *Doctoral thesis*, Universidad de Murcia, Murcia. 211 pp. https://digitum.um.es/jspui/bitstream/10201/3945/1/SabaterMolina.pdf

Sánchez-Tena S, Lizárraga D, Miranda A, Vinardell MP, García-García F, Dopazo J, *et al.* (2013). Grape antioxidant dietary fiber inhibits intestinal polyposis in ApcMin/+ mice: relation to cell cycle and immune response. *Carcinogenesis* 34:1881–1888.

Scharlau D, Borowicki A, Habermann N, Hofmann T, Klenow S, Miene C. *et al.* (2009). Mechanisms of primary cancer prevention by butyrate and other products formed during gut flora-mediated fermentation of dietary fibre. *Mutat Res Rev Mutat Res* 682(1):39–53.

Sequeira AC (2005). Caracterización de propiedades relacionadas con la textura de suspensiones de fibras alimentarias. *Doctoral thesis*, Universitat Politècnica de València, Valencia.

Shah P, Nankova BB, Parab S, La EF (2006). Gamma, Short chain fatty acids induce TH gene expression via ERK-dependent phosphorylation of CREB protein. *Brain Res* 1107:13–23.

Sohn OS, Fiala ES, Requeijo SP, Weisburgerr JH, Gonzalez FJ (2001). Differential effects of CYP2E1 status on the metabolic activation of the colon carcinogens azoxymethane and methylazoxymethanol. *Cancer Res* 61:8435–8440.

Song Y, Liu M, Yang FG, Cui LH, Lu XY, Chen C (2015). Dietary fibre and the risk of colorectal cancer: a case-control study. *Asian Pac J Cancer Prev* 37:47–52.

Sporn MB, Dunlop NM, Newton DL, Smith JM (1976). Prevention of chemical carcinogenesis by vitamin A and its synthetic analogs (retinoids). *Fed Proc* 35(6):1332–1338.

Surh YJ (2003). Cancer chemoprevention with dietary phytochemicals. *Nat Rev Cancer* 3:768–780.

Tantamango YM, Knutsen SF, Beeson L, Fraser G, Sabate J (2011). Association between dietary fiber and incident cases of colon polyps: The Adventist Health Study. *Gastrointestinal Cancer Res* 4:161–167.

Tedelind S, Westberg F, Kjerrulf M, Vidal A (2007). Anti-inflammatory properties of the short-chain fatty acids acetate and propionate: A study with relevance to inflammatory bowel disease. *World J Gastroenterol* 13(20):2826–2832.

Trock B, Lanza E, Greenwald P (1990). Dietary fiber, vegetables, and colon cancer: critical review and meta-analyses of the epidemiologic evidence. *J Natl Cancer Inst* 82:650–661.

Tsai CW, Chen HW, Yang JJ, Sheen LY, Lii CK (2007). Diallyl disulfide and diallyl trisulfide up-regulate the expression of the pi class of glutathione S-transferase via an AP-1-dependent pathway. *J Agric Food Chem* 55:1019–1026.

Ushida K, Hatanaka H, Inoue R, Tsukahara T, Phillips G (2011). Effect of log term ingestion of gum arabic on the adipose tissues of female mice. *Food Hydrocolloids* 25:1344.

Valenzuela A, Maiz A (2006). El rol de la fibra dietética en la nutrición enteral. *Rev Chil Nutr* 33:342–351.

van Duijnhoven FJ, Bueno-De-Mesquita HB, Ferrari P, Jenab M, Boshuizen HC, Ros MM, *et al.* (2009). Fruit, vegetables, and colorectal cancer risk: the European Prospective Investigation into Cancer and Nutrition. *Am J Clin Nutr* 89:1441–1452.

Viladomiua M, Hontecillasa R, Yuanc L, Lua P, Bassaganya-Riera J (2013). Nutritional protective mechanisms against gut inflammation. *J Nutr Biochem* 24:929–939.

Wollowski GR, Pool-Zobel BL (2001). Protective role of probiotics and prebiotics in colon cancer. *Am J Clin Nutr* 73:451–455.

WCR/AICR (World Cancer Research Fund/American Institute for Cancer Research) (2007). *Food, Nutrition, Physical Activity, and the Prevention of Cancer: a Global Perspective.* AICR, Washington, DC, 537 pp.

WCR/AICR (2011). *Continuous Update Project Report. Food, Nutrition, Physical Activity, and the Prevention of Colorectal Cancer.* AICR, Washington, DC, 40 pp.

Yadav UC, Ramana KV, Awasthi YC, Srivastava SK (2008). Glutathione level regulates HNE-induced genotoxicity in human erythroleukemia cells. *Toxicol Appl Pharmacol* 227:257–264.

Yeum K-J, Russell R, Aldini G (2010). Antioxidant activity and oxidative stress: an overview. In *Biomarkers for Antioxidant Defense and Oxidative Damage: Principles and Practical Application* (eds. G Aldini, K-J Yeum, E Niki, RM Russel). Blackwell Publishing, Iowa, pp. 1–19.

Zamora-Ponce E, Lagos-Muñoz P, Rivera-Camaño P, Fernández-Romer J (2009). Un modelo experimental inducible en ratón para conducir estudios en quimioprevención y anticarcinogénesis. *Theoria* 17:71–86.

Zeng H, Briske-Anderson M (2005). Prolonged butyrate treatment inhibits the migration and invasion potential of HT1080 tumor cells. *J Nutr* 135:291–295.

Zeng H, Lazarova DL, Bordonaro M (2014). Mechanisms linking dietary fiber, gut microbiota and colon cancer prevention. *World J Gastrointest Oncol* 6:41–51.

Zeng H, Claycombe KJ, Reindl KM (2015). Butyrate and deoxycolic acid play common and distinct roles in HCT116 human colon cell proliferation. *J Nutr Biochem* May 15.

Zimmerman MA, Singh N, Martin PM, Thangaraju M, Ganapathy V, Waller JL, *et al.* (2012). Butyrate supresses colonic inflammation through HDAC-1 dependent Fas upregulation and Fas-mediated apoptosis of T cells. *Am J Physiol Gastrointest Liver Physiol* 302:G1405–G1415.

8

The Role of Fibers and Bioactive Compounds in Gut Microbiota Composition and Health

Émilie A. Graham[1], Jean-François Mallet[2], Majed Jambi[2], Nawal Alsadi[2] and Chantal Matar[3]

[1] *Faculty of Health Sciences, University of Ottawa, Ottawa, Ontario, Canada*
[2] *Faculty of Medicine, University of Ottawa, Ottawa, Ontario, Canada*
[3] *Faculty of Health Sciences and Faculty of Medicine, University of Ottawa, Ottawa, Ontario, Canada*

8.1 The Influence of Gut Microbiota in Health and Disease

Maintenance of health and protection against disease is greatly influenced by the interactions between the human immune system and the 10^{14} microbes residing on our gut mucosa, collectively known as our *gut microbiota* (Zhang *et al.*, 2015). The gut microbiota is now recognized as an important "organ" within the body that is involved in metabolic, immune, and endocrine functions. Emerging studies are pointing out the importance of microbiota in preventing disease, maintaining homeostasis, and even promoting longevity (Biteau *et al.*, 2010; Buela *et al.*, 2015; Rera *et al.*, 2011). Genomic analysis has revealed the great diversity of microbiota and its sensitivity to environmental changes, such as diet (David *et al.*, 2014; Lang *et al.*, 2014). In fact, the gut microbiota mostly consists of friendly, commensal bacteria, but is also home to archaea, eukaryotes, and viruses (Sankar *et al.*, 2015). Some of the main phyla in the gut include *Bacteroidetes, Firmicutes, Actinobacteria, Cyanobacteria, Fusobacteria, Proteobacteria,* and *Verrucomicrobia*, with the first two being the most numerous (Sankar *et al.*, 2015). From these phyla, there are many common species, including *Lactobacillus* and *Bacteroides* (Figure 8.1). These microbes play an important role in our everyday body functions, such as by producing vitamin K and biotin, regulating gut motility, transforming bile acid and steroids, metabolizing indigestible fibers such as cellulose, absorbing minerals, and managing toxins and mutagens (Sankar *et al.*, 2015; Zhang *et al.*, 2015). In addition, some microbes produce short-chain fatty acids (SCFAs) that provide energy to the colonic mucosa and peripheral body tissues, as well as influence colonic water absorption and fecal pH (Zhang *et al.*, 2015).

The shift in gut bacteria phyla dynamics is dependent on many factors. The microbial species acquired in infancy remain stable over time, but there is an increase in the diversity of bacterial species with age, starting at around

Dietary Fiber Functionality in Food and Nutraceuticals: From Plant to Gut, First Edition.
Edited by Farah Hosseinian, B. Dave Oomah and Rocio Campos-Vega.
© 2017 John Wiley & Sons Ltd. Published 2017 by John Wiley & Sons Ltd.

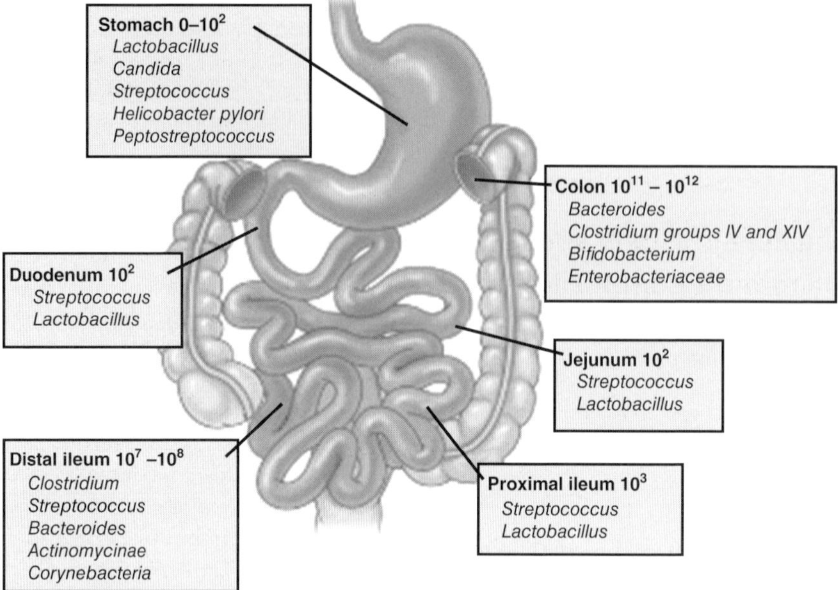

Figure 8.1 The gut microbiota is composed of a diverse number of bacterial species. Source: Sartor (2008). Reproduced with permission of Elsevier.

the age of 1 year, when solid foods are introduced to the diet (O'Toole, 2012; Palmer *et al.*, 2007). As we enter later stages of life, diversity decreases and individual differences increase (Claesson *et al.*, 2011). Bacterial composition starts being influenced early in life by delivery and feeding methods, and is influenced throughout life by factors such as geographical environment, diet, age, and prebiotic, probiotic, and antibiotic uptake (Garmendia *et al.*, 2012; Gueimonde and Collado, 2012; Kemppainen *et al.*, 2015; O'Toole, 2012; Tap *et al.*, 2015). It is important to manage these factors in order to maintain *gut homeostasis*; a balance between tolerating beneficial microbes and implementing proinflammatory responses toward harmful microbes that invade the body (Runtsch *et al.*, 2014).

If the balance is shifted in favor of the harmful microbes, or a *dysbiosis* of the microbial composition occurs, this can lead to an array of inflammatory-related illnesses, including chronic diseases such as obesity, inflammatory bowel disease, diabetes, inflammaging, and cancer to name a few (Claesson *et al.*, 2012; Devkota and Chang, 2015; Giongo *et al.*, 2011; Huycke *et al.*, 2002; Ley *et al.*, 2006). The mechanisms by which these diseases manifest as a result of dysbiosis will be discussed in detail later in this chapter. Dysbiosis can be driven by dietary changes or habits. For instance, human populations that consume less fiber in their diet have a greater incidence of inflammatory diseases, such as type 2 diabetes and colon cancer (Maslowski and Mackay, 2011). Another study showed that artificial sweeteners can lead to glucose intolerance by causing dysbiosis in the gut microbiota (Suez *et al.*, 2014). More precisely, it was demonstrated that individuals consuming large amounts of meat have bacteria of the genus *Bacteroides* more dominantly in their microbiota compared to individuals who consume a plant-based diet, in whom *Prevotella* is the dominant genus (David *et al.*, 2014). This pattern of microbiota disturbance in high meat consumers is linked to the prevalence of chronic disease in these individuals (David *et al.*, 2014; Wang *et al.*, 2008).

Gut homeostasis is maintained by optimal host–commensal interactions communicating through gut-associated lymphoid tissues (GALT) (Runtsch *et al.*, 2014). There are two lines of defense protecting against dysbiosis: the mechanical barrier and the immune barrier. The mechanical barrier is composed of polarized intestinal epithelial cells, enterocytes, and mucus lined in a single layer. The immune barrier consists of GALT, such as Peyer's patches and mesenteric lymph nodes, immunoglobulin A (IgA), lymphocytes, macrophages, neutrophils, and natural killer cells that mostly lie within the lamina propria layer of the intestinal mucosa (Zhang *et al.*, 2015). Commensal bacteria work with the host immune system to protect from invading microbes by competing with pathogenic microbes for nutrients and attachment sites on the mucosal wall (Barthel *et al.*, 2003; Biedermann and Rogler, 2015). Furthermore, they chemically prevent invasion by producing lactate and short-chain fatty acids (SCFAs) that lower colon pH and produce toxic or carcinogenic metabolites through fermentation that prevent the growth, or eliminate, invading pathogenic bacteria (Puertollano *et al.*, 2014; Zhong *et al.*, 2015). Moving to a more molecular level, the host immune system and commensal bacteria use *pathogen-associated molecular patterns (PAMPs)* and corresponding messengers to communicate with each other (Peterson *et al.*, 2015). For instance, when pathogens bind to pattern recognition receptors (PRRs) (e.g., Toll-like receptors (TLRs), nucleotide-binding oligomerization domain-like receptors (NOD-like receptors)) located on bacterial cell wall components (lipopolysaccharides (LPS) and peptidoglycan (PGN)), this can activate nuclear factor κB (NFκB), thus inducing the production of inflammatory *cytokines* (e.g., TNFα, interleukin-1B (IL-1B), and antimicrobial peptides) that send messages to the lymphocytes and natural killer cells that defend against these foreign microbes (Peterson *et al.*, 2015; Zhang *et al.*, 2015). This complex system will be further elucidated with examples as we explore the environmental factors that maintain gut homeostasis and diseases that may result from dysbiosis later in this chapter.

Nutrition plays a major role in the interactions between the gut microbiota and host immune system starting at the molecular level and results in either a healthy homeostatic microflora, or dysbiosis and an unhealthy body state (Figure 8.2). In this chapter, we will explore dietary compounds that promote a healthy gut microbiota composition, epidemiological studies looking at demographics that may influence the composition, and how fibers and bioactive compounds can protect against diseases resulting from dysbiosis in the gut microbiota.

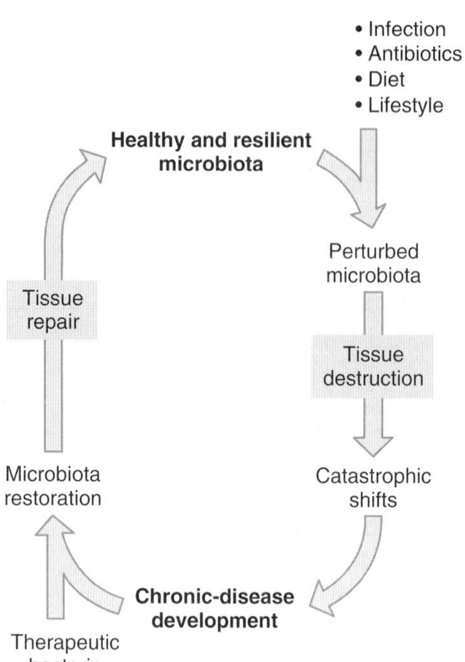

Figure 8.2 Environmental factors can cause inflammation and dysbiosis in the gut. Source: de Vos *et al.* (2013). Reproduced with permission of Elsevier.

8.2 Bioactive Substances and Fiber Promoting a Healthy Gut

How does our environment and diet influence our gut microbiota composition? One possible mechanism is through *epigenetics*: heritable changes to gene activity not attributable to changes in the DNA sequence (Hullar and Fu, 2014). Changes in gene activity may be due to DNA methylation, histone modification, or microRNA upregulation/downregulation (Teegarden *et al.*, 2012). These alterations work to either increase protein activity or limit it, changing important molecular pathways in the body. More specifically, *nutritional epigenetics* is the study of how nutritional compounds influence epigenetics. For example, curcumin (found in turmeric) suppresses histone acetylation by deactivating the histone acetyl transferase enzyme and also targets miR-21, preventing colorectal cancer metastasis (Mudduluru *et al.*, 2011; Vahid *et al.*, 2015). Other dietary compounds, such as fiber, polyphenols, and saponins, play an important role in maintaining gut microbiota homeostasis by influencing epigenetic mechanisms. An overview on the role of these compounds in health and disease will be given by reporting data from *in vitro, in vivo,* and clinical studies.

8.2.1 Fiber

Dietary fiber plays an important role in shaping our gut microbiota. Importantly, a high intake of fiber has been shown to lower the risk of several diseases, including obesity, type 2 diabetes, cardiovascular disease, and cancer to name a few (Cho *et al.*, 2013; Huang *et al.*, 2015; Kaczmarczyk *et al.*, 2012; Kunzmann *et al.*, 2015). Fiber supplementation is broken down into four categories: solubility, fermentability, viscosity, and gel forming ability (McRorie, 2015). Fiber solubility is its ability to dissolve in water or remain in clumps (Lattimer and Haub, 2010). For fibers that fit into this first category, viscosity refers to those that thicken when hydrated (Dikeman and Fahey, 2006). Gel formation is the ability of these viscous soluble fibers to form cross-links when hydrated (McRorie, 2015). The classification that these fibers fall under affects their fermentability by gut bacteria and, hence, their metabolite availability to the host. *Insoluble fibers* are poorly fermented, whereas *soluble fibers* are easily fermented (McRorie, 2015). Fibers that are able to be fermented are those that change the composition of the gut microbiota (Slavin, 2013). Additional classifications include dietary fibers and functional fibers. *Functional fibers* are synthesized or extracted from non-digestible forms of carbohydrates, whereas fruits and vegetables have *dietary fibers* that are non-digestible carbohydrates in their natural form (Slavin, 2013).

It is believed that fiber works partly by reducing the absorption of macronutrients and the contact time of carcinogens within the intestinal tract (Kaczmarczyk *et al.*, 2012). It is also believed that the digestion of dietary fiber by commensal bacteria in the gut creates metabolites that influence epigenetics. The better known metabolites for this influence are SCFAs. SCFAs include acetate, butyrate, and propionate, which are produced by the fermentation of dietary fiber by commensal gut bacteria (Kasubuchi *et al.*, 2015). In particular, SCFAs (butyrate and propionate) have been shown to epigenetically regulate gene expression by inhibiting histone deacetylase (Arpaia *et al.*, 2013; Cousens *et al.*, 1979; Kasubuchi *et al.*, 2015). Insoluble fibers, such as wheat bran, are non-fermentable, but soluble fibers like inulin can be fermented into SCFAs (Stewart *et al.*, 2009). Many studies have evaluated the influence of different types of fiber on gut microbiota at all levels, including *in vitro*, *in vivo*, and clinical studies.

8.2.1.1 *In Vitro* Studies

Although research on fiber has progressed to human subjects to date, it is valuable to go back and look at the fundamental influences of fiber on bacteria at the *in vitro* level. One study investigated the melanoidins derived from bread and their influence on gut microbiota species (Helou *et al.*, 2015). They found that bread melanoidins were partially digested by amylases and proteases and that the melanoidins reduced *Enterobacteria* spp. (Helou *et al.*, 2015). Since pathogenic *Enterobacteria* have been associated with inflammation, this suggests that bread melanoidins may play an anti-inflammatory role (Stecher *et al.*, 2013). A second study instead focused on inulin, a carbohydrate found in plants, and its effects on batch fermentation of human fecal microbiota (Jung *et al.*, 2015). Administration of inulin increased the ratio of *Lactobacillus* or *Bifidobacteria* to *Enterobacteria*, and increased butyrate production, both previously shown to be in favor of human gut health (Geirnaert *et al.*, 2015; Jung *et al.*, 2015; Ringel-Kulka *et al.*, 2015; Walter, 2008). These studies demonstrated potential anti-inflammatory response modulation by functional fibers.

8.2.1.2 *In Vivo* Studies

Numerous animal studies have reported the effects of fibers on gut microbiota. For instance, feeding rabbits four different diets of dietary neutral detergent fiber induced changes in the phyla *Bacteroidetes*, *Proteobacteria*, and *Verrucomicrobia*, with the latter two being influenced by age as well (Zhu *et al.*, 2015). This indicates that fiber positively influences the gut microbiota composition in rabbits. Another study used rats as an animal model and focused on whole grain barley and barley malt (Zhong *et al.*, 2015). Specifically, the male rats were fed barley or malt for 4 weeks and their fecal microbiota composition was analyzed (Zhong *et al.*, 2015). The barley group had increased abundance of *Verrucomicrobia* and *Actinobacteria*, but lower numbers of *Firmicutes* and *Deferribacteres* than the control group, whereas the malt group had higher abundance of *Turicibacter* and *Roseburia* (Zhong *et al.*, 2015). *Turicibacter* and *Roseburia* are butyric acid-producing bacteria with probiotic-like effects and thus may exert a protective effect against inflammatory diseases such as inflammatory bowel disease (IBD) (Geirnaert *et al.*, 2015; Zhong *et al.*, 2015). In the same vein, it has been demonstrated that soluble-resistant maltodextrin improved glucose tolerance in the mice and favored a higher abundance of probiotic-associated bacteria, such as *Lactobacillus* and *Bifidobacterium*, and reduced *Alistipes* and *Bacteroides*, which are associated with high fat/protein diets (David *et al.*, 2014; He *et al.*, 2015). These studies suggest that different types of fiber have diverse, but beneficial influences on gut microbiota composition.

8.2.1.3 Clinical Studies

Different clinical studies have consolidated the beneficial effects of fibers on microbiota and subsequently of health outcomes. During a 6-week nutritional trial, 19 healthy adults given a diet supplemented with dietary fiber were followed and their gut microbiotas were examined (Tap *et al.*, 2015). The study found that a high fiber diet enhanced gut microbiota richness and stability in all of the participants (Tap *et al.*, 2015). Furthermore, the dietary fiber was observed to modulate glycan metabolism pathways by influencing the expression of genes encoding carbohydrate-active enzymes (Tap *et al.*, 2015). Moreover, in a double-blind, placebo-controlled, and randomized study conducted on 21 healthy male participants, it was discovered that increased polydextrose or soluble corn fiber intake altered the *Bacteroidetes:Firmicutes* ratio in favor of the phylum *Bacteroidetes* (Holscher *et al.*, 2015). Polydextrose is a non-viscous functional fiber derived from glucose and sorbitol, and soluble corn fiber comes from cornstarch (Slavin, 2013). Previously, polydextrose was found to decrease *Bacteroides* and increase *Bifidobacterium* and *Lactobacillus* (Jie *et al.*, 2000).

This supports previous study, since both *Bacteroides* spp. and *Bifidobacteria* spp. are members of the phylum *Bacteroidetes*. Although the species *Bacteroides thetaiotaomicron* is known to be a symbiont, many *Bacteroides* spp. are known to be pathobionts, such as *Bacteroides fragilis* (Hoffmann *et al.*, 2015; Wu *et al.*, 2007). On the other hand, *Bifidobacteria* spp. are believed to be probiotic in nature (Masco *et al.*, 2005). In support of Holscher *et al.*'s observations, it was shown that the intake of the functional fiber inulin increased the levels of *Bifidobacterium adolescentis* and *Faecalibacterium prausnitzii* in a sample of 12 adults (Ramirez-Farias *et al.*, 2009). *F. prausnitzii* has a lower abundance in patients with IBD and has been shown to have anti-inflammatory effects (Lopez-Siles *et al.*, 2015; Miquel *et al.*, 2015). Members of the genus *Bifidobacterium*, including *B. adolescentis*, also exhibit anti-inflammatory effects (Okada *et al.*, 2009). A randomized, double-blind study examining the effects of fiber on quality of life (QOL) for 59 tube-feeding older adults living at home compared to healthy adult controls found that scores on the Gastrointestinal Quality of Life Index improved with the number of fecal *Bifidobacteria*, and fiber-enriched tube feeding increased the number of *Bifidobacteria* (Wierdsma *et al.*, 2009). This supports the findings of Ramirez-Farias *et al.* that fiber increased the abundance of *Bifidobacteria* spp. Finally, a study on infants showed an increase in *Bifidobacteria* spp. and *Lactobacillus* spp. when galacto-oligosaccharides were added to their formula (Ben *et al.*, 2008). Moreover, adding galacto-oligosaccharides and fructo-oligosaccharides to infant formula was found to be beneficial for their mucosal immunity development by increasing levels of IgA measured in their feces (Scholtens *et al.*, 2008). Taken together, these studies on human subjects promote the use of dietary fiber in gut microbiota health through the life cycles, from infancy, adulthood, to advanced age.

In addition to fiber, a healthy diet encompassing a wide range of phytonutrient-rich fruit and vegetables is an important source of functionally active compounds that act on enrichment and modulation of the microbiota and, subsequently, on regulating immune/metabolic/endocrine systemic responses. An overview of different compounds and their particular impact on microbiota is addressed in the following paragraphs.

8.2.2 Polyphenols

Dietary polyphenols consist of new bioactive products that may be effective for the prevention of degenerative and chronic diseases, chiefly cardiovascular disease and cancer. These compounds are secondary metabolites of plants and are naturally occurring compounds containing multiple phenolic functionalities (Kozikowski *et al.*, 2003). Polyphenols are commonly found in fruits, vegetables, grape seeds, tea, coffee, and red wine (Scalbert *et al.*, 2005). Until the mid-1990s, most studies focused on antioxidant vitamins, carotenoids, and minerals, despite the wide distribution of phenols in plants (Halliwell, 1996). In recent decades, polyphenols have become an important and interesting scientific subject because of their many biological activities, including antioxidant, anticarcinogenic, and antimicrobial activities. Chemically, they are classified into different groups based on the number of phenol rings and on the structural elements binding these rings together. Mainly, these polyphenols are divided into four classes: phenolic acids, flavonoids, stilbenes, and lignans. Phenolic acids, which account for about a third of the polyphenolic compounds in our diet, are divided into hydroxyl benzoic and hydroxyl cinnamic acids. The most abundant polyphenols in the human diet are flavonoids (Spencer *et al.*, 2008). Flavonoids can modulate the gut microbiota by affecting the adhesion of bacteria to intestinal cells (Bustos *et al.*, 2012).

The degree of structural complexity and polymerization of dietary polyphenols influences their bioavailability. Many recent studies have focused on the metabolism of polyphenols by bacterial and human enzymes in the gut and their bioavailability (Gross *et al.*, 2010). Bioavailability is dependent upon the biotransformation carried out in the host microbiota by means of demethylation, dehydroxylation, and decarboxylation in the gut (Possemiers *et al.*, 2011). To understand the role and effect of polyphenols on human health, it is crucial to study the metabolism of polyphenols by gut microbiota.

The gut microbiota plays a fundamental role in bioavailability, and therefore, the biological activity of phenolic metabolites, especially in food that contains high molecular weight polyphenols (Cardona *et al.*, 2013). These high molecular weight polyphenols are extensively degraded by microbiota into a series of absorbable, low molecular weight phenolic metabolites (Cardona *et al.*, 2013). In fact, the two-way relationship between polyphenols and microbiota is quite complex. Since individuals have diverging gut microbiota profiles, they likely have different capacities for polyphenol bioconversion. There are two major interactions between the gut microbiota and polyphenols. Under complex metabolism, polyphenols interact with human and microbial enzymes that lead to the excretion of polyphenol metabolites and catabolic products. Alternatively, polyphenols and their metabolites can modulate the gut microbiota composition by different mechanisms, suggesting that some phenolic compounds have the potential to be applied as antimicrobial agents against human infections (Selma *et al.*, 2009). Although polyphenol–microbiota interactions are complex, more studies promise to give a clearer picture of food functionality through a better understanding of the microbiota–food component interaction (Valdés *et al.*, 2015). Again, we will briefly examine *in vitro*, *in vivo*, and clinical evidence supporting polyphenol–microbiota interactions.

8.2.2.1 *In Vitro* Studies

Recent studies have demonstrated that different patterns of polyphenol dietary intake that supply gut bacteria may modulate the composition of the microbiota populations. The modulations can occur through discerning prebiotic effects and antimicrobial activities against gut pathogenic bacteria (Lee *et al.*, 2006). For instance, a study found that polyphenols extracted from wild lowbush blueberries exhibited an antimicrobial effect against cultured pathogenic *Escherichia coli* 0157:H7 (Lacombe *et al.*, 2013). Furthermore, polyphenols can work by increasing beneficial bacteria. Polyphenols were shown to increase favorable *Bifidobacteria* in the feces of participants consuming wild blueberry juice (Guglielmetti *et al.*, 2013). Finally, a study looked at the influence of pomegranate juice and extract on multiple gut bacterial species, and observed an increase in *Bifidobacteria* spp. and *Lactobacillus* spp., but a decrease in *B. fragilis* group, *Clostridium*, and *Enterobacteriaceae* (Li *et al.*, 2015). This supports the theory that polyphenols from multiple natural sources lead gut microbiota composition toward homeostasis.

8.2.2.2 *In Vivo* Studies

To further support the above *in vitro* evidence, many investigations of polyphenols have been conducted *in vivo*. Cranberry extract was found to increase *Akkermansia* spp. in mice, along with lowering intestinal inflammation and oxidative stress (Anhê *et al.*, 2015). *Akkermansia muciniphila* is a mucin degrader residing in the mucus layer of the intestinal tract and has been shown to have protective effects against obesity-linked metabolic syndrome (Derrien *et al.*, 2008; Everard *et al.*, 2013). In another study, grape seed polyphenol extract was orally administered to rats and it was observed that gut microbiota converted the extract polyphenols into phenolic acids and increased concentrations of two of these phenolic acids in the brain (D. Wang *et al.*, 2015). This demonstrates that gut microbiota increases bioavailability and bioactivity of dietary polyphenols, which, in this case, could be beneficial for brain health such as in preventing Alzheimer's disease.

8.2.2.3 Clinical Studies

There have been few studies on human participants focusing on the influence of polyphenol intake on gut microbiota composition and related metabolic parameters. First, a trial with randomly assigned, healthy volunteers investigated the effects of palm date consumption on gut microbiota and colon cancer risk (Eid *et al.*, 2015). Palm date contains both fiber and polyphenols. Although their findings were limited, there were significant reductions in stool ammonia, suggesting a reduction in genotoxicity (Eid *et al.*, 2015). A second study examined the effects of a combination containing inulin, beta-glucan, blueberry anthocyanins, and blueberry polyphenols on gut microbiota (Rebello *et al.*, 2015). Again, there was no significant change in gut microbiota composition, but there was an increase in satiety and improved blood glucose tolerance. These two studies suggest that more clinical research is needed to demonstrate the influence of polyphenols on gut microbiota composition in human subjects. Alternatively, studies have supported the increased bioavailability of polyphenolic compounds by gut microbiota. One study on healthy male volunteers found that black tea polyphenols were processed by gut microbiota and their catabolites, catechins, were significantly increased in participants' plasma (van Duynhoven *et al.*, 2014). Another study found that gut microbiota processed ellagitannins and ellagic acid from pomegranate into urolithins and other bioactive metabolites, which successfully integrated into the colon tissue (Nuñez-Sánchez *et al.*, 2014). In summary, the gut microbiota breaks down phenolic compounds into bioactive and bioavailable compounds that can play important roles in human health and disease.

8.2.3 Saponins

Saponins have been less explored in the literature in comparison to fibers and polyphenols, however, there are still some intriguing findings on their influences on gut microbiota. Saponins are phytochemicals produced mainly by plants, but also by lower marine mammals and bacteria (Elekofehinti, 2015). Some of the most popular saponin extracts are from ginseng, also called ginsenosides (Kim *et al.*, 2015). Several studies have examined the effects of ginsenosides on gut microbiota and especially on various illnesses such as fatigue and diabetes (Elekofehinti, 2015; Oh *et al.*, 2015). The mechanisms of action of these saponins are not definite, but there is some evidence that it might inhibit histamine, prostaglandin, and histone deacetylase (Lande *et al.*, 2015). We will examine the evidence supporting the influence of saponins on health and the importance of its metabolism by the gut microbiota.

8.2.3.1 *In Vitro* Studies

A search on PubMed did not reveal many recent *in vitro* articles directly linking saponins to gut microbiota. However, one study demonstrated that particular saponins from the *Rhizoma paridis* root had anticancer activities in breast, liver, and prostate cancer cells (Long *et al.*, 2015). In particular, two saponins were associated with apoptosis and prevention of cell cycle progression in liver cancer cells (Long *et al.*, 2015). Another study took fecal samples from a Chinese man and examined the effects of American ginseng extract on his microbiota (Wan *et al.*, 2013). The researchers found that the bacteria digested the American ginseng into metabolites such as 20S-ginsenoside Rg3, ginsenoside F2, and compound K (Wan *et al.*, 2013). Therefore, the gut microbiota may play an important role in saponin metabolism bioactivity.

8.2.3.2 *In Vivo* Studies

Many studies have used animal models to examine the effects of saponins on gut microbiota and on many different illnesses. One study was interested in the effects of ginsenosides on fatigue (Oh *et al.*, 2015). Using mice as a model, the study found that orally administered protopanaxadiol-type and protopanaxatriol-type ginsenosides prevented a rise in corticosterone, lactate, lactate dehydrogenase (LDH), and creatinine levels, besides the typically seen reduction in glucose level when the mice went through fatigue-inducing tests (Oh *et al.*, 2015). This suggests that these saponins may help prevent fatigue in mice. Another study using rats as a model found that panaxadiol saponins can help with regaining kidney function after acute kidney injury, specifically by inhibiting oxidative stress and reducing the production and release of tumor necrosis factor and IL-6 (potentially acting as an anti-inflammatory agent) (Chen *et al.*, 2015a). Furthermore, some studies were focused on the maintenance of gut microbiota homeostasis by saponins. The saponin clematichinenoside (found in some traditional Chinese medicines) has been shown to have anti-inflammatory effects in rats (Peng *et al.*, 2012). However, it is poorly absorbed orally, limiting its bioavailability (D. Wang *et al.*, 2012). Therefore, some researchers were then interested in its metabolites and found a few produced by rat microflora via deglycosylation (Li *et al.*, 2013), thus consolidating the hypothesis that Chinese traditional medicines may require processing by gut microbiota to gain bioactivity. Similarly, a study on mice found that saponins from soybeans fermented by *Lactobacillus pentosus* var. *plantarum* C29 increased the protective effect of regular soybean against scopolamine-induced memory impairment and also elevated the expression of brain-derived neurotrophic factor and inhibited acetylcholinesterase activity (Yoo and Kim, 2015). In addition, ginsenoside administered to rats was metabolized by gut microbiota to different products, including compound K (Xu *et al.*, 2014). Together, these studies imply that saponin metabolites produced by gut microbiota may have many important health benefits.

8.2.3.3 Clinical Studies

Clinical trials with various saponins have been performed in relation to different diseases. For example, anemic participants given lemongrass tea, measured to have saponins as a component, were observed to have enhanced erythropoiesis (Ekpenyong *et al.*, 2015). Thus, saponins may help with the treatment of anemia. Also, a ginsenoside was found to have anti-angiotensin and anti-leukemia effects in acute leukemia patients (Zeng *et al.*, 2014). Furthermore, a randomized, double-blind, crossover trial found that Korean red ginseng reduced blood pressure in its participants (Jovanovski *et al.*, 2014). How does gut microbiota play a role? Again, the metabolism of saponins, particularly to compound K, may increase its bioactivity. An analysis of human fecal samples revealed that samples containing higher proportions of *Bacteroides* and *Bifidobacterium* had more potently metabolized saponins (Kim *et al.*, 2013). The study proposes that gut microbiota composition influences the metabolism of ginsenosides. As seen in the *in vivo* experiments, ginsenoside metabolism may be important for increasing the bioavailability of the compound. One of its metabolites, ginsenoside compound K, has been shown to have many beneficial properties, including anticarcinogenic, anti-inflammation, anti-allergic, and anti-diabetic effects (Joh *et al.*, 2011; Kim *et al.*, 2014; Shin and Kim, 2005; Zhang *et al.*, 2013).

Fibers and bioactive compounds such as polyphenols and saponins have been shown to have many positive influences on human health. Gut microbiota plays a pivotal role in the bioactivity of these compounds through metabolism and these dietary compounds play an equally important role in shaping our gut microbiota composition and altering its homeostasis. As the chapter progresses, we will examine how important gut microbiota homeostasis is to our health by its involvement in different chronic diseases across different demographics. Furthermore, we will examine how diet can lead to gut microbiota dysbiosis or maintain homeostasis.

8.3 Survey of Epidemiological Studies

The gut microbiota not only varies intra-individually and inter-individually, but also between populations of individuals. Microbiota composition may be influenced by diet, age, sex, and geographical location (Sankar *et al.*, 2015). Therefore, it is important to examine age and geographically related effects on the microbiota.

8.3.1 Age

8.3.1.1 Pediatric Microbiota Composition

Newborns, in particular, have a very different microbiota composition in comparison to adults. Newborns start off with a high proportion of *Proteobacteria*, which compete with *Firmicutes* in the first month of life (Del Chierico *et al.*, 2015). Infant gut microbiota composition is influenced by many factors, including maternal diet, vaginal or C-section delivery, and breast or bottle feeding.

Studies have pointed out the influence of breastfeeding and maternal diet on infant microbiota composition. Maternal milk is important for infant gut microbiota development, providing the symbiotic *Lactobacillus* spp. and promoting the growth of *Bifidobacteria* spp. (Arroyo *et al.*, 2010; Makino *et al.*, 2011). Interestingly, one study found that Tanzanian women consuming yogurt during pregnancy increased the abundance of symbiotic *Bifidobacterium* and decreased that of pathogenic *Enterobacteriaceae* in infant stools after birth (Bisanz *et al.*, 2015). Maternal diet can also have an effect on the health of the mother and child over the pregnancy term. A study conducted in Norway found that mothers who ate more organic vegetables during pregnancy have a lower risk of pre-eclampsia with a suggested possible mechanism through gut microbiota composition (Torjusen *et al.*, 2014). This suggests that feeding methods during pregnancy have an important influence on infant gut microbiota development in two very different countries.

Delivery method also influences infant gut microbiota composition. A study looking at Canadian infants at 4 months old observed that cesarean-delivered infants had lower gut microbiota richness than vaginally born infants, as well as a lower abundance in *Escherichia–Shigella* and *Bacteroides* species (Azad *et al.*, 2013). A delivery method comparison was also made on South Indian infants at 6 months old, and it was similarly found that cesarean-delivered infants experienced delayed colonialization of some bacterial species (Kabeerdoss *et al.*, 2013).

Finally, breast milk-fed and formula-fed infants have differences in their gut microbiota composition. The same study on Canadian infants at 4 months old additionally found that formula-fed infants had greater gut microbiota richness with a high level of *Clostridium difficile* (Azad *et al.*, 2013). A similar study performed on Chinese infants found that breastfed infants had a greater abundance of *Actinobacteria* and *Firmicutes* and lower levels of *Proteobacteria*, whereas *Proteobacteria* were the dominant group in formula-fed infants (Fan *et al.*, 2013). Furthermore, in a study on non-human subjects, rhesus macaques, it was discovered that breastfed infants had a greater T-cell development than bottle-fed infants, suggesting that feeding method possibly influences the immune system through gut microbiota composition (Ardeshir *et al.*, 2014). These three studies suggest that although formula-fed infants may have a greater abundance of some gut bacteria, this method of feeding seems to promote pathobionts, which could negatively influence the developing immune system. Therefore, breastfeeding should likely be the preferred option for infant gut microbiota health.

8.3.1.2 The Influence of Diet and the Role of Fibers in an Aging Population

Gut microbiota may explain the increased susceptibility to immunosenescence, "inflammaging," and infection in older adults (Claesson *et al.*, 2012; Kinross and Nicholson, 2012). Microbiota composition changes with age with more emphasis on interindividual variation in older adults than in younger adults (Claesson *et al.*, 2012). Further, gut microbiota gene count decreases with age (Jeffery *et al.*, 2015). Changes with aging such as loss of teeth and muscle bulk that may lead to a nutritionally imbalanced diet, as well as gastric atrophy that may cause reduced vitamin and mineral absorption may lead to the reduced microbiota diversity seen with age (Dali-Youcef and Andrès, 2009; Ervin, 2008; Russell, 1992; Solemdal *et al.*, 2012). Another important factor may be prescription drugs taken by older adults, such as laxatives and antibiotics, which commonly have side-effects such as malabsorption, diarrhea, and constipation (Triantafyllou *et al.*, 2010). This lack of diversity may account for the greater susceptibility to some age-related illnesses. With knowledge of how the microflora influences these illnesses, we can better understand how fiber and nutraceuticals may be able to counter some of these aging effects.

Immunosenescence, the gradual loss of cell functions of the immune system, may be able to establish a causal link between dysbiosis and deteriorated health in older adults (Kinross and Nicholson, 2012). Again, this may be partly due to a reduced number of bacterial residents that promote healthy immune reactions. If the "good" *symbionts*, which have a mutualistic relationship with the host immune system and produce SCFAs (that exert anti-inflammatory and immunomodulatory effects), are reduced in number and the "bad" *pathobionts*, potentially pathogenic bacteria that make up a minor portion of the gut microbiota, increase in number, the imbalance influences the immune system (Biagi *et al.*, 2012). In particular, *Streptococcus* spp., *Staphylococcus* spp., *Enterococcus* spp., and *Enterobacteria* spp. are known to be opportunistic pathogens (Peterson *et al.*, 2015). Immunosenescence may lead to greater inflammation due to foreign and self-antibodies enhancing proinflammatory cytokines (Sato *et al.*, 2015). More inflammation in the gut can then be responsible for the phenomenon of inflammaging seen in older adults.

Inflammaging, or minor chronic systemic inflammation, increases with age (Ostan *et al.*, 2015). Although inflammation can be a positive response to invasive bacteria or viruses, inflammaging can lead to tissue degeneration and may activate age-related diseases such as type 2 diabetes, frailty, cancer, cardiovascular diseases, and some types of arthritis (Barbieri *et al.*, 2003; Baylis *et al.*, 2014; Chen *et al.*, 2015b; Jones *et al.*, 2015; Larsen *et al.*, 2007) (Figure 8.3). The process of inflammaging involves an increase in the production of proinflammatory cytokines such as *interleukins* (IL-6 and IL-1) that send signals leading to an inflammatory response where lymphocytes and natural killer cells increase in number and attack invaders (Ostan *et al.*, 2015; Pérez Martínez *et al.*, 2014).

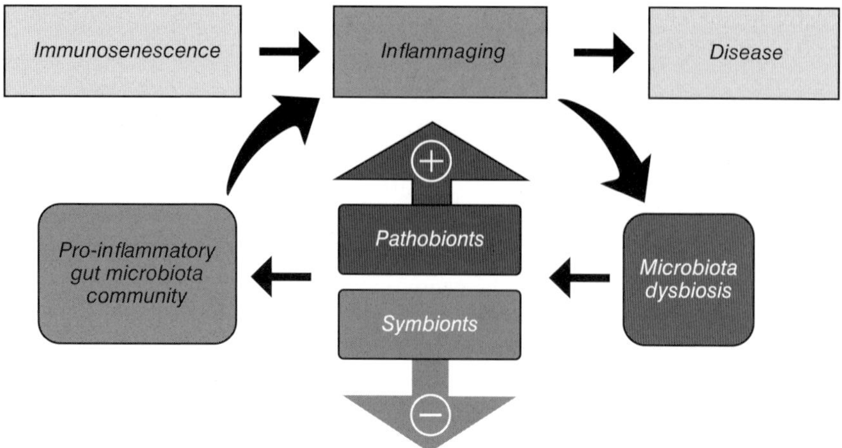

Figure 8.3 Immunosenescence in aging causes inflammaging, leading to gut microbiota dysbiosis, which further increases inflammation and promotes disease in older adults. Source: Data from Biagi *et al.* (2012).

Older adults may experience greater inflammation due to a reduced quantity of anti-inflammatory bacterial residents in the gut, such as *Bifidobacterium* spp., *F. prausnitzii*, and some *Clostridium* members as well as an elevated number of proinflammatory and pathogenic species such as *Streptococcus* spp., *Enterococcus* spp., and *Enterobacteria* spp. (Claesson *et al.*, 2012; Peterson *et al.*, 2015). However, it should be noted that the microbiota composition in older adults appears to be both country dependent and different between old adults and very old adults (above age 70) (Biagi *et al.*, 2012). For instance, *Firmicutes/Bacteroidetes* ratios were lower in Irish older adults in comparison to young adults, however, this difference was not seen in Italian older adults (Claesson *et al.*, 2011; Mueller *et al.*, 2006). Several bacteria are known to delay inflammaging by downregulating the proinflammatory response at the gut epithelium level, including *Faecalibacterium*, *Bifidobacterium*, and *Lactobacillus*, as well as at the transcription level by *Bacteroides thetaiotaomicron* (Heuvelin *et al.*, 2009; Kelly *et al.*, 2004; Sokol *et al.*, 2008; Tien *et al.*, 2006; van Baarlen *et al.*, 2009). Therefore, these would make good targets for treatments such as probiotics and prebiotics.

An increase in *infection*, the invasion of pathogens into the body that may cause harm, likely occurs for similar reasons to inflammaging. For one, an increase in the number of pathobionts may overgrow and induce inflammation under certain circumstances (Pédron and Sansonetti, 2008). This is further compounded by a lower diversity and reduced mucus production in the colon that allows for easier adherence to the mucosa, thus allowing for an easier access to pathogens (Peterson *et al.*, 2015). Immunosenescence also plays a role since it means fewer T-cells and T-cell activity, along with other immune system impairments, which may increase the risk of infection (Sato *et al.*, 2015). Together, these changes seen with aging in the gut microbiota increase the likelihood of infection.

Another potential mechanism involving inflammaging and gut microbiota is through Toll-like receptors (TLRs). *TLRs* are a key family of microbial sensors in innate and adaptive immunity involved in inflammatory signaling. Dysregulation of TLR signaling causes pathological inflammation underlining not only infection, but also cancer and type 2 diabetes, suggesting that TLR-mediated mechanisms are pivotal in chronic disease. More specifically, it has been reported that probiotic components act as physiological ligands to TLR-2/4 (Vinderola *et al.*, 2005). In alignment with this observation, a recent study demonstrated that in *ex vivo* cell cultures of intestinal epithelial cells (*IECs*), with fermented mushroom extract, slightly increased IL-6 production when compared to the control in IECs (Mallet *et al.*, 2015). The physiological increase of IL-6 by this extract differs from the inflammatory response of IECs to LPS and *E.coli*, signifying that extract components may play a crucial role in the orchestration and priming of the immune response through the TLR-2/4 gate, and by the maintenance of homeostasis in the gut. This prompted naming the IL-6 response to probiotics as "*physiological inflammation*" as opposed to "*infectious inflammation*", inflammation influenced by microbes such as pathogenic *E.coli*, or to "*sterile inflammation*", seen in insulin resistance and cancer. Indeed, sterile inflammation closely resembles infectious inflammation and could be counteracted by probiotics and prebiotics as validated TLR ligands (Tomosada *et al.*, 2013).

As mentioned previously, gut microbiota composition is influenced by geographical and community location. Additionally, microenvironments may influence microbial composition in older adults. One study looking at 178 older adults found correlations between gut microbiota composition and the type of location they were living in, such as in the community, in a day hospital, or in long-term care (Claesson *et al.*, 2012). Further, the microbiota composition of these older adults correlated with frailty, co-morbidity, nutritional status, and inflammatory markers (Claesson *et al.*, 2012). The results showed that older adults living in the community had a more diverse gut microbiota compared to those living in long-term care (Claesson *et al.*, 2012). Further, it was noted that individuals in the long-term care group had higher numbers of serum inflammatory markers such as IL-6 and IL-8 (Kinross and Nicholson, 2012). These data suggest that there is a correlation between the diets provided in the various environments, gut microbial composition, and health; known as the *age-dependent diet–microbiota–health axis* (Kinross and Nicholson, 2012). What was the difference between the diets provided in long-term care and those provided by the day hospital or the community? It was found that 83% of participants in long-term care had high fat/low-fiber diets in comparison to low- to medium-fat/high fiber diets seen in most day hospital and community participants (Kinross and Nicholson, 2012). This suggests that fiber may be an important influence on gut microbiota composition.

A diet high in fiber may be able to reduce inflammation by reducing the number of inflammatory markers and limiting insulin secretion that can cause inflammation (Justo *et al.*, 2015; Ostan *et al.*, 2015; Silveira *et al.*, 2015). Prebiotic fibers such as inulin, lactulose, and galacto-oligosaccharides can be fermented by *Bifidobacteria* spp. and/or *Lactobacillus* spp. (both known to reduce inflammatory responses) in the gut (de Vrese and Schrezenmeir, 2008; Ostan *et al.*, 2015). These bacteria are both symbionts that help maintain homeostasis in the gut (de Vrese and Schrezenmeir, 2008; Ostan *et al.*, 2015). Additionally, fiber has been shown to increase bacterial species diversity and gut microbial composition stability, both of which are important indicators for gut microbial health (Tap *et al.*, 2015). Consequently, fiber may be a particularly important dietary component for older adults.

8.3.2 Sex

Several studies have shown that the gut microbiota in males and females differ in animal models (Bolnick *et al.*, 2014). One study found that male rats had higher basal levels of the proinflammatory cytokines interleukin 6 (IL-6) and cytokine-induced neutrophil chemoattractant-1 (CINC-1) than female rats, whereas females had more regulatory cytokine interleukin 10 (IL-10) (Shastri *et al.*, 2015). Further, when fed oligofructose, female rats showed an increase in *Bacteroidetes* spp. abundance, but males did not demonstrate a similar increase (Shastri *et al.*, 2015). Another study examining the effects of administering *Escherichia coli* to rats found that it caused an increase in female rat body weight but a decrease in male rat food intake and body weight (Tennoune *et al.*, 2015). The study also found differences at the molecular level, with female plasma levels of anti-α-MSH and ACTH immunoglobulin (IgG) being higher than in males in response to the *E. coli* (Tennoune *et al.*, 2015). Accordingly, there may be important sex differences in diet–microbiota–host interactions that should be taken into consideration when treating associated conditions.

8.3.3 Geographical Location

Studies have shown that geographical location influences the types of microbes that reside in the human gut. There are important factors to be considered in connection to geographical location, including culturally unique diets and malnutrition. It is of interest to examine studies conducted in different regions of the world in order to get a better perspective on how the diet influences microbiota composition and resulting health conditions.

8.3.3.1 Global Similarities in Gut Microbiota Composition

Despite differences in climate and food consumption, there are certain species, such as *Bacteroides* spp. that make up the majority of the gut in healthy individuals. As evidence, a study conducted on Chinese participants found that the phylum *Bacteroidetes* (which includes *Bacteroides* spp.) and *Clostridium* spp. were the most common (Gu *et al.*, 2016). Another study conducted in Japan found *Bacteroides* spp., *Blautia* spp., and *Faecalibacterium* spp. to be some of the most common species in their participants (Hisada *et al.*, 2015). Moving to North America, a study conducted in Canada found that *Bacteroides* spp. was the most common, with *Akkermansia, Alistepes, Dialister, Parabacteroids*, and *Prevotella* being frequent in one or more of the healthy participants as well (Raymond *et al.*, 2015). A study in the United States with 316 healthy volunteers found *Bacteroides* spp. to be the predominant species in the gut (Yatsunenko *et al.*, 2012). Finally, a study looking at several European countries found that the examined *Bacteroides/Prevotella* group, *Clostridium coccoides* group, and *Clostridium leptum* subgroup made up most of the gut microbiota compositions

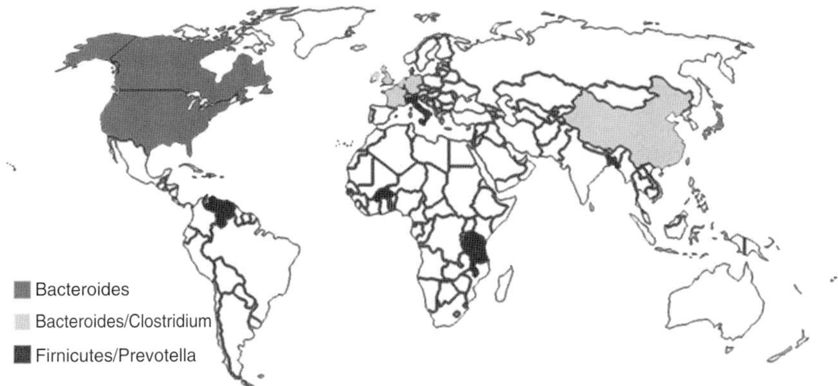

Figure 8.4 There are some similarities and some differences in microbiota composition across different countries. Source: Data from Bisanz *et al.* (2015), Blaut *et al.* (2002), De Filippo *et al.* (2010), Gu *et al.* (2016), Hisada *et al.* (2015), Lin *et al.* (2013), Raymond *et al.* (2015), Yatsunenko *et al.* (2012).

(Blaut *et al.*, 2002). Some other studies have found *Firmicutes* or *Prevotella* to be the prominent species, including studies conducted on Italians, Venezuelans, Malawians, Bangladeshis, Burkinabes, and Tanzanians (Bisanz *et al.*, 2015; De Filippo *et al.*, 2010; Lin *et al.*, 2013; Yatsunenko *et al.*, 2012). Therefore, there are global similarities in gut microbiota composition (Figure 8.4).

8.3.3.2 Geographically and Culturally Influenced Diets

Fermented foods are commonly consumed in many countries in Asia, particularly in Japan and Korea (Battcock and Azam-Ali, 1998; Kim *et al.*, 2011). Fermented milk has been shown to rapidly influence gut microbiota (Veiga *et al.*, 2014). One study, conducted in Japan, was interested in how gut microbiota composition varied seasonally and daily with fermented milk consumption. They found that *Bifidobacterium* spp. was the most influenced by seasonal changes in fermented milk consumption (Hisada *et al.*, 2015). As a result, one could expect some differences in gut microbiota composition in countries where fermented milk is consumed.

Geographical region has a major influence on the availability of certain types of foods. This is particularly important for isolated populations, distant from cities. For instance, the Inuit people living in Greenland have mostly animal-based diets, particularly fish, likely due to the inability to grow many crops in such a cold climate (Fumagalli *et al.*, 2015). Diets high in animal products increase bile-tolerating microorganisms such as *Bacteroides* and decrease bacteria that process plant polysaccharides such as *Firmicutes* (David *et al.*, 2014). A study comparing omnivorous and vegetarian women in India found that omnivorous women had more *Clostridium* bacteria such as *Roseburia* spp. in comparison to the vegetarian group (Kabeerdoss *et al.*, 2012). If one were to compare the microbiota of Inuit people with vegetarians living in India, the composition would likely be quite different.

People living in Western countries are known to consume diets high in fat and sugar. Both high fat and high sugar diets are associated with a decrease in some species of the *Bacteroidetes* phylum and an increase in *Proteobacteria* in mice, which were found to be associated with increased body fat percentage in the mice (Parks *et al.*, 2013; Zhang *et al.*, 2012). Furthermore, diets high in saturated fat and sugar, but low in fiber, have been associated with IBD (Devkota and Chang, 2015). In particular, diets high in saturated fat increase the pathobiont *Bilophila wadsworthia*, which causes an IL-10-mediated immune response, leading to colitis in mice (Devkota and Chang, 2015). Additionally, high protein diets increase *Bacteroides* (from the *Bacteroidetes* phylum), whereas high fiber diets consisting of fruits and vegetables increase beneficial *Firmicutes* and *Prevotella* (Simpson and Campbell, 2015). A diet high in fiber allows for the fermentation of SCFAs, which make the colon more acidic and prevent the invasion of pathobionts (Simpson and Campbell, 2015). High fat/sugar diets in the United States likely explain the higher incidence of IBD in comparison to Europe, Asia, and developing countries (World Gastroenterology Organisation, 2009). Hence, high fat/sugar diets may cause some of the health concerns seen in Western countries.

The Mediterranean diet has been observed to reduce the risk of several types of cancer in epidemiological studies (Estruch *et al.*, 2013; Ostan *et al.*, 2015). The Mediterranean diet consists of many phytochemicals, such as polyphenols, that act as antioxidants and prevent cellular inflammation (Ostan *et al.*, 2015). It is also a diet high in fiber, whose components increase symbiotic *Bifidobacteria* and *Lactobacillus* and influence inflammatory pathways (Guigoz *et al.*, 2002; Kaczmarczyk *et al.*, 2012). A study exploring the effects of a Mediterranean and low-fat diet on metabolic syndrome patients found that a Mediterranean diet might help return healthy gut microbiota to the patients, at least in the short term (Haro *et al.*, 2015). This again supports the idea that fibers and bioactive substances are helpful in modulating gut microbiota homeostasis and preventing related diseases.

8.3.3.3 Malnutrition

Malnutrition is, unfortunately, common in many countries around the world, leading to issues such as childhood obesity and undernourished mothers (Bisanz *et al.*, 2015; Black *et al.*, 2013). Indeed, it has also been demonstrated that higher socioeconomic status is a factor in infant gut microbiota abundance (Kabeerdoss *et al.*, 2013). One study conducted on twin children from Malawi and Bangladesh found that malnutrition led to a decrease in microbiota diversity and an increase in *Acidaminococcus* spp., which corresponded to stunted growth (Gough *et al.*, 2015). Another study showed that severe acute malnutrition in Bangladeshi children led to an immature microbiota composition with a lower diversity of gut microbiota (Subramanian *et al.*, 2014). However, it is possible that intervention at the level of the maternal diet may help improve gut microbiota homeostasis in countries with malnourished children. As mentioned previously, a study found that giving yogurt to pregnant Tanzanian women increased levels of healthier bacteria in their infants' fecal specimens (Bisanz *et al.*, 2015). Since it is at the beginning of life that the critical period of environmental influence has been observed, this could mean improved health for older children and adults in developing countries.

8.3.4 Conclusion

Many demographics play a role in shaping our gut microbiota composition. Gut microbiota composition varies a great deal across the dimension of age and by a smaller amount between the sexes and geographically. Diet can play an important role in all dimensions, such as by influencing species diversity and richness in the elderly and in infants and by altering dominant species between high fat/sugar diets and vegetable and fruit diets. These demographics should be taken into consideration when studying gut microbiota and health.

8.4 Diabetes

Diabetes mellitus is a metabolic disorder characterized by a deficiency in insulin regulatory activity, including hormone synthesis and secretion. Diabetes mellitus is classified as type 1 or type 2, based on the mechanisms of the disease (Gale and Gillespie, 2001). Gut microbial composition differs between individuals with type 2 diabetes and normal flora (Larsen *et al.*, 2010). A study comparing fecal bacterial composition between male participants with type 2 diabetes and controls found that participants with diabetes had lower proportions of *Firmicutes* and *Clostridia* as compared to the controls (Larsen *et al.*, 2010). In addition, the study found that *Bacteroides/Firmicutes* ratios and ratios of the *Bacteroides/Clostridia* group to the *C. coccoides/E. rectale* group correlated positively with blood plasma glucose concentrations in the participants (Larsen *et al.*, 2010). Interestingly, the study did not find the same significant correlation with BMI, suggesting that the change in composition seen is not necessarily due to the confounding variable of obesity-linked insulin resistance (Larsen *et al.*, 2010). It is important to discover which microbiotas are influenced by the disease in order to provide better treatment.

8.4.1 Gut Microbiota and Type 1 Diabetes

Type 1 diabetes is a disability of insulin secretion as a result of the destruction of insulin-delivering pancreatic β-cells by the immune system. It generally begins in youth, normally before 3 years old, driving the ailment to be analyzed mostly in children and adolescents (Parikka *et al.*, 2012). The observation that the occurrence of type 1 diabetes in non-obese diabetic (NOD) mice can be influenced by the microbial environment in animal-housing facilities worldwide suggested that microbiota plays a crucial role in diabetes development (Pozzilli *et al.*, 1993). Studies on mouse and rat models of type 1 diabetes have shown the interaction between the gut microbiota and the innate immune system that adapt the susceptibility toward developing diabetes, indicating that the alterations of bacterial population were responsible for type 1 diabetes modulation at the time of diabetes onset (Roesch *et al.*, 2009; Wen *et al.*, 2008). A clinical study on infant patients who develop type 1 diabetes showed an alteration in microbial diversity of gut microbiota compared to those who do not develop the disease (Giongo *et al.*, 2011). Clinical and experimental studies of type 1 diabetes indicated that a dysfunctional intestinal barrier promotes microbial antigens to destroy β-cells through T-cells (Lee *et al.*, 2010). The NOD mouse model showed that the intestinal barrier permeability allowed for intestinal pathogen infection, resulting in the activation of T-cells and development of insulitis (Lee *et al.*, 2010).

A clinical study examining the intestinal permeability in diabetic patients at different disease stages revealed that the pre-diabetic group displayed a greater intestinal permeability rate compared to the diabetic group (Bosi *et al.*, 2006). This suggests that the induction of the permeability was accelerated at the onset of the disease that led to the exposure of the pathogen infection, resulting in the autoimmune distraction of β-cells (Vaarala, 2008). Studying gut mucosa from patients with type 1 diabetes identified that the stimulation of TNFα and IFNγ levels were associated with celiac disease in patients with type 1 diabetes, indicating an existing link between the gut immune system and type 1 diabetes (Westerholm-Ormio *et al.*, 2003). In celiac disease, the zonulin, a protein that regulates intercellular tight junctions (Fasano *et al.*, 1995) and the innate immunity of the gut (El Asmar *et al.*, 2002) is involved in the intestinal barrier dysfunction in type 1 diabetes (Meddings *et al.*, 1999; Watts *et al.*, 2005). In an animal study, the level of zonulin was increased in the intestinal intralumina of diabetic-prone rat model of type 1 diabetes compared to control diabetic-resistant rats. These elevations corresponded with hyperpermeability in the small intestine, followed by the production of autoantibodies against pancreatic β-cells, thus increasing the levels of blood glucose. However, a zonulin inhibitor was shown to inhibit intestinal hyperpermeability and reduce the onset of diabetes development in biobreeding diabetes-prone (BBDP) rats by 70% (Watts *et al.*, 2005). Clinical studies examining patients with type 1 diabetes and their relatives revealed significantly higher induction of zonulin serum levels compared to either controls or their relatives, which are correlated with the degree of intestinal barrier permeability. Moreover, the pre-diabetic patients also had elevated serum zonulin levels in 7 of 10 specimens (Sapone *et al.*, 2006).

The Toll protein has a role in the innate immune system, thus loss-of-function mutation in the Toll gene showed a defect in the immune response that enhances the susceptibility to pathogen infection (Anderson *et al.*, 1985). The MyD88 adaptor protein is used by many TLRs for induction of inflammatory cytokines such as TNFα and IL-12 through all TLRs (Takeda and Akira, 2004). TLRs are part of the interleukin 1 receptor (IL-1R) superfamily (known as, the Toll/IL-1R (TIR) domain) (Bowie and O'Neill, 2000). TLRs protect against pathogens by triggering protective responses through cytokines and chemokines, thus limiting pathogen spreading (Bowie and O'Neill, 2000; Kawai and Akira, 2010). Wen *et al.* (2008) analyzed the impact of MyD88 gene disturbance on type 1 diabetes. They found that germ-free MyD88-negative NOD mice colonized with a defined microbiota were shielded from diabetes onset in comparison with mice without the microbiota. These discoveries demonstrate that the association of the intestinal organisms with the innate immune system is a basic epigenetic variable adjusting type 1 diabetes inclination.

8.4.2 Gut Microbiota and Type 2 Diabetes

Type 2 diabetes is a chronic metabolic disorder encompassing insulin-resistant activity and a defect in insulin secretion (Donath and Shoelson, 2011). The microbiota has also been linked to type 2 diabetes. Bacterial LPS, cell wall components of Gram-negative bacteria, can trigger an inflammatory state. Infusing mice with LPS led to increased insulin resistance, fasting glycemia, inflammation, and increased body weight. Furthermore, having a high-fat diet increased the number of LPS-containing microbiota in the mouse gut (Cani *et al.*, 2007a, 2007b). Similarly, a high-fat diet induced intestinal permeability by inhibiting the expression of proteins involved in epithelial tight junctions, including zonulin and occludin (Cani *et al.*, 2008). Levels of plasma LPS, inflammatory cytokines, and oxidative stress markers were reduced in association with reduced intestinal permeability and ameliorated tight junction integrity compared to controls upon treating mice with prebiotic supplementation (Cani *et al.*, 2009). The prebiotic supplementation enhanced the bowel mass and mucosal integrity regulation by endogenous intestinotrophic proglucagon-derived peptide production, which also stimulated enterocyte proliferation and prevented apoptosis (Estall and Drucker, 2006). Gut microbiota regulated gut permeability through the endocannabinoid (eCB) system and LPS regulatory loop (Blüher *et al.*, 2006; Muccioli *et al.*, 2010). eCB is made up of lipid mediators, which are produced from membrane phospholipids or triglycerides, and contribute to body weight and metabolic regulation by specific gut microbes (Cota *et al.*, 2003; Di Marzo and Matias, 2005; Geurts *et al.*, 2014). Blockage of cannabinoid receptor 1 in obese mice lowered the expression of tight junction proteins, including zonulin and occludin, and decreased plasma LPS levels, thus enhancing gut barrier function (Blüher *et al.*, 2006; Muccioli *et al.*, 2010).

The metabolic effect of polyphenols on mice fed a high-fat/high-sucrose diet was investigated using a cranberry extract. This study showed that cranberry extract supplementation enhanced insulin sensitivity by increasing insulin tolerance, reducing insulin resistance, and decreasing hyperinsulinemia in association with an increase in the gut microbiota species (Anhê *et al.*, 2015). Likewise, dietary grape polyphenols altered the gut microbial community structure in the intestine, decreasing intestinal and systemic inflammation, and improving metabolic outcomes (Roopchand *et al.*, 2015).

8.5 Infertility

Microbiotas not only reside in the gut, but can also be found on other mucosal membranes, such as in the female and male reproductive tracts and in semen. Changes in vaginal and semen microbiota compositions may lead to infections, inflammation, and, as a result, infertility (Hou *et al.*, 2013; Mastromarino *et al.*, 2014).

Most women with healthy vaginal microbiomes have mostly lactobacilli populating them (Rönnqvist *et al.*, 2006). Lactobacilli are symbionts that prevent the invasion of pathobionts and seem to be associated with a lower vaginal pH, which further prevents bacterial infections (Rönnqvist *et al.*, 2006). Bacterial vaginosis is a condition that can lead to late miscarriage and premature birth and is caused by an imbalance of the vaginal microbiota (Mastromarino *et al.*, 2014). Some pathobionts found in women with bacterial vaginosis include *Gardnerella vaginalis*, *Atopobium vaginae*, *Prevotella*, *Veillonella*, and *Megasphaera* (Fredricks *et al.*, 2005). In terms of possible treatments, one study found that orally administered probiotics containing *Lactobacillus* spp. was able to normalize the vaginal microbial composition of women with bacterial vaginosis more than the placebo group (Vujic *et al.*, 2013).

Men can also have a microbiota dysbiosis leading to fertility issues. A study looking at semen samples found that low-quality samples had higher levels of *Prevotella* and *Pseudomonas* than the normal samples, and higher quality semen had a greater proportion of *Lactobacillus* (Weng *et al.*, 2014). As seen in bacterial vaginosis, it is preferable to have higher proportions of *Lactobacillus*, which prevents pathobionts from becoming more populous. Another study looking at sperm samples found that a prevalence of *Anaerococcus* was also related to poorer sperm quality (Hou *et al.*, 2013). A study examining infertile couples found that women having sexual intercourse with men with inflammatory prostatitis, or inflammation of the prostate, experienced drastic changes in vaginal microbial composition (Borovkova *et al.*, 2011). Inflammatory prostatitis tends to result from a urinary tract infection, which is often caused by uropathogens such as *Escherichia coli*, *Enterococcus faecalis*, *Ureaplasma urealyticum*, *Chlamydia trachomatis*, *Mycoplasma hominis*, *Candida albicans*, and *Trichomonas vaginalis* (Hou *et al.*, 2013; Nickel *et al.*, 2008). These uropathogens can also lead to sperm abnormalities, such as decreased sperm motility and mitochondrial potential and increased apoptosis (Benchimol *et al.*, 2007; Burrello *et al.*, 2009; Fraczek *et al.*, 2012; Hosseinzadeh *et al.*, 2001; Ouzounova-Raykova *et al.*, 2015; Villegas *et al.*, 2005). Another study found that leukocytospermia, higher than normal levels of peroxidase-positive leukocytes in semen, could cause fertility problems in men (Korrovits *et al.*, 2006). The total concentration and diversity of bacteria were observed to be higher in the leukocytospermia patients in comparison to the controls and, in particular, *Corynebacteria* levels were greater in the leukocytospermia patients (Korrovits *et al.*, 2006). Therefore, changes in microbiota composition along the male reproductive tract may lead to poorer quality sperm and possibly infertility.

Although there are few studies looking at the effects of diet on female or male reproductive tract microbiomes, one review suggested that changes to the gut microbiome in terms of amino acid metabolism could influence female and male reproductive health (Dai *et al.*, 2015). Amino acid metabolism by gut bacteria produces nitrogenous products that may play a role in cell proliferation regulation in the uterus, placenta, and embryo/fetus (Kong *et al.*, 2014; Wang *et al.*, 2014). It is likely that changes in the gut microbiota may influence changes in reproductive tract microbiota as well. It would be interesting to see more studies connecting the diet not only to gut microbiota, but also to microbiota found in other mucosal membranes and fluids of the human body.

8.6 Mental Health and Gut Microbiota

Many recent studies have explored the association between gut microbiota and the central nervous system, otherwise known as the *gut–microbiota–brain axis.* It is already well-established that psychiatric symptoms such as stress and anxiety often come hand in hand with gastrointestinal disorders, such as irritable bowel syndrome and inflammatory bowel disorder (Moloney *et al.*, 2015; Reber *et al.*, 2011). Then there is the well-known case of *Taxoplasmic gondii*, found in cat litter, which has been shown to affect self-control and increase risky behavior in infected humans (Flegr *et al.*, 2000, 1996). What is the connection between the gut and the brain? One suggestion is that the immune system acts as a connection between psychological imbalance and gastrointestinal dysbiosis (Dunlop *et al.*, 2003; Wouters *et al.*, 2015). This is likely since it is also known that stress can influence the immune system (Dunlop *et al.*, 2003; Rehm *et al.*, 2012; Wouters *et al.*, 2015).

Indeed, as mentioned in the introduction, commensal bacteria communicate with the host immune system via PAMPs and TLRs and are involved in inflammatory pathways. One study looking at women with alexithymia, defined as the inability to understand and express emotions, found reduced ratios of IL-2/IL-10 (Th1/Th2) and CD4/CD8 T-cells and decreased IL-2 and IL-4 production in affected women compared to the controls (Guilbaud *et al.*, 2009). A second study examining the influence of stress on the immune system in mice found that the Th1/Th2 cytokine balance was reduced through the IL-10/STAT3 pathway (Hu *et al.*, 2014). The IL-10/STAT3 pathway involves TLR-4, which is also involved with the intestinal symbiont regulation of mucosal integrity (Venkatesh *et al.*, 2014). Furthermore, a couple of studies have shown that administration of probiotics that increase the Th1/Th2 ratio in humans and mice led to a decreased infection rate (Sharma *et al.*, 2014; Tan *et al.*, 2011). All of this evidence points to a possible gut–immune–brain pathway through a Th1/Th2 ratio balance.

These findings suggest that the gut–microbiota–brain axis has multiple mechanisms by which it can influence mental health and disease (Figure 8.5). In this section of the chapter, we will examine how the gut–brain axis is involved in illnesses such as anxiety, depression, autism, and dementia.

8.6.1 Mood, Stress, and Depression

Gut microbiota dysbiosis may lead to a higher risk of depression and anxiety (Foster and McVey Neufeld, 2013). Several animal studies have examined the influence of the gut–microbiota–brain axis on stress, particularly in germ-free mice (Foster and McVey Neufeld, 2013). A review summarized a few of these findings, showing that lower levels of *Bacteroides* and *Porphyromonadaceae*, and higher levels of *Clostridium, Odoribacter, Alistipes,* and *Coriobacteriaceae* increase stress levels in an animal model (Liu *et al.*, 2015). In addition, oral administration of pathogenic bacteria has been shown to increase anxiety-like behavior in animal models (Goehler *et al.*, 2008; Lyte *et al.*, 2006). These findings

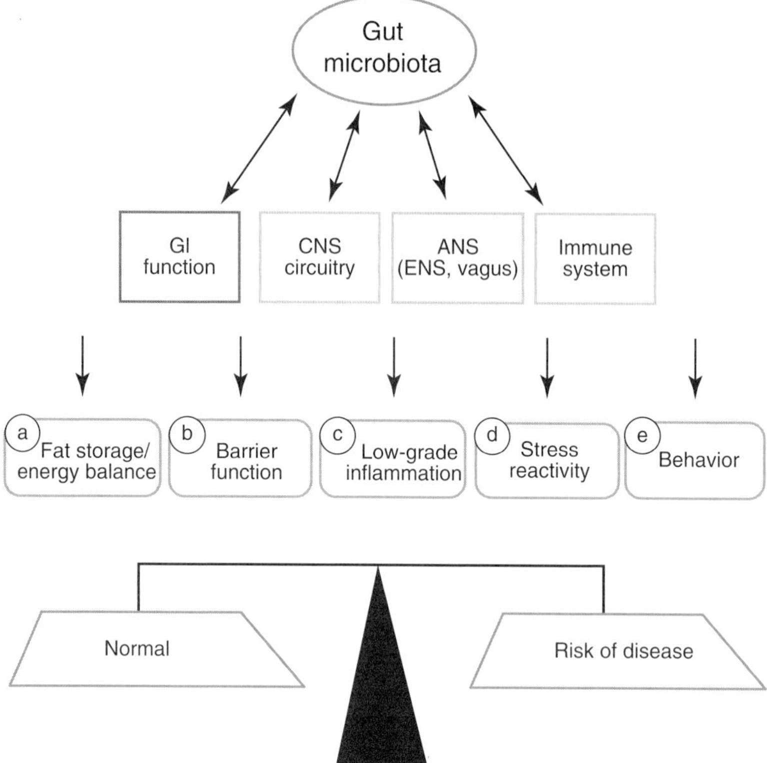

Figure 8.5 The gut microbiota influences health balance in our bodies, including mental health and behavior. Source: Foster and McVey Neufeld (2013). Reproduced with permission from Elsevier.

support the suggestion that the gut–microbiota–brain axis has an influence on mood disorders.

Some of these studies have also examined how these bacteria influence pathways related to depression and anxiety. The hypothalamic–pituitary–adrenal (HPA) axis has a central role in stress regulation (Kino, 2015; Weidenfeld *et al.*, 2015). It is also known that depression is often a result of HPA axis dysregulation (Barden, 2004). One study of HPA axis in germ-free mice found a direct connection between microbiota and HPA reactivity by observing an increased corticosteroid and adrenocorticotrophin response to stress in comparison to normal mice (Sudo *et al.*, 2004). This study showed that germ-free mice are a good model for studying the connection between microbiota and mood disorders. Another study reported that the influence of microbiota on stress behaviors may have a critical period of effect, since germ-free mice exposed to microbiota early in life expressed a normalized stress response, but exposed adult germ-free mice remained more stressed than control mice (Clarke *et al.*, 2013). Thus, maintaining a healthy gut microbiota at a young age may prove to be important for later mental health.

Probiotics could possibly help with anxiety and depression based on observations made in animal models and humans. One study found that adding *Bifidobacterium infantis* to the water of adult rats reduced depressive symptoms caused by maternal separation during their neonatal period in a similar way to another group of rats given the antidepressant citalopram (Desbonnet *et al.*, 2010). A study performed on rats and healthy human volunteers found that administration of some symbionts (*Lactobacillus helveticus* and *Bifidobacterium longum*) reduced anxiety-like symptoms in rats and improved psychology in human volunteers based on questionnaires examining stress, anxiety, and depression (Messaoudi *et al.*, 2011). This suggests that diet may play an important role on mental health by influencing gut microbiota composition.

8.6.2 Autism Spectrum Disorders

Autism spectrum disorders (ASDs) include various symptoms such as reduced verbal communication, difficulty in socializing, repetitive behaviors, a need for particular daily routines, and an increased response to external stimuli (Rosenfeld, 2015). These disorders occur in approximately 1 in 68 children (Government of Canada, 2012). Although the exact cause is unknown, the rate of co-morbidity with gastrointestinal disorders has been reported to be as high as 91.4%, with a few other studies reporting rates above 50% (Buie *et al.*, 2010). Furthermore, the age of autism onset is usually between ages 1 to 3, which is the age of transition between an unstable and stable adult-like microbiome (Buie, 2015). It is therefore of interest to consider the microbiome as a potential factor in ASD and autism development.

A number of studies have examined the changes of microbiota composition in individuals with ASD, particularly in children. *Desulfovibrio*, known to be a pathobiont, was found in high levels in children with ASD as well as autistic children (Finegold, 2011). The same study found that the microbiota dysbiosis may be linked to the home environment, since non-ASD siblings had intermediate levels of *Desulfovibrio* (Finegold, 2011). An earlier study found a similar occurrence, with ASD children having high levels of *Clostridium* spp. and siblings having intermediate levels in comparison to normal unrelated children (Parracho *et al.*, 2005). The elevation of *Clostridium* spp. has been observed in other studies as well (Song *et al.*, 2004; Williams *et al.*, 2011). Feces of children with ASDs exhibited an elevation in *Sutterella* spp. and *Ruminococcus torques* (L. Wang *et al.*, 2013). Other dysregulated species composition may include *Akkermansia muciniphila, Bifidobacterium, Prevotella, Copprococcus,* and *Veillonellaceae* (Kang *et al.*, 2013; Wang *et al.*, 2011). It is thus apparent that there are alterations in gut microbial composition in ASD children.

The dysbiosis in certain bacterial species seen in ASD and autism patients may lead to some of the metabolic disturbances observed in these patients, such as increased oxalate, homocysteine, and para-cresol levels, tryptophan deficiency, and changes in organic and fatty acid levels, creatinine metabolism, and porphyrin metabolism (El-Ansary *et al.*, 2011; Heyer *et al.*, 2012; Kałużna-Czaplińska *et al.*, 2010, 2011; Konstantynowicz *et al.*, 2012; Longo *et al.*, 2011; L. Wang *et al.*, 2012). Some of the microorganisms mentioned above may be responsible for these metabolic disturbances. For instance, an increase in *Clostridium* spp. colonization may lead to increased para-cresol levels (Altieri *et al.*, 2011). Also, enteric SCFAs produced by *Clostridium* spp., *Bacteroides* spp., and *Desulfovibrio* spp. have been shown to alter metabolism, behavior, neuroinflammation, and epigenetics in animal models and to produce changes similar to those seen in ASD patients (Finegold, 2011; Foley *et al.*, 2014; Macfabe, 2012; MacFabe *et al.*, 2011). SCFAs have been found to be elevated in autism patients (L. Wang *et al.*, 2012). More research will surely divulge more important pathways connecting gut microbiota dysbiosis and ASD, allowing for the determination of possible targets for treatment.

Probiotics may possibly treat some ASD and autism symptoms in the future. One study on a mouse model for autism found that oral treatment with the commensal bacteria *Bacteroides fragilis* improved mouse communicative, stereotypic, and anxiety-related behaviors (Hsiao *et al.*, 2013). This bacteria is known to work with the host immune system and to correct Th1/Th2 imbalances (Mazmanian *et al.*, 2005). A review summarized probiotics consisting of *Bifidobacterium* spp., *Lactobacillus* spp., *Bacteroides* spp., and galacto-oligosaccharides studied for the treatment of ASD symptoms in humans and animal models (Liu *et al.*, 2015). Probiotics may prove to be a possible treatment to reduce symptoms such as stress and anxiety.

8.6.3 Dementia

The root causes of dementia are still unknown, but many theories exist. One is that dysbiosis in the gut may lead to neuroinflammation and cognitive dysfunction (Daulatzai, 2015). Indeed, inflammation of the brain is a key characteristic of Alzheimer's disease (Azizi *et al.*, 2015). The innate immune system recognizes bacteria in the gut by the LPS on their cell surface and sends signals that can lead to systemic inflammation (Cunningham and Hennessy, 2015; Daulatzai, 2015). Furthermore, dementia cases increase with age at the same time that inflammaging occurs, supporting another connection between inflammation and neurodegeneration. Another hypothesis suggests that oral bacteria weaken the blood–brain barrier with aging through an innate proinflammatory response, influencing the pathogenesis of Alzheimer's disease (Shoemark and Allen, 2015). A second study using mice as an animal model found that a reduced number of microbiota can lead to increased permeability of the blood–brain barrier by influencing tight junction proteins occludin and claudin-5 (Braniste *et al.*, 2014). Consequently, both oral and gut microbiota may influence the development of dementia, particularly Alzheimer's disease.

Alzheimer's disease is often termed "type 3 diabetes" because it has been associated with insulin resistance in the brain (Xiang *et al.*, 2015). Low-grade inflammation can lead to insulin resistance through pathways such as the IL-1 cytokine family pathway (Ballak *et al.*, 2015) and, as mentioned above, inflammaging is a low-grade inflammation occurring particularly in older adults that may result from a change in gut microbiota composition with age. This suggests a possible connection between gut microbiota, inflammaging, diabetes, and Alzheimer's disease.

Polyphenols may be helpful in the prevention of Alzheimer's disease when digested by gut microbiota. A study using rats as a model found that gut microbiota digests grape seed polyphenol extract and produce phenolic acids, including 3-hydroxybenzoic acid and 3-(3′-hydroxyphenyl) propionic acid, which may interfere with neurotoxic β-amyloid aggregates involved in Alzheimer's disease (D. Wang *et al.*, 2015). Another study looking at polyphenols *in vitro* and *in vivo*, by administering bilberry anthocyanoside extracts to cells and mice, found that they detoxified Aβ-amyloid aggregations and prevented cognitive degeneration in the mice (Yamakawa *et al.*, 2016). Hence, polyphenols may be useful in slowing down the progression of Alzheimer's disease.

8.7 Cancer of the Gastrointestinal Tract and Extragastrointestinal Organs

8.7.1 Gastrointestinal Tract Cancer

The mucosa of the gastrointestinal tract contains many glandular epithelial cells that produce all the acid, mucus, and compounds to ensure digestive and protective functions. The vast majority of cancers found in the digestive tract (95% of gastric cancers and almost all of the colorectal cancers) are adenocarcinomas composed of cancerous epithelial cells originating from glandular tissues (Bosman *et al.*, 2010; Schwartz, 1996).

8.7.1.1 Inflammation

Chronic inflammation causes a number of diseases related to the gastrointestinal tract. For example, the irritable bowel syndrome (IBS) is caused by an abnormally high inflammation level that results in tissue damage, preventing the absorption of nutrients and water in the intestine and causing severe pain (Yamamoto-Furusho and Podolsky, 2007). Inflammation is also an integral part of the cancer microenvironment. It regulates the growth of the tumor and its vascularization and prevents apoptosis (Coussens and Werb, 2002). Inflammation also recruits immune cells and creates a loop effect, generating a microenvironment favorable to tumor progression (Keibel *et al.*, 2009).

Toll-like receptors are part of the innate and adaptive immunity and are capable of recognizing patterns conserved in a variety of microorganisms, providing a quick and effective response to possible infections. TLR binding can lead to the activation of NFκB. NFκB is activated by a large number of stressors, including infection, ultraviolet radiation, and cytokines, and promotes an inflammatory and anti-apoptotic state (Cao and Karin, 2003). Dysregulation of TLR signaling causes pathological inflammation, leading not only to infection but also cancer (Abreu, 2010; Huang *et al.*, 2005). Epithelial cells in the colon express a large number of TLRs since they form one of the primary barriers against infection, and sensing the microbes present in the gastrointestinal tract is important for modulating inflammation (Abreu, 2010). Microbial-associated inflammation resembles neoplasia-associated inflammation in that it triggers similar inflammatory and oncogenic pathways (i.e., PI3K, STAT3). TLR-4 activates NFκB and ERK and

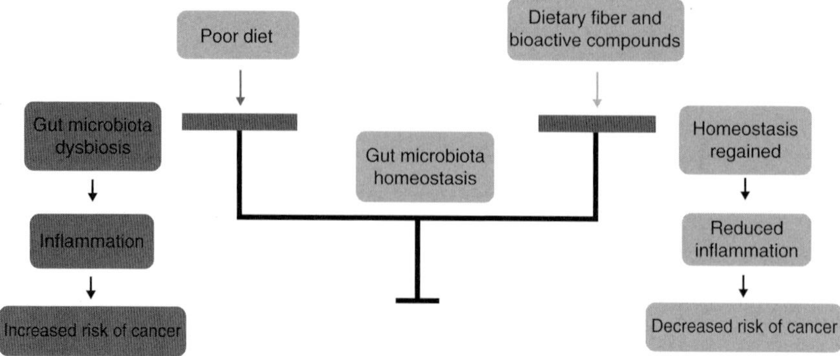

Figure 8.6 Environmental influences such as a poor diet can lead to gut microbiota dysbiosis, increasing inflammation and cancer risk. However, intake of dietary fiber and bioactive compounds may help return homeostasis, leading to a decreased risk. Source: Data from Keibel *et al.* (2009), Ostan *et al.* (2015).

promotes the production of IL-6, permitting tumor cells to evade the immune system (Seya *et al.*, 2010). TLR-2 and TLR-4 are involved in mounting a correct response to *H. pylori* infection and it has been suggested that their upregulation by the infection might cause cancer (de Oliveira and Silva, 2012). Chronic inflammation is regulated by gut microbiota homeostasis, and in this way, diet can influence cancer risk (Figure 8.6).

8.7.1.2 Colon Cancer

Colorectal cancer is the third most commonly diagnosed cancer in both men and women, and is the fourth leading cause of cancer-related death worldwide (Ferlay *et al.*, 2013). Colorectal cancer is often asymptomatic and is found after the tumors have invaded distant sites such as the peritoneal wall, the liver, or the lungs.

There are a number of gut microbiota bacterial species that have been associated with colon cancer. A metabolic analysis discovered an increase in *Clostridium leptum* and *C. coccoides* subgroups in volunteers with colorectal cancer in comparison to healthy participants (Scanlan *et al.*, 2008). Additionally, the species *Escherichia coli* is suspected to promote cancer activity in the colon (Arthur *et al.*, 2014). On another note, *Prevotella* spp. may play a preventative role due to the ability to produce SCFAs, such as butyrate and propionate (Ericsson *et al.*, 2015). Symbiotic microbiota can, therefore, have important protective effects against colon cancer.

A homeostatic microbiota can reduce the presence of mutagens by different mechanisms, prevent mutagens from acting on the intestinal cells regulating oxidizing agents, or by transforming and neutralizing the mutagens (Rafter, 2004). Another possible chemopreventative mechanism could be the competition between probiotics and pathogenic bacteria, by reducing the numbers of toxin-producing bacteria, probiotics reduce the overall level of damaging compounds in the lumen of the intestine (Lamprecht *et al.*, 2012; Wutzke *et al.*,

2010). For instance, the ingestion of yogurt can reduce the concentration of proneoplasia β-glucuronidase and nitroreductase and reduce the incidence of colorectal cancer (de Moreno de LeBlanc and Perdigón, 2005, 2004).

Dietary fiber and bioactive compounds may also have chemopreventative effects on colorectal cancer. The link between fiber consumption and colorectal cancer has been debated many times. Some studies show no links between colorectal cancer and fiber intake (Kunzmann *et al.*, 2015), others found a very low effect of fiber on people who eat a low amount of fat and a high level of fiber, but the results are not significant events when following groups of vegetarians (Gilsing *et al.*, 2015; Lanza *et al.*, 2007). However, fibers may contribute to the chemoprevention of colon cancer, possibly through fermentation by the microbiota and the production of butyrate that can, in turn, protect from colorectal cancer (Encarnação *et al.*, 2015). Clinical studies have also shown that polyphenols combined with fiber (in palm dates) may reduce colon cancer risk (Eid *et al.*, 2015). Furthermore, the polyphenol resveratrol was shown to prevent tumor growth and liver metastasis in mice with colon cancer (Narayanan *et al.*, 2015) (Figure 8.7). Similar results were seen with saponins in colon cancer-bearing mice, with a reduced tumor initiation and progression after the administration of American ginseng (C. Yu *et al.*, 2015). Although more studies need to be completed, there is some promising evidence supporting a positive influence of dietary fiber and bioactive compounds on colon cancer.

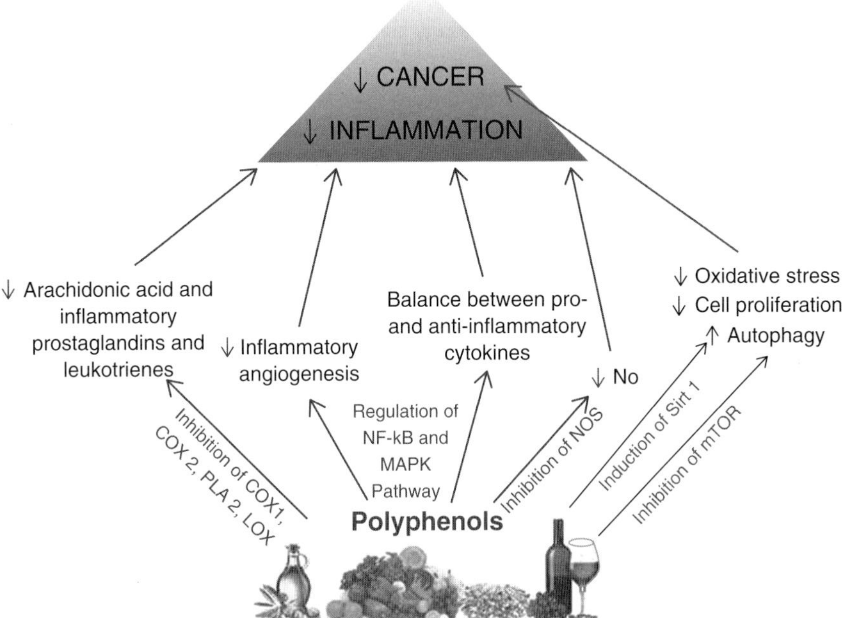

Figure 8.7 Polyphenols may play an important role in reducing inflammation and cancer risk and improving cancer prognosis through several molecular pathways. Source: Ostan *et al.* (2015).

8.7.1.3 Gastric Cancer

Gastric cancer is the fifth most prevalent cancer worldwide and the third leading cause of cancer-related death (Stewart *et al.*, 2014). It is often found late in the progression of the disease, but proper screening can significantly reduce the incidence of death (Ro *et al.*, 2015). *Helicobacter pylori* is a major risk factor and is found in 60–90% of patients with gastric cancer; however, a large portion of people infected with *H. pylori* do not develop gastric cancer (de Souza *et al.*, 2014; Kusters *et al.*, 2006; Uemura *et al.*, 2001). Other factors raising the risk of gastric cancer are a high salt diet and smoking (D'Elia *et al.*, 2012; La Torre *et al.*, 2009). A relationship between gut microbiota composition and *H. pylori* invasion has been demonstrated. Specifically, a study found that participants testing positive for *H. pylori* had a higher proportion of *Proteobacteria, Spirochetes*, and *Acidobacteria*, but a decreased abundance of *Actinobacteria, Bacteroidetes*, and *Firmicutes* (Maldonado-Contreras *et al.*, 2011). This suggests that a dysbiosis of microbiota composition in the gastrointestinal tract could give an opportunity for *H. pylori* to invade the stomach mucosa. Alternatively, gut microbiota can influence *H. pylori* via T-cells, namely, proinflammatory helper T-cells 1 and 17 (Th1 and Th17), which play important roles in modulating *H. pylori* infection (Shi *et al.*, 2010). Gut microbiota dysbiosis has been shown to influence T-cell activity in the immune system (B. Yu *et al.*, 2015). It is likely that the bacteria exert their influence via the metabolites they produce, such as butyrate and propionate (Arpaia *et al.*, 2013). Therefore, gut microbiota may indirectly lead to some cases of *H. pylori*-associated gastric cancer.

Research has shown that diet impacts stomach cancer risk (Hu *et al.*, 2015). Fat, saturated fat, and cholesterol intakes have all been associated with an increase in stomach cancer risk, and, interestingly, fiber was inversely associated (Hu *et al.*, 2015). This suggests that fiber may have beneficial effects on stomach cancers. Alternatively, saponins have been shown to inhibit gastric cancer cell proliferation and invasion, and cause apoptosis in gastric cancer cell lines (Fang *et al.*, 2015; Lin *et al.*, 2014; T. Wang *et al.*, 2013). As a final point, the polyphenol quercetin was found to prevent proliferation in gastric cancer cells (Borska *et al.*, 2012). Fiber and bioactive substances play a role in reducing stomach cancer risk and may be helpful at the treatment stage as well.

8.7.2 Extragastrointestinal Organ Cancer

Although colon cancer is the most commonly influenced by gut microbiota due to proximity, other cancers have been shown to be influenced by gut microbiota dysbiosis. These include, but are not limited to, pancreatic cancer and liver cancer. Gut bacteria could lead to cancer via three different mechanisms: chronic inflammation (such as inflammaging), immune evasion, and immune suppression (Compare and Nardone, 2011). One important pathway involved with immune suppression includes regulatory T-cells. When regulatory T-cell numbers are too high, immune responses are suppressed and this allows for tumor growth in the body (Compare and Nardone, 2011). This can happen when gut microbiota dysbiosis is extended, implicating gut microbiota as a factor in cancer progression throughout the body.

8.7.2.1 Pancreatic Cancer

Pancreatic cancer has a high fatality rate and one of the worst prognoses worldwide due to ineffective screening methods and limited treatments (Komura *et al.*, 2015; Zambirinis *et al.*, 2014). Inflammation plays an important role in pancreatic cancer, both as a risk factor and consequence (Chang *et al.*, 2015; Komura *et al.*, 2015). In fact, the bacteria that make up the gut microbiota are very involved in inflammation pathways. Bacteria PRRs such as NOD-like receptors, when bound by their ligands, activate a pathway associated with inflammasomes (Franchi *et al.*, 2012). These inflammasomes have been connected to the development of pancreatitis, or inflammation of the pancreas (Hoque *et al.*, 2011). Pancreatitis has been associated with some cases of pancreatic cancer (Loncle *et al.*, 2015). One possible pathway is through signaling via the cytokine IL-17 to the pancreatitis mediator REG3β (Loncle *et al.*, 2015). Therefore, we may be able to prevent some cases of pancreatic cancer by targeting gut microbiota.

A meta-analysis of 13 case–control studies found that dietary fiber intake significantly reduced pancreatic cancer risk (C.-H. Wang *et al.*, 2015). Further, an *in vitro* study found that catechin and inositol hexaphosphate found in green tea and high fiber foods inhibited the growth of pancreatic cancer cells (McMillan *et al.*, 2007). On another note, polyphenols have been shown to target pancreatic cancer stem cells, and therefore, may help prevent recurrence of the disease (Aravindan *et al.*, 2015). Another *in vitro* study even suggested that ginsenosides may be beneficial in controlling pancreatic cancer (Guo *et al.*, 2014). Consequently, diet may have some influence on pancreatic cancer through gut microbiota and possibly other pathways.

8.7.2.2 Liver Cancer

The main causes of hepatocellular carcinoma, or liver cancer, are usually attributed to alcoholism, autoimmunity, and hepatitis B and C infections (Sherman, 2010). The gut microbiota could be implicated in a number of these risks. For instance, a study on mice found that intestinal colonization with *Helicobacter hepaticus* stimulated hepatitis C transgene-induced hepatocellular carcinoma (HCC) without moving to the liver (Fox *et al.*, 2010). *H. hepaticus* activated Th1-type adaptive immunity in the lower bowel and liver (Fox *et al.*, 2010). *H. hepaticus* has been connected to lower bowel inflammation and cancer in other studies as well (Cahill *et al.*, 1997; Fox *et al.*, 2011; Ihrig *et al.*, 1999). Furthermore, the interaction between gut microbiota and host immune system can promote liver disease during autoimmunity (Henao-Mejia *et al.*, 2013). A large study in Ireland found that primary sclerosing cholangitis (PSC), an autoimmune liver disease, was significantly associated with an inflamed colon (O'Toole *et al.*, 2012). It was suggested that TLRs in the Kupffer cells of the liver respond to endotoxins from the gut microbiota and produce chemical signals that cause liver disease (Henao-Mejia *et al.*, 2013). Also of interest, patients with chronic liver disease were observed to have elevated levels of LPS (PAMPs) in their plasma (Lin *et al.*, 1995). As mentioned previously, LPS are found on the surfaces of Gram-negative bacteria and produce harmful endotoxins (Janssen and Kersten, 2015). These findings all connect the gut microbiota to liver disease and cancer.

Again, dietary fiber and bioactive substances appear to play a role in reducing liver cancer risk and ameliorating prognosis. A large-scale European study found an inverse relationship between total fiber intake and liver cancer (Bradbury *et al.*, 2014). Additionally, an *in vivo* study supported this finding by showing that dietary fiber protected the liver of rats by reducing fatty degeneration of their hepatocytes and infiltration of leukocytes into the portal vein when injected with a carcinogen (Lahouar *et al.*, 2014). Furthermore, several recent *in vitro* and *in vivo* studies support the protective effects of polyphenols and saponins on liver cancer (Long *et al.*, 2015; Man *et al.*, 2014; Stadlbauer *et al.*, 2015; Sur *et al.*, 2016; Weerawatanakorn *et al.*, 2015). Overall, dietary fiber and bioactive substances play an important role in modulating liver cancer and associated risks.

8.7.3 Last Remarks

Gut microbiota is not limited to influencing cancer in the intestinal tract. Their influence is extended to the entire body because of their communications with the host through the immune system. Accordingly, targeting gut microbiota through dietary factors can benefit the body as a whole. Through multiple mechanisms, dietary fiber and bioactive substances, such as polyphenols and saponins, can in some cases reduce risk, help with treatment, and improve prognosis for multiple different cancers.

8.8 Conclusion

The relationship between dietary fiber, bioactive substances, gut microbiota, and disease is gaining importance in disease prevention and outcome. Recent *in vitro*, *in vivo*, clinical, and epidemiological studies support the diet–microbiota–health axis hypothesis. The gut microbiota is influenced by fiber, polyphenols, saponins, and their metabolites to prevent many chronic diseases through different pathways, such as nutritional epigenetics. Insoluble, non-fermentable fibers are important for easier gastrointestinal transit, whereas soluble, fermentable fibers produce bioactive metabolites, such as butyrate, that play important roles in gut health maintenance through epigenetic mechanisms. Polyphenol metabolism in the gut influences bacterial adhesion to the gut wall. Although the mechanism of saponin influence is uncertain, there is some evidence that it might work by inhibiting histamine, prostaglandin, and histone deacetylase. All of these compounds have direct or indirect effects on microbiota by conferring an equilibrium between pathobionts and symbionts. More clinical studies should be carried out to further substantiate the effect of dietary fiber and bioactive compounds on mechanisms of gut microbiota maintenance.

Additionally, important demographics such as age, sex, and geographical region may influence gut microbiota composition. Infants are born with higher proportions of *Proteobacteria* and their gut microbiota composition changes after being introduced to solid foods. Older adults have diminished diversity in their gut, which can lead to inflammaging and related health problems. Male and female animal models have demonstrated differing reactions in gut microbial composition to dietary compounds. Lastly, geographical location influences gut microbiota composition, depending on the availability of food in different regions. Therefore, these demographics should be taken into account when considering disease prevention and treatment.

Finally, diet influences the risk and progression of diseases such as diabetes, infertility, mental health disorders, and cancer. There is evidence that gut microbiota composition plays an important role in both type 1 and type 2 diabetes. Research has shown that bioactive compounds such as polyphenols from cranberry extract may improve insulin sensitivity. Changes in gut microbiota composition, such as increases in pathobionts, in vaginal membranes and semen may lead to infertility. Additional studies examining whether diet-induced microbiota dysbiosis may influence inflammation and sustain the infertility state need to be conducted. The diet influences many mental health disorders, including depression, anxiety, autism, and dementia by continually altering the balance between dysbiosis and symbiosis. For example, polyphenols from bilberry extract have been shown to detoxify Aβ-amyloid aggregations and prevent cognitive degeneration in mice. Another major chronic illness influenced by the diet is cancer. Research has shown that diet induces microbiota changes that significantly contribute to prevention in oncology. For example, a dietary intervention showed that a few months of Mediterranean diet are sufficient to favorably modify the metabolic/endocrine characteristics of breast cancer survivors. Fiber has been inversely associated with stomach cancer risk and *in vitro* studies of saponin have demonstrated it to inhibit gastric cancer cell proliferation and invasion. The polyphenol resveratrol, found in red wine, has been shown to prevent tumor growth and liver metastasis in mice with colon cancer. These findings make it clear that though more research needs to be completed in many areas, there is astounding evidence supporting the influence of dietary fiber and bioactive compounds on gut microbiota and human health. In conclusion, diet in general and fibers, in particular, contribute to the maintenance of effective symbiosis and communication between the host and its gut microbiota, thus adding to the effective equilibrium and protection in this microcosmos.

References

Abreu, M.T. (2010). Toll-like receptor signalling in the intestinal epithelium: how bacterial recognition shapes intestinal function. *Nat. Rev. Immunol.* 10, 131–144. doi: 10.1038/nri2707

Altieri, L., Neri, C., Sacco, R., Curatolo, P., Benvenuto, A., Muratori, F., *et al.* (2011). Urinary p-cresol is elevated in small children with severe autism spectrum disorder. *Biomarkers* 16, 252–260. doi: 10.3109/1354750X.2010.548010

Anderson, K.V., Jürgens, G., Nüsslein-Volhard, C. (1985). Establishment of dorsal-ventral polarity in the Drosophila embryo: genetic studies on the role of the Toll gene product. *Cell* 42, 779–789.

Anhê, F.F., Roy, D., Pilon, G., Dudonné, S., Matamoros, S., Varin, T.V., *et al.* (2015). A polyphenol-rich cranberry extract protects from diet-induced obesity, insulin resistance and intestinal inflammation in association with increased *Akkermansia* spp. population in the gut microbiota of mice. *Gut* 64, 872–883. doi: 10.1136/gutjnl-2014-307142

Aravindan, S., Ramraj, S.K., Somasundaram, S.T., Herman, T.S., Aravindan, N. (2015). Polyphenols from marine brown algae target radiotherapy-coordinated EMT and stemness-maintenance in residual pancreatic cancer. *Stem Cell Res. Ther.* 6, 182. doi: 10.1186/s13287-015-0173-3

Ardeshir, A., Narayan, N.R., Méndez-Lagares, G., Lu, D., Rauch, M., Huang, Y., *et al.* (2014). Breast-fed and bottle-fed infant rhesus macaques develop distinct gut microbiotas and immune systems. *Sci. Transl. Med.* 6, 120. doi: 10.1126/scitranslmed.3008791

Arpaia, N., Campbell, C., Fan, X., Dikiy, S., van der Veeken, J., deRoos, P., *et al.* (2013). Metabolites produced by commensal bacteria promote peripheral regulatory T-cell generation. *Nature* 504, 451–455. doi: 10.1038/nature12726

Arroyo, R., Martín, V., Maldonado, A., Jiménez, E., Fernández, L., Rodríguez, J.M. (2010). Treatment of infectious mastitis during lactation: antibiotics versus oral administration of Lactobacilli isolated from breast milk. *Clin. Infect. Dis.* 50, 1551–1558. doi: 10.1086/652763

Arthur, J.C., Gharaibeh, R.Z., Mühlbauer, M., Perez-Chanona, E., Uronis, J.M., McCafferty, J., *et al.* (2014). Microbial genomic analysis reveals the essential role of inflammation in bacteria-induced colorectal cancer. *Nat. Commun.* 5, 4724. doi: 10.1038/ncomms5724

Azad, M.B., Konya, T., Maughan, H., Guttman, D.S., Field, C.J., Chari, R.S., *et al.*, CHILD Study Investigators (2013). Gut microbiota of healthy Canadian infants: profiles by mode of delivery and infant diet at 4 months. *CMAJ Can. Med. Assoc. J.* 185, 385–394. doi: 10.1503/cmaj.121189

Azizi, G., Navabi, S.S., Al-Shukaili, A., Seyedzadeh, M.H., Yazdani, R., Mirshafiey, A. (2015). The role of inflammatory mediators in the pathogenesis of Alzheimer's disease. *Sultan Qaboos Univ. Med. J.* 15, e305–316. doi: 10.18295/squmj.2015.15.03.002

Ballak, D.B., Stienstra, R., Tack, C.J., Dinarello, C.A., van Diepen, J.A. (2015). IL-1 family members in the pathogenesis and treatment of metabolic disease: Focus on adipose tissue inflammation and insulin resistance. *Cytokine* 75, 280–290. doi: 10.1016/j.cyt0.2015.05.005

Barbieri, M., Ferrucci, L., Ragno, E., Corsi, A., Bandinelli, S., Bonafè, M., *et al.* (2003). Chronic inflammation and the effect of IGF-I on muscle strength and power in older persons. *Am. J. Physiol. Endocrinol. Metab.* 284, E481–487. doi: 10.1152/ajpend0.00319.2002

Barden, N. (2004). Implication of the hypothalamic–pituitary–adrenal axis in the physiopathology of depression. *J. Psychiatry Neurosci.* 29, 185–193.

Barthel, M., Hapfelmeier, S., Quintanilla-Martínez, L., Kremer, M., Rohde, M., Hogardt, M., *et al.* (2003). Pretreatment of mice with streptomycin provides a *Salmonella enterica* serovar *Typhimurium* colitis model that allows analysis of both pathogen and host. *Infect. Immun.* 71, 2839–2858.

Battcock, M., Azam-Ali, S. (1998). *Fermented and vegetables.* A global perspective. Introduction. www.fao.org/docrep/x0560e/x0560e05.htm#Fer (accessed 22 September 2015).

Baylis, D., Ntani, G., Edwards, M., Syddall, H., Bartlett, D., Dennison, E., *et al.* (2014). Inflammation, telomere length and grip strength: a 10 year longitudinal study. *Calcif. Tissue Int.* 95, 54–63. doi: 10.1007/s00223-014-9862-7

Benchimol, M., Rosa, I. de A., Fontes, R. da S., Dias, Â.J.B. (2007). Trichomonas adhere and phagocytose sperm cells: adhesion seems to be a prominent stage during interaction. *Parasitol. Res.* 102, 597–604. doi: 10.1007/s00436-007-0793-3

Ben, X.-M., Li, J., Feng, Z.-T., Shi, S.-Y., Lu, Y.-D., Chen, R., *et al.* (2008). Low level of galacto-oligosaccharide in infant formula stimulates growth of intestinal Bifidobacteria and Lactobacilli. *World J. Gastroenterol.* 14, 6564–6568.

Biagi, E., Candela, M., Fairweather-Tait, S., Franceschi, C., Brigidi, P. (2012). Ageing of the human metaorganism: the microbial counterpart. *Age* 34, 247–267. doi: 10.1007/s11357–011–9217–5

Biedermann, L., Rogler, G. (2015). The intestinal microbiota: its role in health and disease. *Eur. J. Pediatr.* 174, 151–167. doi: 10.1007/s00431-014-2476-2

Bisanz, J.E., Enos, M.K., PrayGod, G., Seney, S., Macklaim, J.M., Chilton, S., *et al.* (2015). Microbiota at multiple body sites during pregnancy in a rural Tanzanian population and effects of moringa-supplemented probiotic yogurt. *Appl. Environ. Microbiol.* 81, 4965–4975. doi: 10.1128/AEM.00780-15

Biteau, B., Karpac, J., Supoyo, S., Degennaro, M., Lehmann, R., Jasper, H. (2010). Lifespan extension by preserving proliferative homeostasis in *Drosophila. PLoS Genet.* 6, e1001159. doi: 10.1371/journal.pgen.1001159

Black, R.E., Victora, C.G., Walker, S.P., Bhutta, Z.A., Christian, P., de Onis, M., *et al.*, Maternal and Child Nutrition Study Group (2013). Maternal and child undernutrition and overweight in low-income and middle-income countries. *Lancet* 382, 427–451. doi: 10.1016/S0140-6736(13)60937-X

Blaut, M., Collins, M.D., Welling, G.W., Doré, J., van Loo, J., de Vos, W. (2002). Molecular biological methods for studying the gut microbiota: the EU human gut flora project. *Br. J. Nutr.* 87, S203–S211. doi: 10.1079/BJN/2002539

Blüher, M., Engeli, S., Klöting, N., Berndt, J., Fasshauer, M., Bátkai, S., *et al.* (2006). Dysregulation of the peripheral and adipose tissue endocannabinoid system in human abdominal obesity. *Diabetes* 55, 3053–3060. doi: 10.2337/db06-0812

Bolnick, D.I., Snowberg, L.K., Hirsch, P.E., Lauber, C.L., Org, E., Parks, B., *et al.* (2014). Individual diet has sex-dependent effects on vertebrate gut microbiota. *Nat. Commun.* 5, 4500. doi: 10.1038/ncomms5500

Borovkova, N., Korrovits, P., Ausmees, K., Türk, S., Jõers, K., Punab, M., *et al.* (2011). Influence of sexual intercourse on genital tract microbiota in infertile couples. *Anaerobe* 17, 414–418. doi: 10.1016/j.anaerobe.2011.04.015

Borska, S., Chmielewska, M., Wysocka, T., Drag-Zalesinska, M., Zabel, M., Dziegiel, P. (2012). *In vitro* effect of quercetin on human gastric carcinoma: targeting cancer cells death and MDR. *Food Chem. Toxicol.* 50, 3375–3383. doi: 10.1016/j.fct.2012.06.035

Bosi, E., Molteni, L., Radaelli, M.G., Folini, L., Fermo, I., Bazzigaluppi, E., *et al.* (2006). Increased intestinal permeability precedes clinical onset of type 1 diabetes. *Diabetologia* 49, 2824–2827. doi: 10.1007/s00125-006-0465-3

Bosman, F.T., Carneiro, F., Hruban, R.H., Theise, N.D. (eds.) (2010). *World Health Organization Classification of Tumours,* 4th edn. International Agency for Research on Cancer, Lyon.

Bowie, A., O'Neill, L.A. (2000). The interleukin-1 receptor/Toll-like receptor superfamily: signal generators for pro-inflammatory interleukins and microbial products. *J. Leukoc. Biol.* 67, 508–514.

Bradbury, K.E., Appleby, P.N., Key, T.J. (2014). Fruit, vegetable, and fiber intake in relation to cancer risk: findings from the European Prospective Investigation into Cancer and Nutrition (EPIC). *Am. J. Clin. Nutr.* 100, 394S–398S. doi:10.3945/ajcn.113.071357

Braniste, V., Al-Asmakh, M., Kowal, C., Anuar, F., Abbaspour, A., Tóth, M., *et al.* (2014). The gut microbiota influences blood-brain barrier permeability in mice. *Sci. Transl. Med.* 6, 263ra158. doi: 10.1126/scitranslmed.3009759

Buela, K.-A.G., Omenetti, S., Pizarro, T.T. (2015). Cross-talk between type 3 innate lymphoid cells and the gut microbiota in inflammatory bowel disease. *Curr. Opin. Gastroenterol.* 31, 449–455. doi: 10.1097/MOG.0000000000000217

Buie, T. (2015). Potential etiologic factors of microbiome disruption in autism. *Clin. Ther.* 37, 976–983. doi: 10.1016/j.clinthera.2015.04.001

Buie, T., Campbell, D.B., Fuchs, G.J., Furuta, G.T., Levy, J., VandeWater, J., *et al.* (2010). Evaluation, diagnosis, and treatment of gastrointestinal disorders in individuals with ASDs: A consensus report. *Pediatrics* 125, S1–S18. doi: 10.1542/peds.2009-1878C

Burrello, N., Salmeri, M., Perdichizzi, A., Bellanca, S., Pettinato, G., D'Agata, R., *et al.* (2009). *Candida albicans* experimental infection: effects on human sperm motility, mitochondrial membrane potential and apoptosis. *Reprod. Biomed. Online* 18, 496–501.

Bustos, I., García-Cayuela, T., Hernández-Ledesma, B., Peláez, C., Requena, T., Martínez-Cuesta, M.C. (2012). Effect of flavan-3-ols on the adhesion of potential probiotic lactobacilli to intestinal cells. *J. Agric. Food Chem.* 60, 9082–9088. doi:10.1021/jf301133g

Cahill, R.J., Foltz, C.J., Fox, J.G., Dangler, C.A., Powrie, F., Schauer, D.B. (1997). Inflammatory bowel disease: an immunity-mediated condition triggered by bacterial infection with *Helicobacter hepaticus. Infect. Immun.* 65, 3126–3131.

Cani, P.D., Amar, J., Iglesias, M.A., Poggi, M., Knauf, C., Bastelica, D., *et al.* (2007a). Metabolic endotoxemia initiates obesity and insulin resistance. *Diabetes* 56, 1761–1772. doi: 10.2337/db06-1491

Cani, P.D., Neyrinck, A.M., Fava, F., Knauf, C., Burcelin, R.G., Tuohy, K.M., Gibson, G.R., *et al.* (2007b). Selective increases of bifidobacteria in gut microflora improve high-fat-diet-induced diabetes in mice through a mechanism associated with endotoxaemia. *Diabetologia* 50, 2374–2383. doi: 10.1007/s00125-007-0791-0

Cani, P.D., Bibiloni, R., Knauf, C., Waget, A., Neyrinck, A.M., Delzenne, N.M., *et al.* (2008). Changes in gut microbiota control metabolic endotoxemia-induced inflammation in high-fat diet-induced obesity and diabetes in mice. *Diabetes* 57, 1470–1481. doi: 10.2337/db07-1403

Cani, P.D., Possemiers, S., Van de Wiele, T., Guiot, Y., Everard, A., Rottier, O., *et al.* (2009). Changes in gut microbiota control inflammation in obese mice through a mechanism involving GLP-2-driven improvement of gut permeability. *Gut* 58, 1091–1103. doi: 10.1136/gut.2008.165886

Cao, Y., Karin, M. (2003). NF-kappaB in mammary gland development and breast cancer. *J. Mammary Gland Biol. Neoplasia* 8, 215–223.

Cardona, F., Andrés-Lacueva, C., Tulipani, S., Tinahones, F.J., Queipo-Ortuño, M.I. (2013). Benefits of polyphenols on gut microbiota and implications in human health. *J. Nutr. Biochem.* 24, 1415–1422. doi: 10.1016/j.jnutbi0.2013.05.001

Chang, H.-H., Young, S.H., Sinnett-Smith, J., Chou, C.E.N., Moro, A., Hertzer, K.M., *et al.* (2015). Prostaglandin E2 activates the mTORC1 pathway through an EP4/cAMP/PKA-and EP1/Ca^{2+}-mediated mechanism in the human pancreatic carcinoma cell line PANC-1. *Am. J. Physiol. Cell Physiol.* 309, C639–649. doi: 10.1152/ajpce11.00417.2014

Chen, Y., Du, Y., Li, Y., Wang, X., Gao, P., Yang, G., *et al.* (2015a). Panaxadiol saponin and dexamethasone improve renal function in lipopolysaccharide-induced mouse model of acute kidney injury. *PLoS One* 10. doi: 10.1371/journal.pone.0134653

Chen, Y., Sun, T., Wu, J., Kalionis, B., Zhang, C., Yuan, D., *et al.* (2015b). Icariin intervenes in cardiac inflammaging through upregulation of SIRT6 enzyme activity and inhibition of the NF-kappa B pathway. *BioMed Res. Int.* 2015, 895976. doi: 10.1155/2015/895976

Cho, S.S., Qi, L., Fahey, G.C., Klurfeld, D.M. (2013). Consumption of cereal fiber, mixtures of whole grains and bran, and whole grains and risk reduction in type 2 diabetes, obesity, and cardiovascular disease. *Am. J. Clin. Nutr.* 98, 594–619. doi:10.3945/ajcn.113.067629

Claesson, M.J., Cusack, S., O'Sullivan, O., Greene-Diniz, R., de Weerd, H., Flannery, E., *et al.* (2011). Composition, variability, and temporal stability of the intestinal microbiota of the elderly. *Proc. Natl. Acad. Sci. U.S.A.* 108, 4586–4591. doi: 10.1073/pnas.1000097107

Claesson, M.J., Jeffery, I.B., Conde, S., Power, S.E., O'Connor, E.M., Cusack, S., *et al.* (2012). Gut microbiota composition correlates with diet and health in the elderly. *Nature* 488, 178–184. doi: 10.1038/nature11319

Clarke, G., Grenham, S., Scully, P., Fitzgerald, P., Moloney, R.D., Shanahan, F., *et al.* (2013). The microbiome-gut-brain axis during early life regulates the hippocampal serotonergic system in a sex-dependent manner. *Mol. Psychiatry* 18, 666–673. doi: 10.1038/mp.2012.77

Compare, D., Nardone, G. (2011). Contribution of gut microbiota to colonic and extracolonic cancer development. *Dig. Dis.* 29, 554–561. doi: 10.1159/000332967

Cota, D., Marsicano, G., Lutz, B., Vicennati, V., Stalla, G.K., Pasquali, R., *et al.* (2003). Endogenous cannabinoid system as a modulator of food intake. *Int. J. Obes. Relat. Metab. Disord.* 27, 289–301. doi: 10.1038/sj.ij0.0802250

Cousens, L.S., Gallwitz, D., Alberts, B.M. (1979). Different accessibilities in chromatin to histone acetylase. *J. Biol. Chem.* 254, 1716–1723.

Coussens, L.M., Werb, Z. (2002). Inflammation and cancer. *Nature* 420, 860–867. doi: 10.1038/nature01322

Cunningham, C., Hennessy, E. (2015). Co-morbidity and systemic inflammation as drivers of cognitive decline: new experimental models adopting a broader paradigm in dementia research. *Alzheimers Res. Ther.* 7, 33. doi: 10.1186/s13195-015-0117-2

Dai, Z., Wu, Z., Hang, S., Zhu, W., Wu, G. (2015). Amino acid metabolism in intestinal bacteria and its potential implications for mammalian reproduction. *Mol. Hum. Reprod.* 21, 389–409. doi: 10.1093/molehr/gav003

Dali-Youcef, N., Andrès, E. (2009). An update on cobalamin deficiency in adults. *QJM* 102, 17–28. doi: 10.1093/qjmed/hcn138

Daulatzai, M.A. (2015). Non-celiac gluten sensitivity triggers gut dysbiosis, neuroinflammation, gut-brain axis dysfunction, and vulnerability for dementia. *CNS Neurol. Disord. Drug Targets* 14, 110–131.

David, L.A., Maurice, C.F., Carmody, R.N., Gootenberg, D.B., Button, J.E., Wolfe, B.E., *et al.* (2014). Diet rapidly and reproducibly alters the human gut microbiome. *Nature* 505, 559–563. doi: 10.1038/nature12820

De Filippo, C., Cavalieri, D., Di Paola, M., Ramazzotti, M., Poullet, J.B., Massart, S., Collini, S., Pieraccini, G., Lionetti, P. (2010). Impact of diet in shaping gut microbiota revealed by a comparative study in children from Europe and rural Africa. *Proc. Natl. Acad. Sci. U.S.A.* 107, 14691–14696. doi: 10.1073/pnas .1005963107

Del Chierico, F., Vernocchi, P., Petrucca, A., Paci, P., Fuentes, S., Praticò, G., *et al.* (2015). Phylogenetic and metabolic tracking of gut microbiota during perinatal development. *PLoS One* 10. doi: 10.1371/journal.pone.0137347

D'Elia, L., Rossi, G., Ippolito, R., Cappuccio, F.P., Strazzullo, P. (2012). Habitual salt intake and risk of gastric cancer: a meta-analysis of prospective studies. *Clin. Nutr.* 31, 489–498. doi: 10.1016/j.clnu.2012.01.003

de Moreno de LeBlanc, A., Perdigón, G. (2004). Yogurt feeding inhibits promotion and progression of experimental colorectal cancer. *Med. Sci. Monit.* 10, BR96–104.

de Moreno de LeBlanc, A., Perdigón, G. (2005). Reduction of beta-glucuronidase and nitroreductase activity by yoghurt in a murine colon cancer model. *Biocell* 29, 15–24.

de Oliveira, J.G., Silva, A.E. (2012). Polymorphisms of the TLR2 and TLR4 genes are associated with risk of gastric cancer in a Brazilian population. *World J. Gastroenterol.* 18, 1235–1242. doi: 10.3748/wjg.v18.i11.1235

Derrien, M., Collado, M.C., Ben-Amor, K., Salminen, S., de Vos, W.M. (2008). The Mucin degrader *Akkermansia muciniphila* is an abundant resident of the human intestinal tract. *Appl. Environ. Microbiol.* 74, 1646–1648. doi: 10.1128/AEM .01226–07

Desbonnet, L., Garrett, L., Clarke, G., Kiely, B., Cryan, J.F., Dinan, T.G. (2010). Effects of the probiotic *Bifidobacterium infantis* in the maternal separation model of depression. *Neuroscience* 170, 1179–1188. doi: 10.1016/j.neuroscience. 2010.08.005

de Souza, C.R.T., de Oliveira, K.S., Ferraz, J.J.S., Leal, M.F., Calcagno, D.Q., Seabra, A.D., *et al.* (2014). Occurrence of *Helicobacter pylori* and Epstein-Barr virus infection in endoscopic and gastric cancer patients from Northern Brazil. *BMC Gastroenterol.* 14, 179. doi: 10.1186/1471-230X-14-179

Devkota, S., Chang, E.B. (2015). Interactions between diet, bile acid metabolism, gut microbiota, and inflammatory bowel diseases. *Dig. Dis.* 33, 351–356. doi:10.1159/000371687

de Vos, W.M., Nieuwdorp, M. (2013). Genomics: A gut prediction. *Nature* 498, 48–49. doi: 10.1038/nature12251

de Vrese, M., Schrezenmeir, J. (2008). Probiotics, prebiotics, and synbiotics. *Adv. Biochem. Eng. Biotechnol.* 111, 1–66. doi: 10.1007/10_2008_097

Dikeman, C.L., Fahey, G.C. (2006). Viscosity as related to dietary fiber: a review. *Crit. Rev. Food Sci. Nutr.* 46, 649–663. doi: 10.1080/10408390500511862

Di Marzo, V., Matias, I. (2005). Endocannabinoid control of food intake and energy balance. *Nat. Neurosci.* 8, 585–589. doi: 10.1038/nn1457

Donath, M.Y., Shoelson, S.E. (2011). Type 2 diabetes as an inflammatory disease. *Nat. Rev. Immunol.* 11, 98–107. doi: 10.1038/nri2925

Dunlop, S.P., Jenkins, D., Neal, K.R., Spiller, R.C. (2003). Relative importance of enterochromaffin cell hyperplasia, anxiety, and depression in postinfectious IBS. *Gastroenterology* 125, 1651–1659. doi: 10.1053/j.gastr0.2003.09.028

Eid, N., Osmanova, H., Natchez, C., Walton, G., Costabile, A., Gibson, G., *et al.* (2015). Impact of palm date consumption on microbiota growth and large intestinal health: a randomised, controlled, cross-over, human intervention study. *Br. J. Nutr.* 114, 1226–1236. doi: 10.1017/S0007114515002780

Ekpenyong, C.E., Daniel, N.E., Antai, A.B. (2015). Bioactive natural constituents from lemongrass tea and erythropoiesis boosting effects: potential use in prevention and treatment of anemia. *J. Med. Food* 18, 118–127. doi: 10.1089/jmf.2013.0184

El-Ansary, A.K., Bacha, A.G.B., Al-Ayahdi, L.Y. (2011). Plasma fatty acids as diagnostic markers in autistic patients from Saudi Arabia. *Lipids Health Dis.* 10, 62. doi: 10.1186/1476-511X-10-62

El Asmar, R., Panigrahi, P., Bamford, P., Berti, I., Not, T., Coppa, G.V., *et al.* (2002). Host-dependent zonulin secretion causes the impairment of the small intestine barrier function after bacterial exposure. *Gastroenterology* 123, 1607–1615.

Elekofehinti, O.O. (2015). Saponins: Anti-diabetic principles from medicinal plants – A review. *Pathophysiology* 22, 95–103. doi: 10.1016/j.pathophys.2015.02.001

Encarnação, J.C., Abrantes, A.M., Pires, A.S., Botelho, M.F. (2015). Revisit dietary fiber on colorectal cancer: butyrate and its role on prevention and treatment. *Cancer Metastasis Rev.* 34, 465–478. doi: 10.1007/s10555-015-9578-9

Ericsson, A.C., Akter, S., Hanson, M.M., Busi, S.B., Parker, T.W., Schehr, R.J., *et al.* (2015). Differential susceptibility to colorectal cancer due to naturally occurring gut microbiota. *Oncotarget* 6, 33689–33704. doi: 10.18632/oncotarget.5604

Ervin, R.B. (2008). Healthy Eating Index scores among adults, 60 years of age and over, by sociodemographic and health characteristics: United States, 1999–2002. *Adv. Data* 1–16.

Estall, J.L., Drucker, D.J. (2006). Glucagon-like peptide-2. *Annu. Rev. Nutr.* 26, 391–411. doi: 10.1146/annurev.nutr.26.061505.111223

Estruch, R., Ros, E., Salas-Salvadó, J., Covas, M.-I., Corella, D., Arós, F., *et al.*, PREDIMED Study Investigators (2013). Primary prevention of cardiovascular disease with a Mediterranean diet. *N. Engl. J. Med.* 368, 1279–1290. doi: 10.1056/NEJMoa1200303

Everard, A., Belzer, C., Geurts, L., Ouwerkerk, J.P., Druart, C., Bindels, L.B., *et al.* (2013). Cross-talk between Akkermansia muciniphila and intestinal epithelium controls diet-induced obesity. *Proc. Natl. Acad. Sci. U.S.A.* 110, 9066–9071. doi: 10.1073/pnas.1219451110

Fan W, Huo G, Li X, Yang L, Duan C, Wang T, Chen J. (2013). Diversity of the intestinal microbiota in different patterns of feeding infants by Illumina high-throughput sequencing. *World J. Microbiol. Biotechnol.* 29(12):2365–2372. doi: 10.1007/s11274-013-1404-3

Fang, H., Gong, X., Hong, X., Hua, M., Huang, J. (2015). [Effect of Paridis Rhizoma total saponins on apoptosis of human gastric cancer cell MKN-45 and Fas/FasL signaling pathway]. *Zhongguo Zhong Yao Za Zhi* 40, 1388–1391.

Fasano, A., Fiorentini, C., Donelli, G., Uzzau, S., Kaper, J.B., Margaretten, K., *et al.* (1995). Zonula occludens toxin modulates tight junctions through protein kinase C-dependent actin reorganization, *in vitro. J. Clin. Invest.* 96, 710–720. doi: 10.1172/JCI118114

Ferlay, J., Soerjomataram, I., Ervik, M., Dikshit, R., Eser, S., Mathers, C., *et al.* (2013). *Globocan 2012: Estimated Cancer Incidence, Mortality and Prevalence Worldwide in 2012.* International Agency for Research on Cancer, Lyon, France.

Finegold, S.M. (2011). State of the art; microbiology in health and disease. Intestinal bacterial flora in autism. *Anaerobe* 17, 367–368. doi: 10.1016/j.anaerobe.2011 .03.007

Flegr, J., Zitková, S., Kodym, P., Frynta, D. (1996). Induction of changes in human behaviour by the parasitic protozoan *Toxoplasma gondii. Parasitology* 113 (Pt 1), 49–54.

Flegr, J., Kodym, P., Tolarová, V. (2000). Correlation of duration of latent *Toxoplasma gondii* infection with personality changes in women. *Biol. Psychol.* 53, 57–68.

Foley, K.A., Ossenkopp, K.-P., Kavaliers, M., Macfabe, D.F. (2014). Pre- and neonatal exposure to lipopolysaccharide or the enteric metabolite, propionic acid, alters development and behavior in adolescent rats in a sexually dimorphic manner. *PLoS One* 9, e87072. doi: 10.1371/journal.pone.0087072

Foster, J.A., McVey Neufeld, K.-A. (2013). Gut-brain axis: how the microbiome influences anxiety and depression. *Trends Neurosci.* 36, 305–312. doi: 10.1016/j.tins.2013.01.005

Fox, J.G., Feng, Y., Theve, E.J., Raczynski, A.R., Fiala, J.L.A., Doernte, A.L., *et al.* (2010). Gut microbes define liver cancer risk in mice exposed to chemical and viral transgenic hepatocarcinogens. *Gut* 59, 88–97. doi: 10.1136/gut.2009.183749

Fox, J.G., Ge, Z., Whary, M.T., Erdman, S.E., Horwitz, B.H. (2011). *Helicobacter hepaticus* infection in mice: models for understanding lower bowel inflammation and cancer. *Mucosal Immunol.* 4, 22–30. doi: 10.1038/mi.2010.61

Fraczek, M., Piasecka, M., Gaczarzewicz, D., Szumala-Kakol, A., Kazienko, A., Lenart, S., *et al.* (2012). Membrane stability and mitochondrial activity of human-ejaculated spermatozoa during *in vitro* experimental infection with *Escherichia coli, Staphylococcus haemolyticus* and *Bacteroides ureolyticus. Andrologia* 44, 315–329. doi: 10.1111/j.1439-0272.2012.01283.x

Franchi, L., Muñoz-Planillo, R., Núñez, G. (2012). Sensing and reacting to microbes through the inflammasomes. *Nat. Immunol.* 13, 325–332. doi: 10.1038/ni.2231

Fredricks, D.N., Fiedler, T.L., Marrazzo, J.M. (2005). Molecular identification of bacteria associated with bacterial vaginosis. *N. Engl. J. Med.* 353, 1899–1911. doi: 10.1056/NEJMoa043802

Fumagalli, M., Moltke, I., Grarup, N., Racimo, F., Bjerregaard, P., Jørgensen, M.E., *et al.* (2015). Greenlandic Inuit show genetic signatures of diet and climate adaptation. *Science* 349, 1343–1347. doi: 10.1126/science.aab2319

Gale, E.A., Gillespie, K.M. (2001). Diabetes and gender. *Diabetologia* 44, 3–15. doi: 10.1007/s001250051573

Garmendia, L., Hernandez, A., Sanchez, M.B., Martinez, J.L. (2012). Metagenomics and antibiotics. *Clin. Microbiol. Infect.* 18(Suppl 4), 27–31. doi: 10.1111/j.1469 -0691.2012.03868.x

Geirnaert, A., Wang, J., Tinck, M., Steyaert, A., Van den Abbeele, P., Eeckhaut, V., *et al.* (2015). Interindividual differences in response to treatment with butyrate-producing Butyricicoccus pullicaecorum 25–3T studied in an *in vitro* gut model. *FEMS Microbiol. Ecol.* 91. doi: 10.1093/femsec/fiv054

Geurts, L., Neyrinck, A.M., Delzenne, N.M., Knauf, C., Cani, P.D. (2014). Gut microbiota controls adipose tissue expansion, gut barrier and glucose metabolism: novel insights into molecular targets and interventions using prebiotics. *Benef. Microbes* 5, 3–17. doi: 10.3920/BM2012.0065

Gilsing, A.M.J., Schouten, L.J., Goldbohm, R.A., Dagnelie, P.C., van den Brandt, P.A., Weijenberg, M.P. (2015). Vegetarianism, low meat consumption and the risk of colorectal cancer in a population based cohort study. *Sci. Rep.* 5, 13484. doi: 10.1038/srep13484

Giongo, A., Gano, K.A., Crabb, D.B., Mukherjee, N., Novelo, L.L., Casella, G., *et al.* (2011). Toward defining the autoimmune microbiome for type 1 diabetes. *ISME J.* 5, 82–91. doi: 10.1038/ismej.2010.92

Goehler, L.E., Park, S.M., Opitz, N., Lyte, M., Gaykema, R.P.A. (2008). *Campylobacter jejuni* infection increases anxiety-like behavior in the holeboard: possible anatomical substrates for viscerosensory modulation of exploratory behavior. *Brain. Behav. Immun.* 22, 354–366. doi: 10.1016/j.bbi.2007.08.009

Gough, E.K., Stephens, D.A., Moodie, E.E.M., Prendergast, A.J., Stoltzfus, R.J., Humphrey, J.H., *et al.* (2015). Linear growth faltering in infants is associated with *Acidaminococcus* sp. and community-level changes in the gut microbiota. Microbiome 3, 24. doi: 10.1186/s40168-015-0089-2

Government of Canada (2012). *Autism spectrum disorders.* http://healthycanadians .gc.ca/diseases-conditions-maladies-affections/disease-maladie/autism-eng.php (accessed 28 August 2015).

Gross, G., Jacobs, D.M., Peters, S., Possemiers, S., van Duynhoven, J., Vaughan, E.E., *et al.* (2010). *In vitro* bioconversion of polyphenols from black tea and red wine/grape juice by human intestinal microbiota displays strong interindividual variability. *J. Agric. Food Chem.* 58, 10236–10246. doi: 10.1021/jf101475m

Gu, S., Chen, Y., Zhang, X., Lu, H., Lv, T., Shen, P., *et al.* (2016). Identification of key taxa that favor intestinal colonization of *Clostridium difficile* in an adult Chinese population. *Microbes Infect* 18(1), 30–38. doi: 10.1016/j.micinf.2015.09.008

Gueimonde, M., Collado, M.C. (2012). Metagenomics and probiotics. *Clin. Microbiol. Infect.* 18(Suppl 4), 32–34. doi: 10.1111/j.1469-0691.2012.03873.x

Guglielmetti, S., Fracassetti, D., Taverniti, V., Del Bo', C., Vendrame, S., Klimis-Zacas, D., *et al.* (2013). Differential modulation of human intestinal bifidobacterium populations after consumption of a wild blueberry (*Vaccinium angustifolium*) drink. *J. Agric. Food Chem.* 61, 8134–8140. doi: 10.1021/jf402495k

Guigoz, Y., Rochat, F., Perruisseau-Carrier, G., Rochat, I., Schiffrin, E.J. (2002). Effects of oligosaccharide on the faecal flora and non-specific immune system in elderly people. *Nutr. Res.* 22, 13–25. doi: 10.1016/S0271-5317(01)00354-2

Guilbaud, O., Curt, F., Perrin, C., Chaouat, G., Berthoz, S., Dugré-Le Bigre, C., *et al.* (2009). Decreased immune response in alexithymic women: A cross-sectional study. *Biomed. Pharmacother.* 63, 297–304. doi: 10.1016/j.biopha.2008.08.007

Guo, J.-Q., Zheng, Q.-H., Chen, H., Chen, L., Xu, J.-B., Chen, M.-Y., *et al.* (2014). Ginsenoside Rg3 inhibition of vasculogenic mimicry in pancreatic cancer through downregulation of VE- cadherin/EphA2/MMP9/MMP2 expression. *Int. J. Oncol.* 45, 1065–1072. doi: 10.3892/ij0.2014.2500

Halliwell, B. (1996). Antioxidants in human health and disease. *Annu. Rev. Nutr.* 16, 33–50. doi: 10.1146/annurev.nu.16.070196.000341

Haro, C., Garcia-Carpintero, S., Alcala-Diaz, J.F., Gomez-Delgado, F., Delgado-Lista, J., Perez-Martinez, P., *et al.* (2015). The gut microbial community in metabolic syndrome patients is modified by diet. *J. Nutr. Biochem.* 27, 27–31. doi: 10.1016/j.jnutbi0.2015.08.011

He, B., Nohara, K., Ajami, N.J., Michalek, R.D., Tian, X., Wong, M., *et al.* (2015). Transmissible microbial and metabolomic remodeling by soluble dietary fiber improves metabolic homeostasis. *Sci. Rep.* 5, 10604. doi: 10.1038/srep10604

Helou, C., Denis, S., Spatz, M., Marier, D., Rame, V., Alric, M., *et al.* (2015). Insights into bread melanoidins: fate in the upper digestive tract and impact on the gut microbiota using *in vitro* systems. *Food Funct.* 6(12), 3737–3745. doi: 10.1039/c5f000836k

Henao-Mejia, J., Elinav, E., Thaiss, C.A., Licona-Limon, P., Flavell, R.A. (2013). Role of the intestinal microbiome in liver disease. *J. Autoimmun.* 46, 66–73. doi: 10.1016/j.jaut.2013.07.001

Heuvelin, E., Lebreton, C., Grangette, C., Pot, B., Cerf-Bensussan, N., Heyman, M. (2009). Mechanisms involved in alleviation of intestinal inflammation by bifidobacterium breve soluble factors. *PLoS One* 4, e5184. doi: 10.1371/journal.pone.0005184

Heyer, N.J., Echeverria, D., Woods, J.S. (2012). Disordered porphyrin metabolism: a potential biological marker for autism risk assessment. *Autism Res.* 5, 84–92. doi: 10.1002/aur.236

Hisada, T., Endoh, K., Kuriki, K. (2015). Inter- and intra-individual variations in seasonal and daily stabilities of the human gut microbiota in Japanese. *Arch. Microbiol.* 1–16. doi: 10.1007/s00203-015-1125-0

Hoffmann, T.W., Pham, H.-P., Bridonneau, C., Aubry, C., Lamas, B., Martin-Gallausiaux, C., *et al.* (2015). Microorganisms linked to inflammatory bowel disease-associated dysbiosis differentially impact host physiology in gnotobiotic mice. *ISME J.* doi: 10.1038/ismej.2015.127

Holscher, H.D., Caporaso, J.G., Hooda, S., Brulc, J.M., Fahey, G.C., Swanson, K.S. (2015). Fiber supplementation influences phylogenetic structure and functional capacity of the human intestinal microbiome: follow-up of a randomized controlled trial. *Am. J. Clin. Nutr.* 101, 55–64. doi: 10.3945/ajcn.114.092064

Hoque, R., Sohail, M., Malik, A., Sarwar, S., Luo, Y., Shah, A., *et al.* (2011). TLR9 and the NLRP3 inflammasome link acinar cell death with inflammation in acute pancreatitis. *Gastroenterology* 141, 358–369. doi: 10.1053/j.gastr0.2011.03.041

Hosseinzadeh, S., Brewis, I.A., Eley, A., Pacey, A.A. (2001). Co-incubation of human spermatozoa with *Chlamydia trachomatis* serovar E causes premature sperm death. *Hum. Reprod.* 16, 293–299. doi: 10.1093/humrep/16.2.293

Hou, D., Zhou, X., Zhong, X., Settles, M., Herring, J., Wang, L., *et al.* (2013). Microbiota of the seminal fluid from healthy and infertile men. *Fertil. Steril.* 100, 1261–1269. doi: 10.1016/j.fertnstert.2013.07.1991

Hsiao, E.Y., McBride, S.W., Hsien, S., Sharon, G., Hyde, E.R., McCue, T., *et al.* (2013). Microbiota modulate behavioral and physiological abnormalities associated with neurodevelopmental disorders. *Cell* 155, 1451–1463. doi: 10.1016/j.ce11.2013.11.024

Huang, B., Zhao, J., Li, H., He, K.-L., Chen, Y., Chen, S.-H., *et al.* (2005). Toll-like receptors on tumor cells facilitate evasion of immune surveillance. *Cancer Res.* 65, 5009–5014. doi: 10.1158/0008–5472.CAN-05-0784

Huang, T., Xu, M., Lee, A., Cho, S., Qi, L. (2015). Consumption of whole grains and cereal fiber and total and cause-specific mortality: prospective analysis of 367,442 individuals. *BMC Med.* 13. doi: 10.1186/s12916-015-0294-7

Hu, D., Wan, L., Chen, M., Caudle, Y., LeSage, G., Li, Q., *et al.* (2014). Essential role of IL-10/STAT3 in chronic stress-induced immune suppression. *Brain. Behav. Immun.* 36, 118–127. doi: 10.1016/j.bbi.2013.10.016

Hu, J., La Vecchia, C., Negri, E., de Groh, M., Morrison, H., Mery, L., Canadian Cancer Registries Epidemiology Research Group (2015). Macronutrient intake and stomach cancer. *Cancer Causes Control* 26, 839–847. doi: 10.1007/s10552-015-0557-9

Hullar, M.A.J., Fu, B.C. (2014). Diet, the gut microbiome, and epigenetics. *Cancer J.* 20, 170–175. doi: 10.1097/PPO.0000000000000053

Huycke, M.M., Abrams, V., Moore, D.R. (2002). Enterococcus faecalis produces extracellular superoxide and hydrogen peroxide that damages colonic epithelial cell DNA. *Carcinogenesis* 23, 529–536.

Ihrig, M., Schrenzel, M.D., Fox, J.G. (1999). Differential susceptibility to hepatic inflammation and proliferation in AXB recombinant inbred mice chronically infected with *Helicobacter hepaticus*. *Am. J. Pathol.* 155, 571–582. doi: 10.1016/S0002-9440(10)65152-8

Janssen, A.W.F., Kersten, S. (2015). The role of the gut microbiota in metabolic health. *FASEB J.* 29(8), 3111–3123. doi: 10.1096/fj.14-269514

Jeffery, I.B., Lynch, D.B., O'Toole, P.W. (2015). Composition and temporal stability of the gut microbiota in older persons. *ISME J.* 10(1), 170–182. doi: 10.1038/ismej.2015.88

Jie, Z., Bang-Yao, L., Ming-Jie, X., Hai-Wei, L., Zu-Kang, Z., Ting-Song, W., *et al.* (2000). Studies on the effects of polydextrose intake on physiologic functions in Chinese people. *Am. J. Clin. Nutr.* 72, 1503–1509.

Joh, E.-H., Lee, I.-A., Jung, I.-H., Kim, D.-H. (2011). Ginsenoside Rb1 and its metabolite compound K inhibit IRAK-1 activation – the key step of inflammation. *Biochem. Pharmacol.* 82, 278–286. doi: 10.1016/j.bcp.2011.05.003

Jones, G.W., Bombardieri, M., Greenhill, C.J., McLeod, L., Nerviani, A., Rocher-Ros, V., *et al.* (2015). Interleukin-27 inhibits ectopic lymphoid-like structure development in early inflammatory arthritis. *J. Exp. Med.* doi: 10.1084/jem.20132307

Jovanovski, E., Bateman, E.A., Bhardwaj, J., Fairgrieve, C., Mucalo, I., Jenkins, A.L., *et al.* (2014). Effect of Rg3-enriched Korean red ginseng (*Panax ginseng*) on arterial stiffness and blood pressure in healthy individuals: a randomized controlled trial. *J. Am. Soc. Hypertens.* 8, 537–541. doi: 10.1016/j.jash.2014.04.004

Jung, T.-H., Jeon, W.-M., Han, K.-S. (2015). *In vitro* effects of dietary inulin on human fecal microbiota and butyrate production. *J. Microbiol. Biotechnol.* 25, 1555–1558. doi: 10.4014/jmb.1505.05078

Justo, M.L., Claro, C., Zeyda, M., Stulnig, T.M., Herrera, M.D., Rodríguez-Rodríguez, R. (2015). Rice bran prevents high-fat diet-induced inflammation and macrophage content in adipose tissue. *Eur. J. Nutr.* doi: 10.1007/s00394-015–1015-x

Kabeerdoss, J., Shobana Devi, R., Regina Mary, R., Ramakrishna, B.S. (2012). Faecal microbiota composition in vegetarians: comparison with omnivores in a cohort of young women in southern India. *Br. J. Nutr.* 108, 953–957. doi: 10.1017/S0007114511006362

Kabeerdoss, J., Ferdous, S., Balamurugan, R., Mechenro, J., Vidya, R., Santhanam, S., *et al.* (2013). Development of the gut microbiota in southern Indian infants from birth to 6 months: a molecular analysis. *J. Nutr. Sci.* 2, e18. doi: 10.1017/jns.2013.6

Kaczmarczyk, M.M., Miller, M.J., Freund, G.G. (2012). The health benefits of dietary fiber: beyond the usual suspects of type 2 diabetes mellitus, cardiovascular disease and colon cancer. *Metabolism* 61, 1058–1066. doi: 10.1016/j.metab01.2012.01.017

Kałuzna-Czaplinska, J., Michalska, M., Rynkowski, J. (2010). Determination of tryptophan in urine of autistic and healthy children by gas chromatography/mass spectrometry. *Med. Sci. Monit.* 16, CR488–492.

Kałużna-Czaplińska, J., Michalska, M., Rynkowski, J. (2011). Vitamin supplementation reduces the level of homocysteine in the urine of autistic children. *Nutr. Res.* 31, 318–321. doi: 10.1016/j.nutres.2011.03.009

Kang, D.-W., Park, J.G., Ilhan, Z.E., Wallstrom, G., Labaer, J., Adams, J.B., *et al.* (2013). Reduced incidence of *Prevotella* and other fermenters in intestinal microflora of autistic children. *PLoS One* 8, e68322. doi: 10.1371/journal.pone.0068322

Kasubuchi, M., Hasegawa, S., Hiramatsu, T., Ichimura, A., Kimura, I. (2015). Dietary gut microbial metabolites, short-chain fatty acids, and host metabolic regulation. *Nutrients* 7, 2839–2849. doi: 10.3390/nu7042839

Kawai, T., Akira, S. (2010). The role of pattern-recognition receptors in innate immunity: update on Toll-like receptors. *Nat. Immunol.* 11, 373–384. doi: 10.1038/ni.1863

Keibel, A., Singh, V., Sharma, M.C. (2009). Inflammation, microenvironment, and the immune system in cancer progression. *Curr. Pharm. Des.* 15, 1949–1955.

Kelly, D., Campbell, J.I., King, T.P., Grant, G., Jansson, E.A., Coutts, A.G.P., *et al.* (2004). Commensal anaerobic gut bacteria attenuate inflammation by regulating nuclear-cytoplasmic shuttling of PPAR-gamma and RelA. *Nat. Immunol.* 5, 104–112. doi: 10.1038/ni1018

Kemppainen, K.M., Ardissone, A.N., Davis-Richardson, A.G., Fagen, J.R., Gano, K.A., León-Novelo, L.G., *et al.*, TEDDY Study Group (2015). Early childhood gut microbiomes show strong geographic differences among subjects at high risk for type 1 diabetes. *Diabetes Care* 38, 329–332. doi: 10.2337/dc14-0850

Kim, J., Kang, M., Lee, J.-S., Inoue, M., Sasazuki, S., Tsugane, S. (2011). Fermented and non-fermented soy food consumption and gastric cancer in Japanese and Korean populations: a meta-analysis of observational studies. *Cancer Sci.* 102, 231–244. doi: 10.1111/j.1349-7006.2010.01770.x

Kim, K.-A., Jung, I.-H., Park, S.-H., Ahn, Y.-T., Huh, C.-S., Kim, D.-H. (2013). Comparative analysis of the gut microbiota in people with different levels of ginsenoside Rb1 degradation to compound K. *PLoS One* 8, e62409. doi: 10.1371/journal.pone.0062409

Kim, K., Park, M., Lee, Y.M., Rhyu, M.R., Kim, H.Y. (2014). Ginsenoside metabolite compound K stimulates glucagon-like peptide-1 secretion in NCI-H716 cells via bile acid receptor activation. *Arch. Pharm. Res.* 37, 1193–1200. doi: 10.1007/s12272-014-0362-0

Kim, Y.-J., Zhang, D., Yang, D.-C. (2015). Biosynthesis and biotechnological production of ginsenosides. *Biotechnol. Adv.* 33, 717–735. doi: 10.1016/j.biotechadv.2015.03.001

Kino, T. (2015). Stress, glucocorticoid hormones, and hippocampal neural progenitor cells: implications to mood disorders. *Front. Physiol.* 6, 230. doi: 10.3389/fphys.2015.00230

Kinross, J., Nicholson, J.K. (2012). Gut microbiota: Dietary and social modulation of gut microbiota in the elderly. *Nat. Rev. Gastroenterol. Hepatol.* 9, 563–564. doi: 10.1038/nrgastr0.2012.169

Komura, T., Sakai, Y., Harada, K., Kawaguchi, K., Takabatake, H., Kitagawa, H., *et al.* (2015). Inflammatory features of pancreatic cancer highlighted by monocytes/macrophages and CD4+ T cells with clinical impact. *Cancer Sci.* 106, 672–686. doi: 10.1111/cas.12663

Kong, X., Wang, X., Yin, Y., Li, X., Gao, H., Bazer, F.W., *et al.* (2014). Putrescine stimulates the mTOR signaling pathway and protein synthesis in porcine trophectoderm cells. *Biol. Reprod.* 91, 106. doi: 10.1095/biolreprod.113.113977

Konstantynowicz, J., Porowski, T., Zoch-Zwierz, W., Wasilewska, J., Kadziela-Olech, H., Kulak, W., *et al.* (2012). A potential pathogenic role of oxalate in autism. *Eur. J. Paediatr. Neurol.* 16, 485–491. doi: 10.1016/j.ejpn.2011.08.004

Korrovits, P., Punab, M., Türk, S., Mändar, R. (2006). Seminal microflora in asymptomatic inflammatory (NIH IV category) prostatitis. *Eur. Urol.* 50, 1338–1346. doi: 10.1016/j.eurur0.2006.05.013

Kozikowski, A.P., Tückmantel, W., Böttcher, G., Romanczyk, L.J. (2003). Studies in polyphenol chemistry and bioactivity. 4.(1) Synthesis of trimeric, tetrameric, pentameric, and higher oligomeric epicatechin-derived procyanidins having all-4beta,8-interflavan connectivity and their inhibition of cancer cell growth through cell cycle arrest. *J. Org. Chem.* 68, 1641–1658. doi: 10.1021/j0020393f

Kunzmann, A.T., Coleman, H.G., Huang, W.-Y., Kitahara, C.M., Cantwell, M.M., Berndt, S.I. (2015). Dietary fiber intake and risk of colorectal cancer and incident and recurrent adenoma in the Prostate, Lung, Colorectal, and Ovarian Cancer Screening Trial. *Am. J. Clin. Nutr.* 102, 881–890. doi: 10.3945/ajcn.115.113282

Kusters, J.G., van Vliet, A.H.M., Kuipers, E.J. (2006). Pathogenesis of *Helicobacter pylori* infection. *Clin. Microbiol. Rev.* 19, 449–490. doi: 10.1128/CMR.00054-05

Lacombe, A., Tadepalli, S., Hwang, C.-A., Wu, V.C.H. (2013). Phytochemicals in lowbush wild blueberry inactivate *Escherichia coli* 0157:H7 by damaging its cell membrane. *Foodborne Pathog. Dis.* 10, 944–950. doi: 10.1089/fpd.2013.1504

Lahouar, L., Ghrairi, F., Arem, A.E., Sghaeir, W., Felah, M.E., Salem, H.B., *et al.* (2014). Attenuation of histopathological alterations of colon, liver and lung by dietary fibre of barley Rihane in azoxymethane-treated rats. *Food Chem.* 149, 271–276. doi: 10.1016/j.foodchem.2013.10.101

Lamprecht, M., Bogner, S., Schippinger, G., Steinbauer, K., Fankhauser, F., Hallstroem, S., *et al.* (2012). Probiotic supplementation affects markers of intestinal barrier, oxidation, and inflammation in trained men; a randomized, double-blinded, placebo-controlled trial. *J. Int. Soc. Sports Nutr.* 9, 45. doi: 10.1186/1550-2783-9-45

Lande, A.A., Ambavade, S.D., Swami, U.S., Adkar, P.P., Ambavade, P.D., Waghamare, A.B. (2015). Saponins isolated from roots of *Chlorophytum borivilianum* reduce acute and chronic inflammation and histone deacetylase. *J. Integr. Med.* 13, 25–33. doi: 10.1016/S2095-4964(15)60157-1

Lang, J.M., Eisen, J.A., Zivkovic, A.M. (2014). The microbes we eat: abundance and taxonomy of microbes consumed in a day's worth of meals for three diet types. *PeerJ* 2, e659. doi: 10.7717/peerj.659

Lanza, E., Yu, B., Murphy, G., Albert, P.S., Caan, B., Marshall, J.R., *et al.* (2007). The polyp prevention trial–continued follow-up study: no effect of a low-fat, high-fiber, high-fruit, and-vegetable diet on adenoma recurrence eight years after randomization. *Cancer Epidemiol. Biomarkers Prev.* 16, 1745–1752. doi: 10.1158/1055–9965.EPI-07–0127

Larsen, C.M., Faulenbach, M., Vaag, A., Vølund, A., Ehses, J.A., Seifert, B., *et al.* (2007). Interleukin-1-receptor antagonist in type 2 diabetes mellitus. *N. Engl. J. Med.* 356, 1517–1526. doi: 10.1056/NEJMoa065213

Larsen, N., Vogensen, F.K., van den Berg, F.W.J., Nielsen, D.S., Andreasen, A.S., Pedersen, B.K., *et al.* (2010). Gut microbiota in human adults with type 2 diabetes differs from non-diabetic adults. *PLoS One* 5, e9085. doi: 10.1371/journal.pone .0009085

La Torre, G., Chiaradia, G., Gianfagna, F., De Lauretis, A., Boccia, S., Mannocci, A., *et al.* (2009). Smoking status and gastric cancer risk: an updated meta-analysis of case-control studies published in the past ten years. *Tumori* 95, 13–22.

Lattimer, J.M., Haub, M.D. (2010). Effects of dietary fiber and its components on metabolic health. *Nutrients* 2, 1266–1289. doi: 10.3390/nu2121266

Lee, A.S., Gibson, D.L., Zhang, Y., Sham, H.P., Vallance, B.A., Dutz, J.P. (2010). Gut barrier disruption by an enteric bacterial pathogen accelerates insulitis in NOD mice. *Diabetologia* 53, 741–748. doi: 10.1007/s00125-009-1626-y

Lee, H.C., Jenner, A.M., Low, C.S., Lee, Y.K. (2006). Effect of tea phenolics and their aromatic fecal bacterial metabolites on intestinal microbiota. *Res. Microbiol.* 157, 876–884. doi: 10.1016/j.resmic.2006.07.004

Ley, R.E., Turnbaugh, P.J., Klein, S., Gordon, J.I. (2006). Microbial ecology: human gut microbes associated with obesity. *Nature* 444, 1022–1023. doi: 10.1038/4441022a

Li, F., Wang, D., Xu, P., Wu, J., Liu, L., Liu, X. (2013). Identification of the metabolites of anti-inflammatory compound clematichinenoside AR in rat intestinal microflora. *Biomed. Chromatogr.* 27, 1767–1774. doi: 10.1002/bmc.2991

Lin, A., Bik, E.M., Costello, E.K., Dethlefsen, L., Haque, R., Relman, D.A., *et al.* (2013). Distinct distal gut microbiome diversity and composition in healthy children from Bangladesh and the United States. *PLoS One* 8, e53838. doi: 10.1371/journal.pone.0053838

Lin, R.S., Lee, F.Y., Lee, S.D., Tsai, Y.T., Lin, H.C., Lu, R.H., *et al.* (1995). Endotoxemia in patients with chronic liver diseases: relationship to severity of liver diseases, presence of esophageal varices, and hyperdynamic circulation. *J. Hepatol.* 22, 165–172.

Lin, S.-S., Fan, W., Sun, L., Li, F.-F., Zhao, R.-P., Zhang, L.-Y., Yu, B.-Y., Yuan, S.-T. (2014). The saponin DT-13 inhibits gastric cancer cell migration through down-regulation of CCR5-CCL5 axis. *Chin. J. Nat. Med.* 12, 833–840. doi: 10.1016/S1875-5364(14)60125-4

Liu, X., Cao, S., Zhang, X. (2015). Modulation of gut microbiota-brain axis by probiotics, prebiotics, and diet. *J. Agric. Food Chem.* 63, 7885–7895. doi: 10.1021/acs.jafc.5b02404

Li, Z., Summanen, P.H., Komoriya, T., Henning, S.M., Lee, R.-P., Carlson, E., *et al.* (2015). Pomegranate ellagitannins stimulate growth of gut bacteria *in vitro*: Implications for prebiotic and metabolic effects. *Anaerobe* 34, 164–168. doi: 10.1016/j.anaerobe.2015.05.012

Loncle, C., Bonjoch, L., Folch-Puy, E., Lopez-Millan, M.B., Lac, S., Molejon, M.I., *et al.* (2015). IL17 Functions through the novel REG3β-JAK2-STAT3 inflammatory pathway to promote the transition from chronic pancreatitis to pancreatic cancer. *Cancer Res.* 75, 4852–4862. doi: 10.1158/0008-5472.CAN -15-0896

Long, F.-Y., Chen, Y.-S., Zhang, L., Kuang, X., Yu, Y., Wang, L.-F., *et al.* (2015). Pennogenyl saponins induce cell cycle arrest and apoptosis in human hepatocellular carcinoma HepG2 cells. *J. Ethnopharmacol.* 162, 112–120. doi: 10.1016/j.jep.2014.12.065

Longo, N., Ardon, O., Vanzo, R., Schwartz, E., Pasquali, M. (2011). Disorders of creatine transport and metabolism. *Am. J. Med. Genet. C Semin. Med. Genet.* 157C, 72–78. doi: 10.1002/ajmg.c.30292

Lopez-Siles, M., Martinez-Medina, M., Abellà, C., Busquets, D., Sabat-Mir, M., Duncan, S.H., *et al.* (2015). Mucosa-associated *Faecalibacterium prausnitzii* phylotype richness is reduced in patients with inflammatory bowel disease. *Appl. Environ. Microbiol.* 81, 7582–7592. doi: 10.1128/AEM.02006-15

Lyte, M., Li, W., Opitz, N., Gaykema, R.P.A., Goehler, L.E. (2006). Induction of anxiety-like behavior in mice during the initial stages of infection with the agent of murine colonic hyperplasia *Citrobacter rodentium*. *Physiol. Behav.* 89, 350–357. doi: 10.1016/j.physbeh.2006.06.019

Macfabe, D.F. (2012). Short-chain fatty acid fermentation products of the gut microbiome: implications in autism spectrum disorders. *Microb. Ecol. Health Dis.* 23. doi: 10.3402/mehd.v23i0.19260

MacFabe, D.F., Cain, N.E., Boon, F., Ossenkopp, K.-P., Cain, D.P. (2011). Effects of the enteric bacterial metabolic product propionic acid on object-directed behavior, social behavior, cognition, and neuroinflammation in adolescent rats: Relevance to autism spectrum disorder. *Behav. Brain Res.* 217, 47–54. doi: 10.1016/j.bbr.2010.10.005

Makino, H., Kushiro, A., Ishikawa, E., Muylaert, D., Kubota, H., Sakai, T., *et al.* (2011). Transmission of intestinal *Bifidobacterium longum* subsp. *longum* strains from mother to infant, determined by multilocus sequencing typing and amplified fragment length polymorphism. *Appl. Environ. Microbiol.* 77, 6788–6793. doi: 10.1128/AEM.05346-11

Maldonado-Contreras, A., Goldfarb, K.C., Godoy-Vitorino, F., Karaoz, U., Contreras, M., Blaser, M.J., *et al.* (2011). Structure of the human gastric bacterial community in relation to *Helicobacter pylori* status. *ISME J.* 5, 574–579. doi: 10.1038/ismej.2010.149

Mallet, J.-F., Graham, É., Ritz, B.W., Homma, K., Matar, C. (2015). Active hexose correlated compound (AHCC) promotes an intestinal immune response in BALB/c mice and in primary intestinal epithelial cell culture involving toll-like receptors TLR-2 and TLR-4. *Eur. J. Nutr.* 1–8. doi: 10.1007/s00394-015-0832-2

Man, S., Fan, W., Liu, Z., Gao, W., Li, Y., Zhang, L., Liu, C. (2014). Antitumor pathway of *Rhizoma paridis* saponins based on the metabolic regulatory network alterations in H22 hepatocarcinoma mice. *Steroids* 84, 17–21. doi: 10.1016/j.steroids.2014.03.005

Masco, L., Huys, G., De Brandt, E., Temmerman, R., Swings, J. (2005). Culture-dependent and culture-independent qualitative analysis of probiotic products claimed to contain bifidobacteria. *Int. J. Food Microbiol.* 102, 221–230. doi: 10.1016/j.ijfoodmicr0.2004.11.018

Maslowski, K.M., Mackay, C.R. (2011). Diet, gut microbiota and immune responses. *Nat. Immunol.* 12, 5–9. doi: 10.1038/ni0111–5

Mastromarino, P., Hemalatha, R., Barbonetti, A., Cinque, B., Cifone, M.G., Tammaro, F., *et al.* (2014). Biological control of vaginosis to improve reproductive health. *Indian J. Med. Res.* 140, S91–S97.

Mazmanian, S.K., Liu, C.H., Tzianabos, A.O., Kasper, D.L. (2005). An immunomodulatory molecule of symbiotic bacteria directs maturation of the host immune system. *Cell* 122, 107–118. doi: 10.1016/j.cell.2005.05.007

McMillan, B., Riggs, D.R., Jackson, B.J., Cunningham, C., McFadden, D.W. (2007). Dietary influence on pancreatic cancer growth by catechin and inositol hexaphosphate. *J. Surg. Res.* 141, 115–119. doi: 10.1016/j.jss.2007.03.065

McRorie, J.W. (2015). Evidence-based approach to fiber supplements and clinically meaningful health benefits, Part 1: What to look for and how to recommend an effective fiber therapy. *Nutr. Today* 50, 82–89. doi: 10.1097/NT.0000000000 000082

Meddings, J.B., Jarand, J., Urbanski, S.J., Hardin, J., Gall, D.G. (1999). Increased gastrointestinal permeability is an early lesion in the spontaneously diabetic BB rat. *Am. J. Physiol.* 276, G951–957.

Messaoudi, M., Lalonde, R., Violle, N., Javelot, H., Desor, D., Nejdi, A., *et al.* (2011). Assessment of psychotropic-like properties of a probiotic formulation (*Lactobacillus helveticus* R0052 and *Bifidobacterium longum* R0175) in rats and human subjects. *Br. J. Nutr.* 105, 755–764. doi: 10.1017/S0007114510004319

Miquel, S., Leclerc, M., Martin, R., Chain, F., Lenoir, M., Raguideau, S., *et al.* (2015). Identification of metabolic signatures linked to anti-inflammatory effects of *Faecalibacterium prausnitzii. mBio* 6. doi: 10.1128/mBi0.00300-15

Moloney, R.D., O'Mahony, S.M., Dinan, T.G., Cryan, J.F. (2015). Stress-induced visceral pain: toward animal models of irritable-bowel syndrome and associated comorbidities. *Front. Psychiatry* 6, 15. doi: 10.3389/fpsyt.2015.00015

Muccioli, G.G., Naslain, D., Bäckhed, F., Reigstad, C.S., Lambert, D.M., Delzenne, N.M., *et al.* (2010). The endocannabinoid system links gut microbiota to adipogenesis. *Mol. Syst. Biol.* 6, 392. doi: 10.1038/msb.2010.46

Mudduluru, G., George-William, J.N., Muppala, S., Asangani, I.A., Kumarswamy, R., Nelson, L.D., *et al.* (2011). Curcumin regulates miR-21 expression and inhibits invasion and metastasis in colorectal cancer. *Biosci. Rep.* 31, 185–197. doi: 10.1042/BSR20100065

Mueller, S., Saunier, K., Hanisch, C., Norin, E., Alm, L., Midtvedt, T., *et al.* (2006). Differences in fecal microbiota in different European study populations in relation to age, gender, and country: a cross-sectional study. *Appl. Environ. Microbiol.* 72, 1027–1033. doi: 10.1128/AEM.72.2.1027-1033.2006

Narayanan, N.K., Kunimasa, K., Yamori, Y., Mori, M., Mori, H., Nakamura, K., *et al.* (2015). Antitumor activity of melinjo (*Gnetum gnemon* L.) seed extract in human and murine tumor models *in vitro* and in a colon-26 tumor-bearing mouse model *in vivo*. *Cancer Med.* 4, 1767–1780. doi: 10.1002/cam4.520

Nickel, J.C., Roehrborn, C.G., O'Leary, M.P., Bostwick, D.G., Somerville, M.C., Rittmaster, R.S. (2008). The relationship between prostate inflammation and lower urinary tract symptoms: Examination of baseline data from the REDUCE Trial. *Eur. Urol.* 54, 1379–1384. doi: 10.1016/j.eururo.2007.11.026

Nuñez-Sánchez, M.A., García-Villalba, R., Monedero-Saiz, T., García-Talavera, N.V., Gómez-Sánchez, M.B., Sánchez-Álvarez, C., *et al.* (2014). Targeted metabolic profiling of pomegranate polyphenols and urolithins in plasma, urine and colon tissues from colorectal cancer patients. *Mol. Nutr. Food Res.* 58, 1199–1211. doi: 10.1002/mnfr.201300931

Oh, H.A., Kim, D.-E., Choi, H.J., Kim, N.J., Kim, D.-H. (2015). Anti-fatigue effects of 20(S)-protopanaxadiol and 20(S)-protopanaxatriol in mice. *Biol. Pharm. Bull.* 38, 1415–1419. doi: 10.1248/bpb.b15-00230

Okada, Y., Tsuzuki, Y., Hokari, R., Komoto, S., Kurihara, C., Kawaguchi, A., *et al.* (2009). Anti-inflammatory effects of the genus *Bifidobacterium* on macrophages by modification of phospho-I kappaB and SOCS gene expression. *Int. J. Exp. Pathol.* 90, 131–140. doi: 10.1111/j.1365-2613.2008.00632.x

Ostan, R., Lanzarini, C., Pini, E., Scurti, M., Vianello, D., Bertarelli, C., *et al.* (2015). Inflammaging and cancer: a challenge for the Mediterranean diet. *Nutrients* 7, 2589–2621. doi: 10.3390/nu7042589

O'Toole, A., Alakkari, A., Keegan, D., Doherty, G., Mulcahy, H., O'Donoghue, D. (2012). Primary sclerosing cholangitis and disease distribution in inflammatory bowel disease. *Clin. Gastroenterol. Hepatol.* 10, 439–441. doi: 10.1016/j.cgh.2011.11.010

O'Toole, P.W. (2012). Changes in the intestinal microbiota from adulthood through to old age. *Clin. Microbiol. Infect.* 18 (Suppl 4), 44–46. doi: 10.1111/j.1469-0691.2012.03867.x

Ouzounova-Raykova, V., Rangelov, S., Ouzounova, I., Mitov, I. (2015). Detection of *Chlamydia trachomatis*, *Ureaplasma urealyticum* and *Mycoplasma hominis* in infertile Bulgarian men with multiplex real-time polymerase chain reaction. *APMIS* 123, 586–588. doi: 10.1111/apm.12391

Palmer, C., Bik, E.M., DiGiulio, D.B., Relman, D.A., Brown, P.O. (2007). Development of the human infant intestinal microbiota. *PLoS Biol.* 5, e177. doi: 10.1371/journal.pbi0.0050177

Parikka, V., Näntö-Salonen, K., Saarinen, M., Simell, T., Ilonen, J., Hyöty, H., *et al.* (2012). Early seroconversion and rapidly increasing autoantibody concentrations predict prepubertal manifestation of type 1 diabetes in children at genetic risk. *Diabetologia* 55, 1926–1936. doi: 10.1007/s00125-012-2523-3

Parks, B.W., Nam, E., Org, E., Kostem, E., Norheim, F., Hui, S.T., *et al.* (2013). Genetic control of obesity and gut microbiota composition in response to high-fat, high-sucrose diet in mice. *Cell Metab.* 17, 141–152. doi: 10.1016/j.cmet.2012.12.007

Parracho, H.M.R.T., Bingham, M.O., Gibson, G.R., McCartney, A.L. (2005). Differences between the gut microflora of children with autistic spectrum disorders and that of healthy children. *J. Med. Microbiol.* 54, 987–991. doi: 10.1099/jmm.0.46101–0

Pédron, T., Sansonetti, P. (2008). Commensals, bacterial pathogens and intestinal inflammation: an intriguing ménage à trois. *Cell Host Microbe* 3, 344–347. doi: 10.1016/j.chom.2008.05.010

Peng, C., Perera, P.K., Li, Y.-M., Fang, W.-R., Liu, L.-F., Li, F.-W. (2012). Anti-inflammatory effects of *Clematis chinensis* Osbeck extract(AR-6) may be associated with NF-κB, TNF-α, and COX-2 in collagen-induced arthritis in rat. *Rheumatol. Int.* 32, 3119–3125. doi: 10.1007/s00296-011-2083-8

Pérez Martínez, G., Bäuerl, C., Collado, M.C. (2014). Understanding gut microbiota in elderly's health will enable intervention through probiotics. *Benef. Microbes* 5, 235–246. doi: 10.3920/BM2013.0079

Peterson, C.T., Sharma, V., Elmén, L., Peterson, S.N. (2015). Immune homeostasis, dysbiosis and therapeutic modulation of the gut microbiota. *Clin. Exp. Immunol.* 179, 363–377. doi: 10.1111/cei.12474

Possemiers, S., Bolca, S., Verstraete, W., Heyerick, A. (2011). The intestinal microbiome: A separate organ inside the body with the metabolic potential to influence the bioactivity of botanicals. *Fitoterapia* 82, 53–66. doi: 10.1016/j.fitote.2010.07.012

Pozzilli, P., Signore, A., Williams, A.J., Beales, P.E. (1993). NOD mouse colonies around the world – recent facts and figures. *Immunol. Today* 14, 193–196. doi: 10.1016/0167-5699(93)90160-M

Puertollano, E., Kolida, S., Yaqoob, P. (2014). Biological significance of short-chain fatty acid metabolism by the intestinal microbiome. *Curr. Opin. Clin. Nutr. Metab. Care* 17, 139–144. doi: 10.1097/MCO.0000000000000025

Rafter, J. (2004). The effects of probiotics on colon cancer development. *Nutr. Res. Rev.* 17, 277–284. doi: 10.1079/NRR200484

Ramirez-Farias, C., Slezak, K., Fuller, Z., Duncan, A., Holtrop, G., Louis, P. (2009). Effect of inulin on the human gut microbiota: stimulation of *Bifidobacterium adolescentis* and *Faecalibacterium prausnitzii*. *Br. J. Nutr.* 101, 541–550. doi: 10.1017/S0007114508019880

Raymond, F., Ouameur, A.A., Déraspe, M., Iqbal, N., Gingras, H., Dridi, B., *et al.* (2015). The initial state of the human gut microbiome determines its reshaping by antibiotics. *ISME J.* 10, 707–720. doi: 10.1038/ismej.2015.148

Rebello, C.J., Burton, J., Heiman, M., Greenway, F.L. (2015). Gastrointestinal microbiome modulator improves glucose tolerance in overweight and obese subjects: A randomized controlled pilot trial. *J. Diabetes Complications* 29, 1272–1276. doi: 10.1016/j.jdiacomp.2015.08.023

Reber, S.O., Peters, S., Slattery, D.A., Hofmann, C., Schölmerich, J., Neumann, I.D., *et al.* (2011). Mucosal immunosuppression and epithelial barrier defects are key events in murine psychosocial stress-induced colitis. *Brain Behav. Immun.* 25, 1153–1161. doi: 10.1016/j.bbi.2011.03.004

Rehm, K.E., Xiang, L., Elci, O.U., Griswold, M., Marshall, Jr., G.D. (2012). Variability in laboratory immune parameters is associated with stress hormone receptor polymorphisms. *Neuroimmunomodulation* 19, 220–228. doi: 10.1159/000334711

Rera, M., Bahadorani, S., Cho, J., Koehler, C.L., Ulgherait, M., Hur, J.H., *et al.* (2011). Modulation of longevity and tissue homeostasis by the *Drosophila* PGC-1 homolog. *Cell Metab.* 14, 623–634. doi: 10.1016/j.cmet.2011.09.013

Ringel-Kulka, T., Kotch, J.B., Jensen, E.T., Savage, E., Weber, D.J. (2015). Randomized, double-blind, placebo-controlled study of synbiotic yogurt effect on the health of children. *J. Pediatr.* 166, 1475–1481. e1–3. doi: 10.1016/j.jpeds .2015.02.038

Roesch, L.F.W., Lorca, G.L., Casella, G., Giongo, A., Naranjo, A., Pionzio, A.M., *et al.* (2009). Culture-independent identification of gut bacteria correlated with the onset of diabetes in a rat model. *ISME J.* 3, 536–548. doi: 10.1038/ismej.2009.5

Rönnqvist, P.D., Forsgren-Brusk, U.B., Grahn-Håkansson, E.E. (2006). Lactobacilli in the female genital tract in relation to other genital microbes and vaginal pH. *Acta Obstet. Gynecol. Scand.* 85, 726–735. doi: 10.1080/00016340600578357

Roopchand, D.E., Carmody, R.N., Kuhn, P., Moskal, K., Rojas-Silva, P., Turnbaugh, P.J., *et al.* (2015). Dietary polyphenols promote growth of the gut bacterium *Akkermansia muciniphila* and attenuate high-fat diet-induced metabolic syndrome. *Diabetes* 64, 2847–2858. doi: 10.2337/db14-1916

Rosenfeld, C.S. (2015). Microbiome disturbances and autism spectrum disorders. *Drug Metab. Dispos. Biol. Fate Chem.* 43, 1557–1571. doi: 10.1124/dmd .115.063826

Ro, T.H., Mathew, M.A., Misra, S. (2015). Value of screening endoscopy in evaluation of esophageal, gastric and colon cancers. *World J. Gastroenterol.* 21, 9693–9706. doi: 10.3748/wjg.v21.i33.9693

Runtsch, M.C., Round, J.L., O'Connell, R.M. (2014). MicroRNAs and the regulation of intestinal homeostasis. *Front. Genet.* 5, 347. doi: 10.3389/fgene.2014.00347

Russell, R.M. (1992). Changes in gastrointestinal function attributed to aging. *Am. J. Clin. Nutr.* 55, 1203S–1207S.

Sankar, S.A., Lagier, J.-C., Pontarotti, P., Raoult, D., Fournier, P.-E. (2015). The human gut microbiome, a taxonomic conundrum. *Syst. Appl. Microbiol.* 38, 276–286. doi: 10.1016/j.syapm.2015.03.004

Sapone, A., de Magistris, L., Pietzak, M., Clemente, M.G., Tripathi, A., Cucca, F., *et al.* (2006). Zonulin upregulation is associated with increased gut permeability in subjects with type 1 diabetes and their relatives. *Diabetes* 55, 1443–1449.

Sartor, R.B. (2008). Microbial influences in inflammatory bowel diseases. *Gastroenterology* 134(2), 577–594. doi.org/10.1053/j.gastro.2007.11.059

Sato, S., Kiyono, H., Fujihashi, K. (2015). Mucosal immunosenescence in the gastrointestinal tract: a mini-review. *Gerontology* 61, 336–342. doi: 10.1159/000368897

Scalbert, A., Manach, C., Morand, C., Rémésy, C., Jiménez, L. (2005). Dietary polyphenols and the prevention of diseases. *Crit. Rev. Food Sci. Nutr.* 45, 287–306. doi: 10.1080/1040869059096

Scanlan, P.D., Shanahan, F., Clune, Y., Collins, J.K., O'Sullivan, G.C., O'Riordan, M., *et al.* (2008). Culture-independent analysis of the gut microbiota in colorectal cancer and polyposis. *Environ. Microbiol.* 10, 789–798. doi: 10.1111/j.1462-2920 .2007.01503.x

Scholtens, P.A.M.J., Alliet, P., Raes, M., Alles, M.S., Kroes, H., Boehm, G., *et al.* (2008). Fecal secretory immunoglobulin A is increased in healthy infants who receive a formula with short-chain galacto-oligosaccharides and long-chain fructo-oligosaccharides. *J. Nutr.* 138, 1141–1147.

Schwartz, G.K. (1996). Invasion and metastases in gastric cancer: *in vitro* and *in vivo* models with clinical correlations. *Semin. Oncol.* 23, 316–324.

Selma, M.V., Espín, J.C., Tomás-Barberán, F.A. (2009). Interaction between phenolics and gut microbiota: role in human health. *J. Agric. Food Chem.* 57, 6485–6501. doi: 10.1021/jf902107d

Seya, T., Shime, H., Ebihara, T., Oshiumi, H., Matsumoto, M. (2010). Pattern recognition receptors of innate immunity and their application to tumor immunotherapy. *Cancer Sci.* 101, 313–320. doi: 10.1111/j.1349-7006 .2009.01442.x

Sharma, R., Kapila, R., Dass, G., Kapila, S. (2014). Improvement in Th1/Th2 immune homeostasis, antioxidative status and resistance to pathogenic *E. coli* on consumption of probiotic *Lactobacillus rhamnosus* fermented milk in aging mice. Age (Dordr.) 36, 9686. doi: 10.1007/s11357-014-9686-4

Shastri, P., McCarville, J., Kalmokoff, M., Brooks, S.P.J., Green-Johnson, J.M. (2015). Sex differences in gut fermentation and immune parameters in rats fed an oligofructose-supplemented diet. *Biol. Sex Differ.* 6, 13. doi: 10.1186/s13293-015 -0031-0

Sherman, M. (2010). Epidemiology of hepatocellular carcinoma. *Oncology* 78 (Suppl 1), 7–10. doi: 10.1159/000315223

Shin, Y.-W., Kim, D.-H. (2005). Antipruritic effect of ginsenoside rb1 and compound k in scratching behavior mouse models. *J. Pharmacol. Sci.* 99, 83–88.

Shi, Y., Liu, X.-F., Zhuang, Y., Zhang, J.-Y., Liu, T., Yin, Z., *et al.* (2010). *Helicobacter pylori*-induced Th17 responses modulate Th1 cell responses, benefit bacterial growth, and contribute to pathology in mice. *J. Immunol.* 1950 184, 5121–5129. doi: 10.4049/jimmunol.0901115

Shoemark, D.K., Allen, S.J. (2015). The microbiome and disease: reviewing the links between the oral microbiome, aging, and Alzheimer's disease. *J. Alzheimers Dis.* 43, 725–738. doi: 10.3233/JAD-141170

Silveira, A.L.M., Ferreira, A.V.M., Oliveira, M.C. de, Rachid, M.A., Sousa, L.F. da C., Martins, F. dos S., *et al.* (2015). Preventive rather than therapeutic treatment with high fiber diet attenuates clinical and inflammatory markers of acute and chronic DSS-induced colitis in mice. *Eur. J. Nutr.* 1–13. doi: 10.1007/s00394-015-1068-x

Simpson, H.L., Campbell, B.J. (2015). Review article: dietary fibre-microbiota interactions. *Aliment. Pharmacol. Ther.* 42, 158–179. doi: 10.1111/apt.13248

Slavin, J. (2013). Fiber and prebiotics: mechanisms and health benefits. *Nutrients* 5, 1417. doi: 10.3390/nu5041417

Sokol, H., Pigneur, B., Watterlot, L., Lakhdari, O., Bermúdez-Humarán, L.G., Gratadoux, J.-J., *et al.* (2008). *Faecalibacterium prausnitzii* is an anti-inflammatory commensal bacterium identified by gut microbiota analysis of Crohn disease patients. *Proc. Natl. Acad. Sci. U.S.A.* 105, 16731–16736. doi: 10.1073/pnas.0804812105

Solemdal, K., Sandvik, L., Møinichen-Berstad, C., Skog, K., Willumsen, T., Mowe, M. (2012). Association between oral health and body cell mass in hospitalised elderly. *Gerodontology* 29, e1038–1044. doi: 10.1111/j.1741-2358.2011.00607.x

Song, Y., Liu, C., Finegold, S.M. (2004). Real-time PCR quantitation of clostridia in feces of autistic children. *Appl. Environ. Microbiol.* 70, 6459–6465. doi: 10.1128/AEM.70.11.6459-6465.2004

Spencer, J.P.E., Abd El Mohsen, M.M., Minihane, A.-M., Mathers, J.C. (2008). Biomarkers of the intake of dietary polyphenols: strengths, limitations and application in nutrition research. *Br. J. Nutr.* 99, 12–22. doi: 10.1017/S0007114507798938

Stadlbauer, S., Rios, P., Ohmori, K., Suzuki, K., Köhn, M. (2015). Procyanidins negatively affect the activity of the phosphatases of regenerating liver. *PLoS One* 10, e0134336. doi: 10.1371/journal.pone.0134336

Stecher, B., Maier, L., Hardt, W.-D. (2013). "Blooming" in the gut: how dysbiosis might contribute to pathogen evolution. *Nat. Rev. Microbiol.* 11, 277–284. doi: 10.1038/nrmicro2989

Stewart, B.W., Wild, C., International Agency for Research on Cancer, World Health Organization (eds.) (2014). *World Cancer Report 2014*. International Agency for Research on Cancer, Lyon, France.

Stewart, M.L., Savarino, V., Slavin, J.L. (2009). Assessment of dietary fiber fermentation: effect of *Lactobacillus reuteri* and reproducibility of short-chain fatty acid concentrations. *Mol. Nutr. Food Res.* 53 (Suppl 1), S114–120. doi: 10.1002/mnfr.200700523

Subramanian, S., Huq, S., Yatsunenko, T., Haque, R., Mahfuz, M., Alam, M.A., *et al.* (2014). Persistent gut microbiota immaturity in malnourished Bangladeshi children. *Nature* 510, 417–421. doi: 10.1038/nature13421

Sudo, N., Chida, Y., Aiba, Y., Sonoda, J., Oyama, N., Yu, X.-N., *et al.* (2004). Postnatal microbial colonization programs the hypothalamic-pituitary-adrenal system for stress response in mice. *J. Physiol.* 558, 263–275. doi: 10.1113/jphysiol.2004.063388

Suez, J., Korem, T., Zeevi, D., Zilberman-Schapira, G., Thaiss, C.A., Maza, O., *et al.* (2014). Artificial sweeteners induce glucose intolerance by altering the gut microbiota. *Nature* 514, 181–186. doi: 10.1038/nature13793

Sur, S., Pal, D., Mandal, S., Roy, A., Panda, C.K. (2016). Tea polyphenols epigallocatechin gallete and theaflavin restrict mouse liver carcinogenesis through modulation of self-renewal Wnt and hedgehog pathways. *J. Nutr. Biochem.* 27, 32–42. doi: 10.1016/j.jnutbio.2015.08.016

Takeda, K., Akira, S. (2004). TLR signaling pathways. *Semin. Immunol.* 16, 3–9.

Tan, M., Zhu, J.-C., Du, J., Zhang, L.-M., Yin, H.-H. (2011). Effects of probiotics on serum levels of Th1/Th2 cytokine and clinical outcomes in severe traumatic brain-injured patients: a prospective randomized pilot study. *Crit. Care* 15, R290. doi: 10.1186/cc10579

Tap, J., Furet, J.-P., Bensaada, M., Philippe, C., Roth, H., Rabot, S., *et al.* (2015). Gut microbiota richness promotes its stability upon increased dietary fibre intake in healthy adults. *Environ. Microbiol.* 17, 4954–4964. doi: 10.1111/1462-2920.13006

Teegarden, D., Romieu, I., Lelièvre, S.A. (2012). Redefining the impact of nutrition on breast cancer incidence: is epigenetics involved? *Nutr. Res. Rev.* 25, 68–95. doi: 10.1017/S0954422411000199

Tennoune, N., Legrand, R., Ouelaa, W., Breton, J., Lucas, N., Bole-Feysot, C., *et al.* (2015). Sex-related effects of nutritional supplementation of *Escherichia coli*: Relevance to eating disorders. *Nutrition* 31, 498–507. doi: 10.1016/j.nut.2014.11.003

Tien, M.-T., Girardin, S.E., Regnault, B., Le Bourhis, L., Dillies, M.-A., Coppée, J.-Y., *et al.* (2006). Anti-inflammatory effect of *Lactobacillus casei* on *Shigella*-infected human intestinal epithelial cells. *J. Immunol.* 176, 1228–1237.

Tomosada, Y., Villena, J., Murata, K., Chiba, E., Shimazu, T., Aso, H., *et al.* (2013). Immunoregulatory effect of bifidobacteria strains in porcine intestinal epithelial cells through modulation of ubiquitin-editing enzyme A20 expression. *PLoS One* 8, e59259. doi: 10.1371/journal.pone.0059259

Torjusen, H., Brantsæter, A.L., Haugen, M., Alexander, J., Bakketeig, L.S., Lieblein, G., *et al.* (2014). Reduced risk of pre-eclampsia with organic vegetable consumption: results from the prospective Norwegian Mother and Child Cohort Study. *BMJ Open* 4, e006143. doi: 10.1136/bmjopen-2014-006143

Triantafyllou, K., Vlachogiannakos, J., Ladas, S.D. (2010). Gastrointestinal and liver side effects of drugs in elderly patients. *Best Pract. Res. Clin. Gastroenterol.* 24, 203–215. doi: 10.1016/j.bpg.2010.02.004

Uemura, N., Okamoto, S., Yamamoto, S., Matsumura, N., Yamaguchi, S., Yamakido, M., *et al.* (2001). Helicobacter pylori infection and the development of gastric cancer. *N. Engl. J. Med.* 345, 784–789. doi: 10.1056/NEJMoa001999

Vaarala, O. (2008). Leaking gut in type 1 diabetes. *Curr. Opin. Gastroenterol.* 24, 701–706. doi: 10.1097/MOG.0b013e32830e6d98

Vahid, F., Zand, H., Nosrat–Mirshekarlou, E., Najafi, R., Hekmatdoost, A. (2015). The role dietary of bioactive compounds on the regulation of histone acetylases and deacetylases: A review. *Gene* 562, 8–15. doi: 10.1016/j.gene.2015.02.045

Valdés, L., Cuervo, A., Salazar, N., Ruas-Madiedo, P., Gueimonde, M., González, S. (2015). The relationship between phenolic compounds from diet and microbiota: impact on human health. *Food Funct* 6, 2424–2439. doi: 10.1039/C5FO00322A

van Baarlen, P., Troost, F.J., van Hemert, S., van der Meer, C., de Vos, W.M., de Groot, P.J., *et al.* (2009). Differential NF-kappaB pathways induction by *Lactobacillus plantarum* in the duodenum of healthy humans correlating with immune tolerance. *Proc. Natl. Acad. Sci. U.S.A.* 106, 2371–2376. doi: 10.1073/pnas.0809919106

van Duynhoven, J., van der Hooft, J.J.J., van Dorsten, F.A., Peters, S., Foltz, M., Gomez-Roldan, V., *et al.* (2014). Rapid and sustained systemic circulation of conjugated gut microbial catabolites after single-dose black tea extract consumption. *J. Proteome Res.* 13, 2668–2678. doi: 10.1021/pr5001253

Veiga, P., Pons, N., Agrawal, A., Oozeer, R., Guyonnet, D., Brazeilles, R., *et al.* (2014). Changes of the human gut microbiome induced by a fermented milk product. *Sci. Rep.* 4, 6328. doi: 10.1038/srep06328

Venkatesh, M., Mukherjee, S., Wang, H., Li, H., Sun, K., Benechet, A.P., *et al.* (2014). Symbiotic bacterial metabolites regulate gastrointestinal barrier function via the xenobiotic sensor PXR and Toll-like receptor 4. *Immunity* 41, 296–310. doi: 10.1016/j.immuni.2014.06.014

Villegas, J., Schulz, M., Soto, L., Sanchez, R. (2005). Bacteria induce expression of apoptosis in human spermatozoa. *Apoptosis* 10, 105–110. doi: 10.1007/s10495-005-6065-8

Vinderola, G., Matar, C., Perdigón, G. (2005). Role of intestinal epithelial cells in immune effects mediated by gram-positive probiotic bacteria: involvement of toll-like receptors. *Clin. Diagn. Lab. Immunol.* 12, 1075–1084. doi: 10.1128/CDLI.12.9.1075-1084.2005

Vujic, G., Jajac Knez, A., Despot Stefanovic, V., Kuzmic Vrbanovic, V. (2013). Efficacy of orally applied probiotic capsules for bacterial vaginosis and other vaginal infections: a double-blind, randomized, placebo-controlled study. *Eur. J. Obstet. Gynecol. Reprod. Biol.* 168, 75–79. doi: 10.1016/j.ejogrb.2012.12.031

Walter, J. (2008). Ecological role of lactobacilli in the gastrointestinal tract: implications for fundamental and biomedical research. *Appl. Environ. Microbiol.* 74, 4985–4996. doi: 10.1128/AEM.00753-08

Wang, C.-H., Qiao, C., Wang, R.-C., Zhou, W.-P. (2015). Dietary fiber intake and pancreatic cancer risk: a meta-analysis of epidemiologic studies. *Sci. Rep.* 5. doi: 10.1038/srep10834

Wang, D., Li, F., Li, P., Zhang, J., Liu, L., Xu, P., *et al.* (2012). Validated LC-MS/MS assay for the quantitative determination of clematichinenoside AR in rat plasma and its application to a pharmacokinetic study. *Biomed. Chromatogr.* 26, 1282–1285. doi: 10.1002/bmc.2691

Wang, D., Ho, L., Faith, J., Ono, K., Janle, E.M., Lachcik, P.J., *et al.* (2015). Role of intestinal microbiota in the generation of polyphenol-derived phenolic acid mediated attenuation of Alzheimer's disease β-amyloid oligomerization. *Mol. Nutr. Food Res.* 59, 1025–1040. doi: 10.1002/mnfr.201400544

Wang, L., Christophersen, C.T., Sorich, M.J., Gerber, J.P., Angley, M.T., Conlon, M.A. (2011). Low relative abundances of the mucolytic bacterium Akkermansia muciniphila and *Bifidobacterium* spp. in feces of children with autism. *Appl. Environ. Microbiol.* 77, 6718–6721. doi: 10.1128/AEM.05212-11

Wang, L., Christophersen, C.T., Sorich, M.J., Gerber, J.P., Angley, M.T., Conlon, M.A. (2012). Elevated fecal short chain fatty acid and ammonia concentrations in children with autism spectrum disorder. *Dig. Dis. Sci.* 57, 2096–2102. doi: 10.1007/s10620-012-2167-7

Wang, L., Christophersen, C.T., Sorich, M.J., Gerber, J.P., Angley, M.T., Conlon, M.A. (2013). Increased abundance of *Sutterella* spp. and *Ruminococcus torques* in feces of children with autism spectrum disorder. *Mol. Autism* 4, 42. doi: 10.1186/2040-2392-4-42

Wang, T., Xuan, X., Li, M., Gao, P., Zheng, Y., Zang, W., *et al.* (2013). Astragalus saponins affect proliferation, invasion and apoptosis of gastric cancer BGC-823 cells. *Diagn. Pathol.* 8, 179. doi: 10.1186/1746-1596-8-179

Wang, X., Frank, J.W., Xu, J., Dunlap, K.A., Satterfield, M.C., Burghardt, R.C., Romero, J.J., Hansen, T.R., Wu, G., Bazer, F.W. (2014). Functional role of arginine during the peri-implantation period of pregnancy. II. Consequences of loss of function of nitric oxide synthase NOS3 mRNA in ovine conceptus trophectoderm. *Biol. Reprod.* 91, 59. doi: 10.1095/biolreprod.114 .121202

Wang, Y.F., Yancy, W.S., Yu, D., Champagne, C., Appel, L.J., Lin, P.H. (2008). The relationship between dietary protein intake and blood pressure: results from the PREMIER study. *J. Hum. Hypertens.* 22, 745–754. doi: 10.1038/jhh.2008.64

Wan, J.-Y., Liu, P., Wang, H.-Y., Qi, L.-W., Wang, C.-Z., Li, P., *et al.* (2013). Biotransformation and metabolic profile of American ginseng saponins with human intestinal microflora by liquid chromatography quadrupole time-of-flight mass spectrometry. *J. Chromatogr. A* 1286, 83–92. doi: 10.1016/j.chroma .2013.02.053

Watts, T., Berti, I., Sapone, A., Gerarduzzi, T., Not, T., Zielke, R., *et al.* (2005). Role of the intestinal tight junction modulator zonulin in the pathogenesis of type I diabetes in BB diabetic-prone rats. *Proc. Natl. Acad. Sci. U.S.A.* 102, 2916–2921. doi: 10.1073/pnas.0500178102

Weerawatanakorn, M., Lee, Y.-L., Tsai, C.-Y., Lai, C.-S., Wan, X., Ho, C.-T., *et al.* (2015). Protective effect of theaflavin-enriched black tea extracts against dimethylnitrosamine-induced liver fibrosis in rats. *Food Funct.* 6, 1832–1840. doi: 10.1039/c5fo00126a

Weidenfeld, J., Itzik, A., Ovadia, H. (2015). Electrical stimulation of the amygdala modifies the negative feedback effect of glucocorticoids on the adrenocortical responses to stress. *Neuroimmunomodulation* 22, 394–399. doi: 10.1159/000437332

Weng, S.-L., Chiu, C.-M., Lin, F.-M., Huang, W.-C., Liang, C., Yang, T., *et al.* (2014). Bacterial communities in semen from men of infertile couples: metagenomic sequencing reveals relationships of seminal microbiota to semen quality. *PLoS One* 9, e110152. doi: 10.1371/journal.pone.0110152

Wen, L., Ley, R.E., Volchkov, P.Y., Stranges, P.B., Avanesyan, L., Stonebraker, A.C., *et al.* (2008). Innate immunity and intestinal microbiota in the development of type 1 diabetes. *Nature* 455, 1109–1113. doi: 10.1038/nature07336

Westerholm-Ormio, M., Vaarala, O., Pihkala, P., Ilonen, J., Savilahti, E. (2003). Immunologic activity in the small intestinal mucosa of pediatric patients with type 1 diabetes. *Diabetes* 52, 2287–2295.

Wierdsma, N.J., van Bodegraven, A.A., Uitdehaag, B.M.J., Arjaans, W., Savelkoul, P.H.M., Kruizenga, H.M., *et al.* (2009). Fructo-oligosaccharides and fibre in enteral nutrition has a beneficial influence on microbiota and gastrointestinal quality of life. *Scand. J. Gastroenterol.* 44, 804–812. doi: 10.1080/00365520902839675

Williams, B.L., Hornig, M., Buie, T., Bauman, M.L., Cho Paik, M., Wick, I., *et al.* (2011). Impaired carbohydrate digestion and transport and mucosal dysbiosis in the intestines of children with autism and gastrointestinal disturbances. *PLoS One* 6, e24585. doi: 10.1371/journal.pone.0024585

World Gastroenterology Organisation (2009). Inflammatory bowel disease. http: //www.worldgastroenterology.org/guidelines/global-guidelines/inflammatory-bowel-disease-ibd/inflammatory-bowel-disease-ibd-english (accessed 24 September 2015).

Wouters, M.M., Van Wanrooy, S., Nguyen, A., Dooley, J., Aguilera-Lizarraga, J., Van Brabant, W., *et al.* (2015). Psychological comorbidity increases the risk for postinfectious IBS partly by enhanced susceptibility to develop infectious gastroenteritis. *Gut* 65(8):1279–1288. doi: 10.1136/gutjnl-2015–309460

Wu, S., Rhee, K.-J., Zhang, M., Franco, A., Sears, C.L. (2007). Bacteroides fragilis toxin stimulates intestinal epithelial cell shedding and gamma-secretase-dependent E-cadherin cleavage. *J. Cell Sci.* 120, 1944–1952. doi: 10.1242/jcs.03455

Wutzke, K.D., Lotz, M., Zipprich, C. (2010). The effect of pre-and probiotics on the colonic ammonia metabolism in humans as measured by lactose-[(15)N(2)] ureide. *Eur. J. Clin. Nutr.* 64, 1215–1221. doi: 10.1038/ejcn.2010.120

Xiang, Q., Zhang, J., Li, C.-Y., Wang, Y., Zeng, M.-J., Cai, Z.-X., *et al.* (2015). Insulin resistance-induced hyperglycemia decreased the activation of Akt/CREB in hippocampus neurons: Molecular evidence for mechanism of diabetes-induced cognitive dysfunction. *Neuropeptides* 54, 9–15. doi: 10.1016/j.npep.2015.08.009

Xu, R., Peng, Y., Wang, M., Fan, L., Li, X. (2014). Effects of broad-spectrum antibiotics on the metabolism and pharmacokinetics of ginsenoside Rb1: a study on rats' gut microflora influenced by lincomycin. *J. Ethnopharmacol.* 158 Pt A, 338–344. doi: 10.1016/j.jep.2014.10.054

Yamakawa, M.Y., Uchino, K., Watanabe, Y., Adachi, T., Nakanishi, M., Ichino, H., *et al.* (2016). Anthocyanin suppresses the toxicity of Aβ deposits through diversion of molecular forms in *in vitro* and *in vivo* models of Alzheimer's disease. *Nutr. Neurosci.* 19, 32–42. doi: 10.1179/1476830515Y.0000000042

Yamamoto-Furusho, J.-K., Podolsky, D.-K. (2007). Innate immunity in inflammatory bowel disease. *World J. Gastroenterol.* 13, 5577–5580.

Yatsunenko, T., Rey, F.E., Manary, M.J., Trehan, I., Dominguez-Bello, M.G., Contreras, M., *et al.* (2012). Human gut microbiome viewed across age and geography. *Nature* 486, 222–227. doi: 10.1038/nature11053

Yoo, D.-H., Kim, D.-H. (2015). *Lactobacillus pentosus* var. *plantarum* C29 increases the protective effect of soybean against scopolamine-induced memory impairment in mice. *Int. J. Food Sci. Nutr.* 66, 912–918. doi: 10.3109/09637486.2015.1064865

Yu, B., Dai, C., Chen, J., Deng, L., Wu, X., Wu, S., *et al.* (2015). Dysbiosis of gut microbiota induced the disorder of helper T cells in influenza virus-infected mice. *Hum. Vaccines Immunother.* 11, 1140–1146. doi: 10.1080/21645515.2015.1009805

Yu, C., Wen, X.-D., Zhang, Z., Zhang, C.-F., Wu, X., He, X., *et al.* (2015). American ginseng significantly reduced the progression of high-fat-diet-enhanced colon carcinogenesis in Apc (Min/+) mice. *J. Ginseng Res.* 39, 230–237. doi: 10.1016/j.jgr.2014.12.004

Zambirinis, C.P., Pushalkar, S., Saxena, D., Miller, G. (2014). Pancreatic cancer, inflammation, and microbiome. *Cancer J.* 20, 195–202. doi: 10.1097/PPO .0000000000000045

Zeng, D., Wang, J., Kong, P., Chang, C., Li, J., Li, J. (2014). Ginsenoside Rg3 inhibits HIF-1α and VEGF expression in patient with acute leukemia via inhibiting the activation of PI3K/Akt and ERK1/2 pathways. *Int. J. Clin. Exp. Pathol.* 7, 2172–2178.

Zhang, C., Zhang, M., Pang, X., Zhao, Y., Wang, L., Zhao, L. (2012). Structural resilience of the gut microbiota in adult mice under high-fat dietary perturbations. *ISME J.* 6, 1848–1857. doi: 10.1038/ismej.2012.27

Zhang, J., Wang, P., Ouyang, H., Yin, J., Liu, A., Ma, C., *et al.* (2013). Targeting cancer-related inflammation: Chinese herbal medicine inhibits epithelial-to-mesenchymal transition in pancreatic cancer. *PLoS One* 8, e70334. doi: 10.1371/journal.pone.0070334

Zhang, Y.-J., Li, S., Gan, R.-Y., Zhou, T., Xu, D.-P., Li, H.-B. (2015). Impacts of gut bacteria on human health and diseases. *Int. J. Mol. Sci.* 16, 7493–7519. doi: 10.3390/ijms16047493

Zhong, Y., Nyman, M., Fåk, F. (2015). Modulation of gut microbiota in rats fed high-fat diets by processing whole-grain barley to barley malt. *Mol. Nutr. Food Res.* 59, 2066–2076. doi: 10.1002/mnfr.201500187

Zhu, Y., Wang, C., Li, F. (2015). Impact of dietary fiber/starch ratio in shaping caecal microbiota in rabbits. *Can. J. Microbiol.* 1–14. doi: 10.1139/cjm-2015-0201

9

Effect of Processing on the Bioactive Polysaccharides and Phenolic Compounds from *Aloe vera* (*Aloe barbadensis* Miller)

José Rafael Minjares-Fuentes and Antoni Femenia

Department of Chemistry, University of the Balearic Islands, Balearic Islands, Spain

9.1 *Aloe vera*

Aloe vera has enjoyed a long history of providing a myriad of health benefits, being one of the herbal remedies most frequently used throughout the world (Guo and Mei, 2016; Pothuraju *et al.*, 2016). With the recent resurgence of herbal products as part of "the green movement," *Aloe vera* has been witnessing a new renaissance, representing an opportunity to open up new range of products with significant added value and high acceptance by consumers demanding a healthier lifestyle (Vega-Gálvez *et al.*, 2011; Javed and Atta-Ur, 2014; Guo and Mei, 2016). The potential use of *Aloe vera* gel either as a food ingredient or as a functional food is mainly due to its beneficial properties in treating constipation, coughs, ulcers, diabetes, headaches, arthritis, and immune-system deficiencies, which makes this plant an interesting alternative for the food industry (Vogler and Ernst, 1999; Eshun and He, 2004; Javed and Atta-Ur, 2014).

There are more than 400 species of *Aloe*, but without a doubt the most popular and widely used is *Aloe barbadensis* Miller (also called *Aloe vera* Linne and commonly referred to as *Aloe vera*). Other *Aloe* species used in health and medicine include *Aloe arborescens* Miller (a member of the Asphodelacea family), *Aloe perryi* Baker, *Aloe andongensis*, and *Aloe ferox*, among others (Rodríguez *et al.*, 2010; Guo and Mei, 2016).

Aloe vera (*Aloe barbadensis* Miller), a member of the Liliaceae family, is a perennial plant with turgid green leaves joined at the stem in a rosette pattern (Figure 9.1). The *Aloe vera* leaves are formed by a thick epidermis (skin) covered with cuticles surrounding the mesophyll, which can be differentiated into chlorenchyma cells and thinner walled cells forming the parenchyma (Femenia *et al.*, 1999). The epidermis or rind is a thick cuticle accounting for about 20 – 30% by weight of the whole plant leaf. It consists of up to 18 layers of cells interspersed with chloroplasts where carbohydrates, lipids, and proteins are synthesized. The outer leaf pulp, a thin, mucilaginous layer just beneath and adjacent to the thick rind, contains vascular bundles acting as the transport system for the plant. Three types of tubular structures make up the vascular bundles: xylem, which moves water and minerals from the roots to the leaves;

Dietary Fiber Functionality in Food and Nutraceuticals: From Plant to Gut, First Edition.
Edited by Farah Hosseinian, B. Dave Oomah and Rocio Campos-Vega.

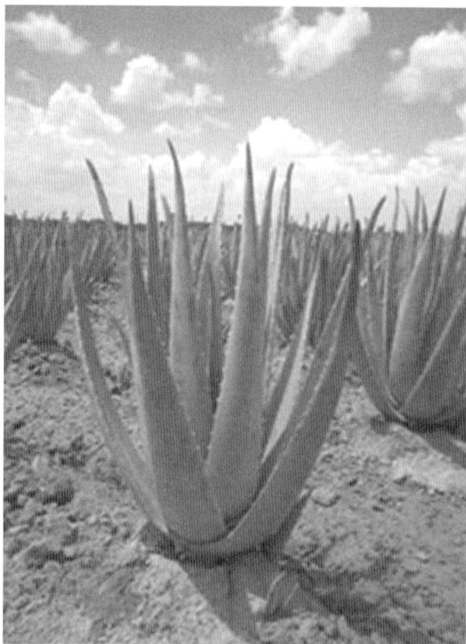

Figure 9.1 *Aloe vera* (*Aloe barbadensis* Miller) plant.

phloem, which takes synthesized minerals to the roots; and the pericyclic tubule, which stores and transports a bitter yellow latex (often referred to as aloe sap) along the margin of the leaf. The parenchyma makes up the majority of the leaf by volume and contains the *Aloe vera* gel. It is referred to as the inner leaf, inner leaf fillet, or aloe fillet (Boudreau and Beland, 2006; Guo and Mei, 2016).

Aloe vera gel consists of about 98.5–99.5% water with the remaining solids containing more than 200 different ingredients, including a combination of polysaccharides and their acetylated derivatives, glycoproteins, phenolic anthraquinones, flavonoids, flavonols, enzymes, minerals, essential and non-essential amino acids, sterols, saponins, and vitamins (Eshun and He, 2004; Rodríguez *et al.*, 2010). The exact chemical composition of an *Aloe* plant depends, however, on the species analyzed (Grindlay and Reynolds, 1986; Reynolds and Dweck, 1999; Ni *et al.*, 2004b; Kim, 2006; Park and Kwon, 2006; Hamman, 2008; Ray and Aswatha, 2013).

Most of the pharmacological properties of *Aloe vera* gel are attributed to the acetylated polysaccharide acemannan present in the gel (Choi and Chung, 2003; Ni *et al.*, 2004a; Rodríguez *et al.*, 2010; Radha and Laxmipriya, 2015; Pothuraju *et al.*, 2016). The acemannan polymer is the main polysaccharide found in *Aloe vera* gel, and it is considered a storage polysaccharide located within the protoplast of the parenchymatous cells (Femenia *et al.*, 1999). The gel also contains a considerable amount of cell wall polysaccharides, such as pectic substances which are the most abundant type of polysaccharides in the cell walls of *Aloe vera* gel (Femenia *et al.*, 2003; Simões *et al.*, 2012).

Processing of *Aloe vera* has become a big industry worldwide due to the use of various processed products in the cosmetic, pharmaceutic, and food fields. In the cosmetic and toiletry industry, *Aloe vera* gel is used as a base for the preparation of creams, lotions, soaps, shampoos, and facial cleaners, whereas in the pharmaceutical industry, the main products based on *Aloe vera* are topical ointments, gel preparations, tablets, and capsules (Eshun and He, 2004; Christaki and Florou-Paneri, 2010). In the food industry, *Aloe vera* is widely used as a source of functional ingredients, especially for the preparation of health food drinks and other beverages, including tea (Christaki and Florou-Paneri, 2010).

9.1.1 Bioactive Compounds of *Aloe vera*

In the last two decades, several scientific reports have been published based on research into the different bioactive compounds present in *Aloe vera*. Most of these studies were related to the beneficial properties attributed to *Aloe vera* and its bioactive polysaccharides, in particular the storage polymer acemannan; cell wall pectins and different phenolic compounds also seem to be key components explaining most of the pharmacological properties of *Aloe vera*.

In this chapter, the most relevant scientific information about the structure and the biological activity of these components, and also the physicochemical modifications of these bioactive compounds during *Aloe vera* processing are summarized.

9.1.1.1 Acemannan

The term acemannan is often used to describe a mannose-rich polymer isolated from *Aloe vera*. According to the scientific literature, acemannan is mainly composed of large amounts of mannose units (Man >60%), which are often partially acetylated, followed by glucose (Glc ~ 20%), and, to a minor extent, galactose (Gal <10%) (Femenia *et al.*, 1999; Talmadge *et al.*, 2004; Chow *et al.*, 2005; Rodríguez-González *et al.*, 2011; Chokboribal *et al.*, 2015; Escobedo-Lozano *et al.*, 2015).

Structurally, acemannan isolated from *Aloe vera* consists of a chain of repeating tetrasaccharide units with a single-branched Gal at C6 of the second acetylated Man residue (Figure 9.2) (Talmadge *et al.*, 2004; Chow *et al.*, 2005; Kim, 2006; Chokboribal *et al.*, 2015). The repeating units of Glc and Man exist in a ratio of 1:3, although ratios of 1:6, 1:15, and 1:22 have also been reported (Gowda *et al.*, 1979; Mandal and Das, 1980b; Chow *et al.*, 2005; Boudreau and Beland, 2006; Campestrini *et al.*, 2013). Acetylation may occur at the C2, C3, or C6 of Man residues with an acetyl:Man ratio of approximately 1:1 or even higher (Fogleman *et al.*, 1992; Manna and McAnalley, 1993; McAnalley, 1993; Talmadge *et al.*, 2004; Hamman, 2008; Simões *et al.*, 2012). Structurally, these acetyl groups are the only non-sugar functional groups present in acemannan and seem to play a key role in the physicochemical properties and biological activity of *Aloe vera* (Ni *et al.*, 2004b; Campestrini *et al.*, 2013; Chokboribal *et al.*, 2015). In general, the molecular weight (MW) of this polysaccharide might range from 30 to 45 kDa, although high MWs have also been reported (>200 kDa) (Femenia *et al.*, 2003; Turner *et al.*, 2004; Im *et al.*, 2005; Chokboribal *et al.*, 2015; Escobedo-Lozano *et al.*, 2015).

The different *Aloe* species, their geographic location (including soil and climate), growth periods, and also the type of extraction and analytical methods applied are probably the main factors that may explain the differences reported

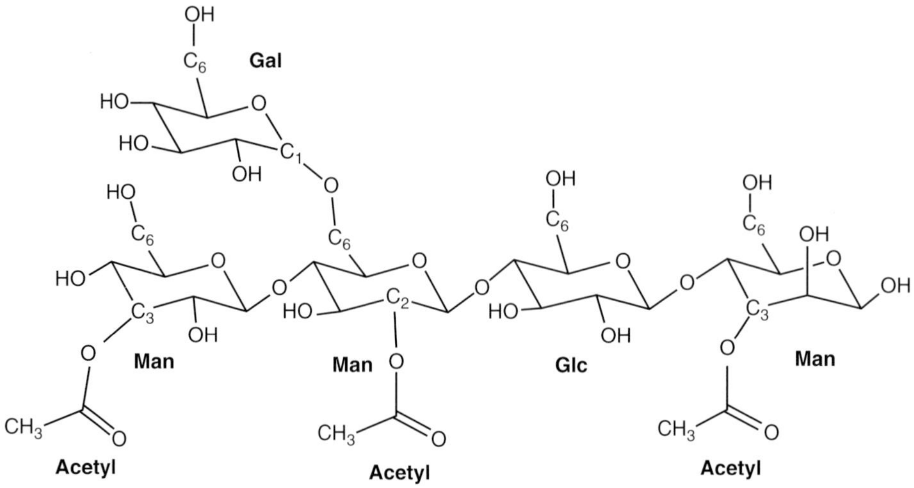

Figure 9.2 Chemical structure of acemannan polymer. Source: Adapted from Chokboribal *et al.* (2015).

about this polysaccharide (Ni *et al.*, 2004a, 2004b; Talmadge *et al.*, 2004; Campestrini *et al.*, 2013; Ray *et al.*, 2013, 2015; Ray and Aswatha, 2013; Bhalang and Tompkins, 2015).

Nevertheless, acemannan is inherently unstable and can be easily degraded by different physicochemical factors, such as high temperature, pH changes, bacterial contamination, or enzymes, such as mannanases, present in the pulp (Kim, 2006; Javed and Atta-Ur, 2014). In some commercial *Aloe* products, the pulp preparation is treated with cellulase, which might also be contaminated with mannanase, promoting the degradation of acemannan (Ni *et al.*, 2004b; Kim, 2006). Furthermore, alkaline pH promotes deacetylation of acemannan, which renders it insoluble (Yaron, 1993; Ni *et al.*, 2004b; Chokboribal *et al.*, 2015). Rheological studies have demonstrated that acemannan is the basis of the pseudoplastic flow behavior of the liquid gel obtained from fresh *Aloe vera* gel. When it is degraded it may become less viscous, exhibiting Newtonian flow properties (Yaron *et al.*, 1992; Yaron, 1993; Ni *et al.*, 2004a; Campestrini *et al.*, 2013). Several studies have shown that the acetyl groups of acemannan are involved in the interaction of this polymer with other biomolecules; therefore, this is a key aspect that should be taken into account when assessing the overall quality of *Aloe vera* processed products (Femenia *et al.*, 2003; Chokboribal *et al.*, 2015).

Acemannan is not only structurally unique but also a characteristic compound of *Aloe* species among other well-known plant mannans, which have distinct side-chains or are unacetylated and insoluble (Ni *et al.*, 2004b). It is also important to point out that the identification and the quantification of acemannan polymer is hard to carry out by colorimetric methods, since they are mainly based on the colored complex formed by the binding between the $\beta(1 \rightarrow 4)$-linked polysaccharides and the dye (Eberendu *et al.*, 2005). The results from these assays could generate confusion since the majority of polysaccharides, including most of the cell wall polymers, are linked by this type of bond.

Acemannan polysaccharide has been reported to be the main bioactive substance present in *Aloe vera* fillet, and to be responsible for most of the beneficial properties attributed to *Aloe vera* (Reynolds, 1985; t'Hart *et al.*, 1989; McAnalley, 1993; Reynolds and Dweck, 1999; Hamman, 2008). Recent studies have revealed that treatment with *Aloe vera* promotes a significant reduction in blood glucose and blood pressure, improving the lipid profile in people with diabetes (Sood *et al.*, 2008; Choudhary *et al.*, 2011; Pothuraju *et al.*, 2016). This biological effect has been attributed to the high molecular weight fractions of acemannan, which are degraded by the intestinal microbiota to form oligosaccharides that inhibit intestinal glucose absorption (Yagi *et al.*, 2001, 2009; Boban *et al.*, 2006; Jain *et al.*, 2007). The epithelial cells lining the gastrointestinal system have mannose-specific receptors, and when taken orally, acemannan can be detected in the blood within 90 minutes (Bhalang and Tompkins, 2015). Also, in a recent *in vitro* study, it was shown that acemannan could decrease the transepithelial electrical resistance of intestinal epithelial cell monolayers (Caco-2), allowing bioactive components to be transported across the intestinal epithelium (Sharma *et al.*, 2015). Nutrigenomic studies have also been conducted to elucidate the mechanism of the hypoglycemic and insulin-sensitizing effects of *Aloe vera*, and the results have shown that acemannan may reduce hepatic fat accumulation and enhance insulin signaling in adipose tissue. This study has provided an explanation of the mechanism that increases insulin sensitivity and decreases blood glucose in diabetic and prediabetic models (Tseng-Crank *et al.*, 2013; Yagi, 2014). On the other hand, clinical studies have demonstrated that acemannan possesses immunomodulatory properties for macrophages and monocytes with minimal systemic toxicity following intraperitoneal or intravenous administration (Karaca *et al.*, 1995; Talmadge *et al.*, 2004; Jettanacheawchankit *et al.*, 2009; Chantarawaratit *et al.*, 2014; Guo and Mei, 2016; Kumar and Tiku, 2016).

From an industrial point of view, the acemannan content could be a good indicator of the overall quality of *Aloe* products; however different aspects such as the structural disposition, MW, and the degree of acetylation should also be considered in order to assess the functional and nutritional properties of *Aloe vera* processed products. In fact, an educated consumer should question any product that has been subjected to excessive and harsh conditions during processing. For instance, the occurrence of low levels of acemannan, as well as a low degree of acetylation, might indicate that the manufacturing stage of a *Aloe* product has been handled roughly (Kim, 2006).

9.1.1.2 Pectic Polysaccharides from *Aloe vera* Gel

Apart from acemannan, pectins are the most abundant polysaccharide present in *Aloe vera* gel. Unlike the storage of acemannan polymer, pectins are formed in the cell walls of the parenchyma (Femenia *et al.*, 1999). In general, pectins are heterogeneous polysaccharides composed primarily of repeating units of $(1 \rightarrow 4)$ α-D-galacturonic acid with intermittent $(1 \rightarrow 2)$-linked rhamnose (Rha) residues, acting as branch points for neutral sugar side-chains (Figure 9.3) (Lim and Cheong, 2015; Sharma *et al.*, 2015). The galacturonic acid units may be

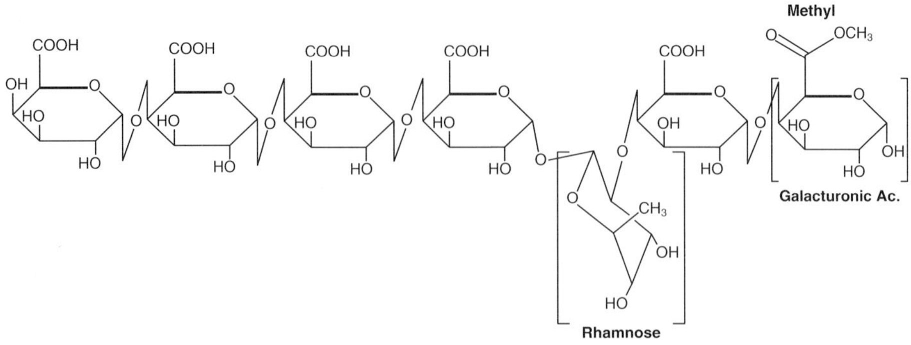

Figure 9.3 Schematic representation of the pectin structure. Source: Adapted from McConaughy *et al.* (2008a).

present in the acid form or may exist as methyl esters with certain degree of methyl ester substitution (DME), which affects their ability to form gels in the presence of multivalent ions such as calcium (Ca^{2+}) (McConaughy *et al.*, 2008b; Gentilini *et al.*, 2014a).

Aloe vera pectins contain a very high percentage of galacturonic acid residues, usually higher than 95% with less than 5% of neutral sugars, with Rha being the most abundant sugar unit. This indicates a structure primarily composed of long galacturonic acid blocks with very few neutral sugar branches (Mandal and Das, 1980a; Femenia *et al.*, 1999; Ni *et al.*, 2004a; McConaughy *et al.*, 2008a, 2008b). Interestingly, in the first studies on *Aloe vera*, pectins were identified as the main polysaccharide present in the *Aloe vera* gel (Ovodova *et al.*, 1975; Mandal and Das, 1980a).

The MW of pectins from *Aloe vera* gel ranges from 200 to 523 kDa, although low MWs have also been observed (McConaughy *et al.*, 2008b; Gentilini *et al.*, 2014a). In addition, *Aloe vera* pectins exhibit a low DME, ranging from 2 to 20% (McConaughy *et al.*, 2008b; Geng *et al.*, 2014; Gentilini *et al.*, 2014a; Lim and Cheong, 2015).

In nature, pectins are degraded by different enzymes such as pectinases and pectinmethylesterases, which can be inactivated when exposed to high temperatures. Furthermore, the application of heat promotes the cleavage of pectic polysaccharides via β-elimination, which is a common reaction during high-temperature processing of low acid foods (Femenia *et al.*, 1998a, 1998b).

With regard to the biological properties of pectins, it has been observed that pectins with MW lower than 400 kDa may exhibit a potent macrophage-activating activity, as determined by increased cytokine production, nitric oxide release, surface molecule expression, and phagocytic activity. Interestingly, a potent antitumor activity *in vivo* has also been reported for this type of polysaccharides (Im *et al.*, 2005; Kaithwas *et al.*, 2014). Recently, it has been documented that pectins containing over 80% of GalA units, as is the case for *Aloe vera* pectins, possess immunostimulatory activity promoting phagocytic activity of the monocyte–macrophage system in mice (Popov and Ovodov, 2013; Wang *et al.*, 2014).

Commonly, pectins are widely used in the food industry as gelling or thickening agents, while in the pharmaceutical industry they are usually used as an excipient due to their non-toxicity, low production costs, and ability to form gels. Because pectins are intact in the upper gastrointestinal tract and then degraded by colonic microflora, pectin-derived drug carriers provide promising potential for colon-specific drug delivery (Liu *et al.*, 2015). Interestingly, *Aloe vera* pectins are an exceptional polysaccharide since these are able to form gels at low polymer (0.2 wt%) and calcium ion (<10 mM) concentrations in comparison with pectins from other sources (McConaughy *et al.*, 2008a, 2008b). The specific intrinsic features together with their high cytocompatibility also make *Aloe vera* pectins a novel and exceptional material in the development of biocomposites for biomedical applications (Gentilini *et al.*, 2014a, 2014b; Tummalapalli *et al.*, 2016).

9.1.1.3 Phenolic Compounds in *Aloe vera*

The *Aloe vera* exudate or latex is distributed within the vascular bundles located between the plant's outer skin (rind) and the pulp. Usually, the exudate is yellow-brownish in color and has a bitter taste. From the exudate, approximately 80 chemical constituents have been isolated by liquid chromatography, the anthraquinone *C*-glycosides, anthrones, chromones, phenyl pyrones, and naphthalene derivatives being the most abundant phenolic compounds (Eshun and He, 2004; Park and Kwon, 2006; Basmatker *et al.*, 2011; Lee *et al.*, 2012; Wu *et al.*, 2013; Guo and Mei, 2016).

The anthrone *C*-glycosides are considered typical constituents of the *Aloe* leaf exudate although they do not, in fact, occur in all species (Kanama *et al.*, 2015). Where they do occur they are usually the main component of the exudate and are mostly represented by aloin. This compound has been found in the majority of *Aloe* species at levels from 0.1 to 6.6% of the leaf dry weight, representing between 3% and 35% of the total exudate (Reynolds, 1985; Kanama *et al.*, 2015). Aloin appears to be exclusive to the leaf exudate, which is also the bitter principle in drug Aloes, and was characterized as the *C*-glycoside of aloe emodin anthrone (Figure 9.4) (Reynolds, 1985, 2004). On the other hand, most of the chromones so far described from *Aloe vera* leaf exudate are derivatives of 8-*C*-glucosyl-7-hydroxy-5-methyl-2-propyl-4-chromone. Variation arises from the degree of oxidation in the propyl side-chain, methylation of the hydroxyl group on C7 and esterification of the glucose moiety (Reynolds, 2004; Machado and Marques, 2010; Zhong *et al.*, 2014; Kanama *et al.*, 2015; Sun *et al.*, 2016). It is noteworthy that *C*-glycosylated compounds represent a class of naturally occurring secondary metabolites that are known to be unique compounds of the *Aloe* genus, not having been reported in other plants (Hutter *et al.*, 1996; Piao *et al.*, 2002; Machado and Marques, 2010).

As in the polysaccharides, the particular species of *Aloe* and also specific geographic and seasonal conditions may affect the presence of different phenolic compounds (Park and Kwon, 2006; Ray *et al.*, 2013). It has been documented that in *Aloe vera*, aloin A and B, 8-*O*-methyl-7-hydroxyaloin A and B, and 10-hydroxyaloin A show a large seasonal variation while chromones such as aloesin and neoaloesin A exhibited relatively small changes (Park and Kwon, 2006; Lee *et al.*, 2012). Moreover, the *C*-glycosylated phenolic compounds of

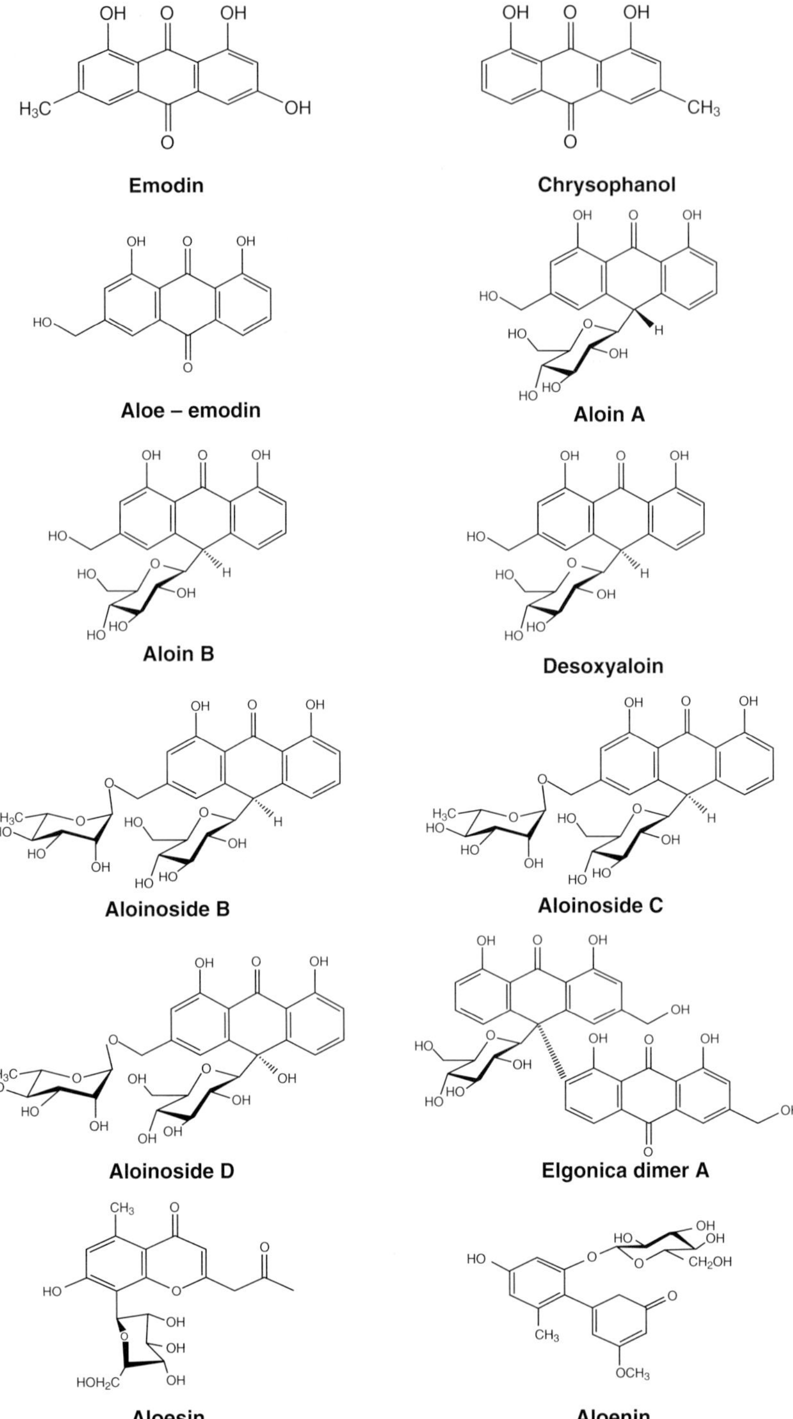

Figure 9.4 Structure of some phenolic compounds from *Aloe vera*. Source: Adapted from Olennikov *et al.* (2013) and Sun *et al.* (2015).

Aloe vera are very sensitive to different physical and chemical factors (Chang *et al.*, 2006). Different studies have demonstrated that the exposure of aloin to alcohol (methanol or ethanol) at low temperature (<6 °C) may result in the formation of aloe emodin, which is associated with a color change from light to dark yellow (Chang *et al.*, 2006; Javed and Atta-Ur, 2014). Furthermore, temperature is another crucial factor for the stability of these metabolites, which undergo a significant decrease when exposed to high temperature (>60 °C) for relatively long times (>6 hours) (Chang *et al.*, 2006).

Several studies have shown that the phenolic compounds from different *Aloe* species possess a wide range of biological activities (Hutter *et al.*, 1996; Lee *et al.*, 2000; Esteban-Carrasco *et al.*, 2001; Park *et al.*, 2011; Zhong *et al.*, 2013; Lucini *et al.*, 2015; Sun *et al.*, 2015, 2016). In particular, aloin and aloe emodin are the main pharmacologically active anthraquinones of *Aloe vera*. It is claimed that they have therapeutic activities including a purgative action, anti-inflammatory activity, antiprotozoal action, antioxidant activity, among others. Interestingly, these components have demonstrated a radical scavenging potential comparable to that of the synthetic antioxidant butylated hydroxytoluene (BHT) (Shahidi *et al.*, 1992; Choi and Chung, 2003; Hu *et al.*, 2003; Shahidi and Naczk, 2003; Wu *et al.*, 2013). In addition, a few phenolic-type substances, derivatives of aloesin, have been isolated from *Aloe vera* gel which exhibit antioxidant activity and may be used as anti-aging agents (Shahidi *et al.*, 1992; Lee *et al.*, 2000; Yagi *et al.*, 2002).

Aloin has been documented for its remarkable potential therapeutic options in cancer, wherein it showed chemoprotective effects against 1,2-dimethylhydrazine-induced preneoplastic lesions in the colon of Wistar rats (Hamiza *et al.*, 2014). Aloin treatment has been demonstrated to inhibit the secretion of vascular endothelial growth factor (VEGF) in cancer cells, causing the inhibition of proliferation and migration of endothelial cells. VEGF is one of the most important pro-angiogenic cytokines known and is well characterized as an inducer of tumor neovascularization (Pan *et al.*, 2013).

Recently, it has been reported that aloe emodin exhibits an antiproliferation effect on some types of cancer cells, such as lung, squamous, glioma, and neuroectodermal cancer cells (Lin *et al.*, 2011; Masaldan and Iyer, 2014). The inhibitory effect of aloe emodin on the activity and gene expression of *N*-acetyltransferase, which plays an initial role in the metabolism of aryl amine carcinogens, was found in human malignant melanoma cells (Lin *et al.*, 2005, 2006). More recently, it has also been observed that aloe emodin exhibits antiviral activity, showing an inhibitory mechanism against influenza A virus with reducing virus-induced cytopathic effect and inhibiting replication of influenza A (Li *et al.*, 2014).

Although these components are highly valued in the pharmaceutical industry, aloin and other hydroxyanthracene derivatives are also irritant laxatives. An excessive dose of aloe latex may be the source of abdominal pain, spasm, and even hepatitis. Furthermore, long-term intake of aloe containing aloin may stimulate electrolyte disturbances, malabsorption, metabolic acidosis, weight loss, hematuria, and albuminuria (Javed and Atta-Ur, 2014). *Aloe vera* gel should not contain aloin as it can be contaminated during the filleting operation; however, mechanical separation is not always perfect and aloe exudate can be easily found in aloe gel (He *et al.*, 2005). Ingredients or foods from *Aloe vera* free of aloin and aloe emodin are considered safer than those having anthraquinones (Buenz, 2008). In European countries, the aloin content regulation limit is 0.1 ppm in food and beverages, whereas the International *Aloe vera* Science Council (IASC) regulation requires an aloin concentration lower than 10 ppm in a 0.5% *Aloe vera* solids solution for oral consumption (Javed and Atta-Ur, 2014).

9.2 Effect of Processing on the Main Bioactive Compounds from *Aloe vera*

Various procedures are involved in the preparation of *Aloe vera* extracts used in the manufacture of cosmetic, pharmaceutical, or food products (He *et al.*, 2005; Ramachandra and Rao, 2008; Ahlawat and Khatkar, 2011). In general, dehydration, to produce powders, and pasteurization, to obtain *Aloe vera* juice, are probably the most common procedures applied in the *Aloe vera* industry.

However, processing may affect the original structure of the different bioactive components present in *Aloe vera*, which may in turn lead to considerable changes, not only in their physicochemical characteristics but also in their physiological and pharmacological properties (Femenia *et al.*, 2003; Eshun and He, 2004; Ramachandra and Rao, 2008; Gulia *et al.*, 2010; Nindo *et al.*, 2010; Ahlawat and Khatkar, 2011; Chokboribal *et al.*, 2015).

9.2.1 Pasteurization

Pasteurization is probably the most common processing technique applied to *Aloe vera* gel in order to reduce or eliminate pathogenic and spoilage microorganisms and deteriorative enzymes (Rodríguez-González *et al.*, 2011). Industrially, treatments based on the use of high temperature and short time (at 85–95 °C for 1–2 minutes) are the most common methods (He *et al.*, 2005). However, no scientific studies have been published about the effects of this type of pasteurization on the main bioactive components of *Aloe vera* gel.

Several reports have shown that polysaccharides present in *Aloe vera* juice may be degraded when the juice is heated. In particular, high degradation of polysaccharides was observed when processes were carried out either at 50 °C or at 90 °C (Chang *et al.*, 2006). According to the authors, the marked degradation of polysaccharides occurring at 90 °C was mainly due to thermal degradation, whereas treatments at lower temperatures (~50 °C) may have been caused by the activation of certain polysaccharide-degrading enzymes, such as polygalacturonase and pectinase, which are responsible for the degradation of pectic polysaccharides (Cohen and Yang, 1995; Femenia *et al.*, 2003). Interestingly, it has been documented that *Aloe vera* polysaccharides achieve their maximal thermal stability when processing is carried out within the temperature range of 65–80 °C (Chang *et al.*, 2006).

Physicochemical modifications promoted by pasteurization treatments performed at 65, 75, and 85 °C, for 15 and 25 minutes, on acemannan and cell wall polymers were evaluated by Rodríguez-González *et al.* (2011). Important changes were detected in pasteurized *Aloe vera* samples depending on the conditions used during the pasteurization process. Thus, with regard to the chemical composition, the yield of bioactive polysaccharide acemannan apparently increased in pasteurized samples, but this effect was attributed to the formation of new hydrogen bonds between mannose-rich oligosaccharides and the high MW chains of acemannan. These physicochemical alterations of the acemannan polymer observed during pasteurization may have important implications for the physiological activities attributed to the *Aloe vera* gel.

With regard to pectic substances, the heat involved in the pasteurization process may promote a considerable degradation of this type of polysaccharide. In fact, pasteurization carried out at 85 °C for 25 minutes caused considerable losses of the galacturonic acid content (~31%), and when pasteurization was carried out at 75 °C, the degradation was significantly lower (~7%). Furthermore, pasteurization at 85 °C also promoted high losses of arabinose and galactose residues, which accompanied by the severe degradation of uronic acids, resulted in the degradation of both unbranched and branched pectin moieties (Rodríguez-González *et al.*, 2011). The degradation of pectic polysaccharides observed at 85 °C was attributed to β-elimination reaction promoted by heating, whereas at temperatures around 65 °C, the degradation of these polysaccharides was associated with enzymatic activity (Chang *et al.*, 2006; Sila *et al.*, 2007; Sila *et al.*, 2009). Pasteurization at 75 °C for 15 minutes was found to be the best condition in order to preserve not only the structure of acemannan and pectic polysaccharides, but also its intrinsic properties, such as the acetylation pattern of acemannan, and the MW and DME of pectins (Rodríguez-González *et al.*, 2011).

On the other hand, studies about the stability of phenolic compounds from *Aloe vera* during pasteurization are scarce. Higher temperatures and longer periods of heat treatment may promote instability of aloin (Chang *et al.*, 2006). In fact, an almost complete degradation of aloin was observed when high temperatures (>80 °C) were applied for 10 hours, whereas the use of a milder temperature (60 °C) promoted a degradation of ~50%. Moreover, the color of *Aloe vera* gel juice changed slightly from whitish to slightly yellow to brownish during thermal processing, suggesting the occurrence of Maillard reactions.

9.2.2 Drying

Although pasteurization is a widely used technique for the preservation of food products, dehydrated products are less bulky, easier to handle, and less susceptible to spoilage in long-term storage than those with high moisture. However, it is important to ensure that quality is not impaired when applying any drying methodology (He *et al.*, 2005; Nindo *et al.*, 2010; Lemmens *et al.*, 2013; Javed and Atta-Ur, 2014).

With regard to the production of *Aloe vera* powders, spray-drying is probably the procedure mostly often applied since it has been shown to have a good retention of the different properties related to the quality of the resulting products, such as flavor, color, and nutrient content (Nindo *et al.*, 2007, 2010; León-Martínez *et al.*, 2011; Caparino *et al.*, 2012; García-Cruz *et al.*, 2013; Medina-Torres *et al.*, 2016).

The effects of convective drying on the main bioactive polymers present in *Aloe vera*, particularly acemannan and pectins, has been documented (Femenia *et al.*, 2003). Convective air-drying was studied in a temperature range from 30 to 80 °C. Overall, drying with hot air promoted significant modifications affecting the bioactive polysaccharides of the *Aloe vera* gel. Thus, acemannan content was significantly reduced as the air temperature increased, with mannose units losses reaching up to 25% when *Aloe vera* gel was dehydrated at 80 °C. A marked degradation of galactose units from acemannan was also observed when drying was carried out at either 70 °C or 80 °C. In fact, the drying procedures promoted a higher degradation of (1,3,4)-linked mannosyl residues than of (1,4)-linked mannosyl units, suggesting the deacetylation of the acemannan backbone, since acetyl groups have been detected at C3 of acemannan Man units (Manna and McAnalley, 1993; McAnalley, 1993). The modification of the acetylation pattern of acemannan polymer as a consequence of processing has been confirmed by several authors using Fourier transform infrared spectroscopy (FTIR) and proton nuclear magnetic resonance (^{1}H NMR) spectroscopy (Diehl and Teichmuller, 1998; Femenia *et al.*, 2003; Nejatzadeh-Barandozi and Enferadi, 2012; Lim and Cheong, 2015). Interestingly, it has also been observed that the apparent MW of acemannan increase when air-drying temperature increases. This could be attributed to the interaction of different Man chains through hydrogen bonding, due to the losses of galactosyl residues and the observed deacetylation process (Femenia *et al.*, 2003). On the other hand, pectic substances from *Aloe vera* gel were the cell wall polymers mostly affected during the drying procedures (Femenia *et al.*, 2003; Lim and Cheong, 2015). Interestingly, drying at 30 °C promoted a degradation rate of ~32% of galacturonic acid units, similar to the degradation observed at 70 °C, whereas drying at 80 °C promoted galacturonic acid losses higher than 50%. Gal and Ara were less affected than galacturonic acid, suggesting that the homogalacturonan backbone was more affected than the pectin side-chains during convective drying (Femenia *et al.*, 2003). The β-elimination process could be responsible for the degradation of pectins observed when drying was performed at high temperatures (>70 °C), whereas at milder temperatures (~50 °C), pectins were probably affected by the activation of different pectic polysaccharide-degrading enzymes (Femenia *et al.*, 1998a).

The effects of spray-drying on the bioactive polymers from *Aloe vera* have also been investigated. Thus, *Aloe vera* powders obtained by spray-drying were mainly composed of Man and Glc, and to a minor extent of Gal and galacturonic acid. However, in comparison to the fresh *Aloe vera*, the spray-drying procedure reduced the Man and Glc contents by around ~10%, whereas Gal and galacturonic acid units were even more affected, observing losses of ~50% and ~21%, respectively. These modifications resulted in a MW reduction of about 20 kDa (Medina-Torres *et al.*, 2016). The degradation of polysaccharides that occurs when spray-drying is applied may be associated with the shear forces produced in the drying chamber and, also, to the high temperatures (>150 °C). Although, spray-drying could promote a high degradation of *Aloe vera* polysaccharides, the acemannan polymer might be preserved if adequate spray-drying conditions, such as inlet temperature (150 °C) and feed flow

(1.5 L/hour), are used (Medina-Torres *et al.*, 2016). The rheological behavior of the reconstituted solution from dried powders could be a good physical indicator of the modifications occurring in the structure of the acemannan polymer, which is responsible for the pseudoplastic behavior of *Aloe vera* (Yaron, 1993; Ni *et al.*, 2004a, 2004b; Campestrini *et al.*, 2013; Lad and Murthy, 2013; Kiran and Rao, 2014; Swami Hulle *et al.*, 2014; Medina-Torres *et al.*, 2016).

With regard to the phenolic compounds, several studies evaluated the stability of these components during *Aloe vera* drying. Thus, anthraquinones and, also, chromones can be degraded almost totally when these phenolic compounds are exposed to high temperature for a long time (>8 hours) (Chang *et al.*, 2006). Recently, it has been observed that aloin (A and B), aloe emodin, aloenin B, aloesin, aloeresin A, and chrysophanol, found in *Aloe vera*, were severely affected by spray-drying, which promoted a considerable degradation of these components when drying air inlet temperature increased from 110 °C to 140 °C (Hendrawati, 2015). Interestingly, aloenin B, aloeresin A, and chrysophanol were not detected in *Aloe vera* powders obtained when temperatures higher than 120 °C were applied (Hendrawati, 2015). In fact, the preservation of aloin during spray-drying has been associated with the combination of high temperature with a short residence time into the drying chamber (Filkova and Mujumdar, 1995; Medina-Torres *et al.*, 2016). In contrast, during oven-drying (at 80 °C), a dramatic reduction of the aloin content, up to ~2 ppm, was attributed to the long drying time applied during this procedure (Gulia *et al.*, 2010).

9.2.3 Ultrasound – An Emergent Technology in *Aloe vera* Processing

In the last decade, the application of emerging technologies has been investigated in order to replace or complement conventional procedures applied during *Aloe vera* processing. Within this context, the application of power ultrasound could play a prominent role.

Ultrasound is defined as sound waves having a frequency that exceeds the hearing limit of the human ear (~20 kHz). It is one of many emerging technologies in the food industry that have been developed to minimize processing, maximize quality, and ensure the safety of food products (Awad *et al.*, 2012). Ultrasound technology is based on the effect produced by the sound waves when crossing a medium. This phenomenon generates waves of compression and rarefaction which forms cavities and/or bubbles known as "cavitation bubbles" (Povey and Mason, 1998). These cavities grow with subsequent cycles of ultrasound and eventually become unstable and collapse, releasing high temperature and pressure. If this collapse occurs within a biological material, ultrasound can affect the physicochemical properties of the components that form the material (Alarcon-Rojo *et al.*, 2015). The benefits derived from the use of ultrasound, in terms of productivity, yield, and selectivity, are based on the reduction of processing time, improvement of the product quality, and reduction of chemical and physical hazards. This means that ultrasound technology can be considered to be environmentally friendly (Patist and Bates, 2008; Soria and Villamiel, 2010; Chemat *et al.*, 2011; Chandrapala *et al.*, 2012; Alarcon-Rojo *et al.*, 2015; Ashokkumar, 2015; Khandpur and Gogate, 2015).

The effects of ultrasound on polysaccharides have been widely investigated by several authors (Kardos and Luche, 2001; Czechowska-Biskup *et al.*, 2005; Bera *et al.*, 2015; Zhu, 2015; Fiamingo *et al.*, 2016; Grassino *et al.*, 2016; Kang *et al.*, 2016). However, its application in the processing of *Aloe vera* is very rare.

Trials carried out in our laboratory have demonstrated that ultrasound could be an excellent alternative technology to assist in the extraction of acemannan from dehydrated *Aloe vera* samples. The ultrasound-assisted extraction (UAE) carried out at low temperature (<30 °C) significantly increased the yield of acemannan, and avoided any thermal degradation. Furthermore, when compared to conventional extraction processes, UAE enhanced the extraction process of acemannan using water as a solvent, obtaining a solvent-free product. High yields of acemannan (>80%) could be obtained by UAE applying extraction times generally less than 10 minutes.

On the other hand, ultrasound applied directly to the fresh gel has been shown to result in a reduction in the acemannan content of ~9%, and the decrease may reach up to ~15% when ultrasound is applied for longer time (>15 minutes). Man units were more affected than Glc and Gal monomers. However, FTIR and ^{1}H NMR spectroscopy revealed that ultrasound promoted minimal changes in the acetylation pattern of acemannan. The modifications observed in the acemannan structure may be attributed to a possible depolymerization process since it has been documented that ultrasound is able to modify the native structure of some polymers, such as starch. The high hydrodynamic shear forces associated with ultrasonic cavitation could be responsible for the breakage of the C−O−C glycosidic linkage, affecting the molecular weight of the polymer (Kang *et al.*, 2016; Zhu, 2015; Bera *et al.*, 2015).

Unlike conventional processing, ultrasound seems to promote a minor degradation of pectic polysaccharides from *Aloe vera* gel. Thus, ultrasound does not cause significant changes in the galacturonic acid content, and other sugars such as Rha, Ara, and Gal are almost unaffected.

The physicochemical modifications observed on the bioactive polysaccharides of *Aloe vera* have been associated with the changes determined in the functional properties of the *Aloe vera* extracts, such as swelling (Sw), water retention (WRC), and fat adsorption (FAC) capacities (Femenia *et al.*, 2003; Rodríguez-González *et al.*, 2011).

Interestingly, it has been observed that appropriate ultrasound treatments could increase the functional properties of the *Aloe vera* extracts, the most remarkable effects being observed in their capacity to absorb organic molecules, such as lipids. Thus, in freeze-dried samples of non-processed *Aloe vera* gel, FAC values can be found between 30 to 40 g oil/g sample, and this value can be increased up to 80 g oil/g sample when ultrasound is applied on *Aloe vera* gel for short times (~6 minutes). Several studies have reported that the efficiency in binding organic molecules might play an important role in the capacity of *Aloe vera* to lower the levels of cholesterol, carcinogens, and other toxic compounds (Elleuch *et al.*, 2011; Rodríguez-González *et al.*, 2011, 2012). Nevertheless, further studies are required to identify the main structural changes in acemannan and pectin polysaccharides promoted by the application of ultrasound.

Recently, Jawade and Chavan (2013) applied ultrasound to assist the extraction of aloin from dehydrated *Aloe vera*. In particular, the effects of particle size (0.4–0.8, 0.8–1.7, 1.7–3.4 mm) and temperature (30–50 °C) were investigated using methanol as a solvent. These authors observed that a particle size lower than 1.6 mm promoted a high extraction rate of aloin, reaching up to 65% in 30 minutes. Aloin was more soluble at medium temperatures (50 °C) than at low temperatures (30 °C). Interestingly, about 90% of the aloin present in *Aloe vera* could be extracted using ultrasound at 50 °C for 40 minutes, whereas when applying the same conditions but without ultrasonic assistance, less than 60% of aloin was extracted. It is well known that the rapid compression and evacuation cycle of ultrasonic waves improves cell disruption and helps the penetration of solvent into the gel matrix, accelerating the mass transfer (Toma *et al.*, 2001). The selection of methanol as a solvent was based on previous studies carried out in *Radix saposhnikoviae* and *Rheum palmatum* L., which demonstrated that anthraquinones exhibited a higher solubility in methanol than in ethanol (Li *et al.*, 2011; Zhao *et al.*, 2011).

9.3 Conclusions

In recent decades, *Aloe vera* has aroused great interest in the food industry as a new source of bioactive compounds for the development of functional ingredients and functional foods. This interest has mainly focused on bioactive polymers, such as acemannan and pectins, and also on the presence of *C*-glycoside phenolic compounds. Interestingly, all these bioactive components possess structural features that make them unique. Acemannan, the major polysaccharide found in the gel, considered by many authors to be the main bioactive component of *Aloe vera* plant, seems to play a key role in most of the health benefits attributed to *Aloe vera*. These beneficial properties could be related to the partially acetylated mannose, which allows the interaction of acemannan with other biomolecules, enhancing its biological activity. On the other hand, pectins from *Aloe vera* gel have also shown interesting properties, mainly based in their specific structural characteristics, which offers a wide range of technological, functional, and biomedical applications. Finally, phenolic compounds from *Aloe vera* plants may also be considered to be important bioactive components, although the majority of these substances, aloin being the most abundant, are found in the exudate. These *C*-glycoside phenolics could also play a key role in the pharmacological activity of *Aloe vera*.

It should be noted that *Aloe vera* extracts are highly susceptible to microbial contamination, and for this reason processing is required in order to extend the shelf-life of *Aloe vera*-derived products. Thermal procedures are the most common methods applied to *Aloe vera* gel, and in particular pasteurization and drying. However, pasteurization may promote important structural modifications, such as the modification of the acetylation pattern of acemannan, or the degradation of the galacturonic acid backbone of pectins. Furthermore, aloin and other phenolic components can be degraded when high temperatures are applied for a long time. It has been observed that drying may cause not only considerable losses of Man units from the acemannan backbone, but also important modification of the degree of acetylation of the Man units from acemannan. Moreover, the homogalacturonan backbone of pectins may also be strongly degraded during the drying procedure. With regard to the phenolic compounds, aloin and aloesin seem to be more stable during dehydration than other compounds such as aloenin B, aloeresin A, and chrysophanol. Due to these potential negative effects promoted by thermal processing on the structure of the main bioactive compounds of *Aloe vera*, the use of non-thermal technologies, such as ultrasound, has been proposed for *Aloe vera* processing.

The extraction process of the main bioactive components in *Aloe vera*, assisted by ultrasound, allows products to be obtained in which the major structural features of acemannan are preserved, including their pattern of acetylation. In addition, the degradation of pectic polysaccharides can also be reduced. It has been shown that ultrasound assistance might improve the extraction of aloin when the process is carried out using mild temperatures and short times.

These results show that ultrasound could be an excellent alternative for *Aloe vera* processing, with the aim of preserving not only the main physicochemical characteristics of the bioactive components, but also their biological activity.

References

Ahlawat, K. and Khatkar, B. (2011). Processing, food applications and safety of aloe vera products: a review. *Journal of Food Science and Technology*, 48, 525–533.

Alarcon-Rojo, A. D., Janacua, H., Rodriguez, J. C., Paniwnyk, L. and Mason, T. J. (2015). Power ultrasound in meat processing. *Meat Science*, 107, 86–93.

Ashokkumar, M. (2015). Applications of ultrasound in food and bioprocessing. *Ultrasonics Sonochemistry*, 25, 17–23.

Awad, T. S., Moharram, H. A., Shaltout, O. E., Asker, D., and Youssef, M. M. (2012). Applications of ultrasound in analysis, processing and quality control of food: a review. *Food Research International*, 48, 410–427.

Basmatker, G., Jais, N., and Daud, F. (2011). *Aloe vera*: a valuable multifunctional cosmetic ingredient. *International Journal of Medicinal and Aromatic Plants*, 1, 338–341.

Bera, S., Mondal, D., Martin, J. T., and Singh, M. (2015). Potential effect of ultrasound on carbohydrates. *Carbohydrate Research*, 410, 15–35.

Bhalang, K. and Tompkins, K. (2015). Polysaccharides from *Aloe vera* and oral ulcerations. *Polysaccharides*, doi: 10.1007/978-3-319-03751-6_75-1

Boban, P. T., Nambisan, B., and Sudhakaran, P. R. (2006). Hypolipidaemic effect of chemically different mucilages in rats: a comparative study. *British Journal of Nutrition*, 96, 1021–1029.

Boudreau, M. D. and Beland, F. A. (2006). An evaluation of the biological and toxicological properties of *Aloe barbadensis* (Miller), *Aloe vera*. *Journal of Environmental Science and Health, Part C*, 24, 103–154.

Buenz, E. J. (2008). Aloin induces apoptosis in Jurkat cells. *Toxicology in Vitro*, 22, 422–429.

Campestrini, L. H., Silveira, J. L. M., Duarte, M. E. R., Koop, H. S., and Noseda, M. D. (2013). NMR and rheological study of *Aloe barbadensis* partially acetylated glucomannan. *Carbohydrate Polymers*, 94, 511–519.

Caparino, O. A., Tang, J., Nindo, C. I., Sablani, S. S., Powers, J. R., and Fellman, J. K. (2012). Effect of drying methods on the physical properties and microstructures of mango (Philippine 'Carabao' var.) powder. *Journal of Food Engineering*, 111, 135–148.

Cohen, J. S. and Yang, T. C. S. (1995). Progress in food dehydration. *Trends in Food Science and Technology*, 6, 20–25.

Chandrapala, J., Oliver, C., Kentish, S., and Ashokkumar, M. (2012). Ultrasonics in food processing. *Ultrasonics Sonochemistry*, 19, 975–983.

Chang, X. L., Wang, C. H., Feng, Y. M., and Liu, Z. P. (2006). Effects of heat treatments on the stabilities of polysaccharides substances and barbaloin in gel juice from *Aloe vera* Miller. *Journal of Food Engineering*, 75, 245–251.

Chantarawaratit, P., Sangvanich, P., Banlunara, W., Soontornvipart, K. and Thunyakitpisal, P. (2014). Acemannan sponges stimulate alveolar bone, cementum and periodontal ligament regeneration in a canine class II furcation defect model. *Journal of Periodontal Research*, 49, 164–178.

Chemat, F., Zill E. H., and Khan, M. K. (2011). Applications of ultrasound in food technology: Processing, preservation and extraction. *Ultrasonics Sonochemistry*, 18, 813–835.

Choi, S. and Chung, M.-H. (2003). A review on the relationship between aloe vera components and their biologic effects. *Seminars in Integrative Medicine*, 1, 53–62.

Chokboribal, J., Tachaboonyakiat, W., Sangvanich, P., Ruangpornvisuti, V., Jettanacheawchankit, S., and Thunyakitpisal, P. (2015). Deacetylation affects the physical properties and bioactivity of acemannan, an extracted polysaccharide from *Aloe vera*. *Carbohydrate Polymers*, 133, 556–566.

Choudhary, M., Kochhar, A., and Sangha, J. (2011). Hypoglycemic and hypolipidemic effect of *Aloe vera* L. in non-insulin dependent diabetics. *Journal of Food Science and Technology*, 51, 90–96.

Chow, J. T., Williamson, D. A., Yates, K. M., and Goux, W. J. (2005). Chemical characterization of the immunomodulating polysaccharide of *Aloe vera* L. *Carbohydrate Research*, 340, 1131–1142.

Christaki, E. V. and Florou-Paneri, P. C. (2010). *Aloe vera*: A plant for many uses. *Journal of Food, Agriculture and Environment*, 8, 245–249.

Czechowska-Biskup, R., Rokita, B., Lotfy, S., Ulanski, P., and Rosiak, J. M. (2005). Degradation of chitosan and starch by 360-kHz ultrasound. *Carbohydrate Polymers*, 60, 175–184.

Diehl, B. and Teichmuller, E. E. (1998). *Aloe vera*, quality inspection and identification. *Agro Food Industry Hi-Tech*, 9, 14–16.

Eberendu, A. R., Luta, G., Edwards, J. A., Mcanalley, B. H., Davis, B., Rodriguez, S., and Ray Henry, C. (2005). Quantitative colorimetric analysis of aloe polysaccharides as a measure of aloe vera quality in commercial products. *Journal of AOAC International*, 88, 684–691.

Elleuch, M., Bedigian, D., Roiseux, O., Besbes, S., Blecker, C., and Attia, H. (2011). Dietary fibre and fibre-rich by-products of food processing: Characterisation, technological functionality and commercial applications: A review. *Food Chemistry*, 124, 411–421.

Escobedo-Lozano, A. Y., Domard, A., Velázquez, C. A., Goycoolea, F. M., and Argüelles-Monal, W. M. (2015). Physical properties and antibacterial activity of chitosan/acemannan mixed systems. *Carbohydrate Polymers*, 115, 707–714.

Eshun, K. and He, Q. (2004). Aloe vera: a valuable ingredient for the food, pharmaceutical and cosmetic industries – a review. *Critical Reviews in Food Science and Nutrition*, 44, 91–96.

Esteban-Carrasco, A., López-Serrano, M., Zapata, J. M., Sabater, B., and Martín, M. (2001). Oxidation of phenolic compounds from *Aloe barbadensis* by peroxidase activity: Possible involvement in defence reactions. *Plant Physiology and Biochemistry*, 39, 521–527.

Femenia, A., Garosi, P., Roberts, K., Waldron, K. W., Selvendran, R. R., and Robertson, J. A. (1998a). Tissue-related changes in methyl-esterification of pectic polysaccharides in cauliflower (*Brassica oleracea* L. var. *botrytis*) stems. *Planta*, 205, 438–444.

Femenia, A., Sánchez, E. S., Simal, S., and Rosselló, C. (1998b). Modification of cell wall composition of apricots (*Prunus armeniaca*) during drying and storage under modified atmospheres. *Journal of Agricultural and Food Chemistry*, 46, 5248–5253.

Femenia, A., Sánchez, E. S., Simal, S., and Rosselló, C. (1999). Compositional features of polysaccharides from *Aloe vera* (*Aloe barbadensis* Miller) plant tissues. *Carbohydrate Polymers*, 39, 109–117.

Femenia, A., García-Pascual, P., Simal, S., and Rosselló, C. (2003). Effects of heat treatment and dehydration on bioactive polysaccharide acemannan and cell wall polymers from *Aloe barbadensis* Miller. *Carbohydrate Polymers*, 51, 397–405.

Fiamingo, A., Delezuk, J. a. D. M., Trombotto, S., David, L., and Campana-Filho, S. P. (2016). Extensively deacetylated high molecular weight chitosan from the multistep ultrasound-assisted deacetylation of beta-chitin. *Ultrasonics Sonochemistry*, 32, 79–85.

Filkova, I. and Mujumdar, A. S. (1995). Industrial spray drying systems. In *Handbook of Industrial Drying* (ed. A. S. Mujumdar). Marcel Dekker, New York.

Fogleman, R. W., Shellenberger, T. E., Balmer, M. F., Carpenter, R. H., and Mcanalley, B. H. (1992). Subchronic oral administration of acemannan in the rat and dog. *Veterinary and Human Toxicology*, 34, 144–147.

García-Cruz, E. E., Rodríguez-Ramírez, J., Méndez Lagunas, L. L., and Medina-Torres, L. (2013). Rheological and physical properties of spray-dried mucilage obtained from *Hylocereus undatus* cladodes. *Carbohydrate Polymers*, 91, 394–402.

Geng, L., Zhou, W., Qu, X., Chen, W., Li, Y., Liu, C., *et al.* (2014). Optimization of the preparation of pectin from aloe using a Box-Behnken design. *Carbohydrate Polymers*, 105, 193–199.

Gentilini, R., Bozzini, S., Munarin, F., Petrini, P., Visai, L., and Tanzi, M. C. (2014a). Pectins from aloe vera: Extraction and production of gels for regenerative medicine. *Journal of Applied Polymer Science*, 131.

Gentilini, R., Munarin, F., Petrini, P., and Tanzi, M. C. (2014b). Pectin gels for biomedical application. In *Pectin: Chemical Properties, Uses and Health Benefits* (ed. P. L. Bush) Nova Science Publishers, New York.

Gowda, C. D., Neelisiddaiah, B., and Anjaneyalu, Y. V. (1979). Structural studies of polysaccharides from aloe vera. *Carbohydrate Research*, 72, 201–205.

Grassino, A. N., Brnčić, M., Vikić-Topić, D., Roca, S., Dent, M., and Brnčić, S. R. (2016). Ultrasound assisted extraction and characterization of pectin from tomato waste. *Food Chemistry*, 198, 93–100.

Grindlay, D. and Reynolds, T. (1986). The *Aloe vera* phenomenon: A review of the properties and modern uses of the leaf parenchyma gel. *Journal of Ethnopharmacology*, 16, 117–151.

Gulia, A., Sharma, H. K., Sarkar, B. C., Upadhyay, A., and Shitandi, A. (2010). Changes in physico-chemical and functional properties during convective drying of aloe vera (*Aloe barbadensis*) leaves. *Food and Bioproducts Processing*, 88, 161–164.

Guo, X. and Mei, N. (2016). Aloe vera – a review of toxicity and adverse clinical effects. *Journal of Environmental Science and Health, Part C*, 34, 77–96.

Hamiza, O., Rehman, M., Khan, R., Tahir, M., Khan, A., Lateef, A., *et al.* (2014). Chemopreventive effects of aloin against 1,2-dimethylhydrazine-induced preneoplastic lesions in the colon of Wistar rats. *Human and Experimental Toxicology*, 33, 148–163.

Hamman, J. (2008). Composition and applications of *Aloe vera* leaf gel. *Molecules*, 13, 1599–1616.

He, Q., Changhong, L., Kojo, E., and Tian, Z. (2005). Quality and safety assurance in the processing of aloe vera gel juice. *Food Control*, 16, 95–104.

Hendrawati, T. Y. (2015). *Aloe vera* powder properties produced from aloe chinensis baker, Pontianak, Indonesia. *Journal of Engineering Science and Technology*, 10, 47–59.

Hu, Y., Xu, J., and Hu, Q. (2003). Evaluation of antioxidant potential of *Aloe vera* (*Aloe barbadensis* Miller) extracts. *Journal of Agricultural and Food Chemistry*, 51, 7788–7791.

Hutter, J. A., Salman, M., Stavinoha, W. B., Satsangi, N., Williams, R. F., Streeper, R. T., *et al.* (1996). Antiinflammatory *C*-glucosyl chromone from *Aloe barbadensis*. *Journal of Natural Products*, 59, 541–543.

Im, S.-A., Oh, S.-T., Song, S., Kim, M.-R., Kim, D.-S., Woo, S.-S., *et al.* (2005). Identification of optimal molecular size of modified Aloe polysaccharides with maximum immunomodulatory activity. *International Immunopharmacology*, 5, 271–279.

Jain, A., Gupta, Y., and Jain, S. K. (2007). Perspectives of biodegradable natural polysaccharides for site-specific drug delivery to the colon. *Journal of Pharmacology and Pharmaceutical Science*, 10, 86–128.

Javed, S. and Atta-Ur, R. (2014). *Aloe vera* gel in food, health products, and cosmetics industry. *Studies in Natural Products Chemistry* 41, 261–285.

Jawade, N. R. and Chavan, A. R. (2013). Ultrasonic-assisted extraction of aloin from aloe vera gel. *Procedia Engineering*, 51, 487–493.

Jettanacheawchankit, S., Sasithanasate, S., Sangvanich, P., Banlunara, W., and Thunyakitpisal, P. (2009). Acemannan stimulates gingival fibroblast proliferation;

expressions of keratinocyte growth factor-1, vascular endothelial growth factor, and type I collagen; and wound healing. *Journal of Pharmacological Sciences*, 109, 525–531.

Kaithwas, G., Singh, P., and Bhatia, D. (2014). Evaluation of in vitro and in vivo antioxidant potential of polysaccharides from *Aloe vera* (*Aloe barbadensis* Miller) gel. *Drug and Chemical Toxicology*, 37, 135–143.

Kanama, S. K., Viljoen, A. M., Kamatou, G. P. P., Chen, W., Sandasi, M., Adhami, H. R., *et al.* (2015). Simultaneous quantification of anthrones and chromones in Aloe ferox ("Cape aloes") using UHPLC-MS. *Phytochemistry Letters*, 13, 85–90.

Kang, N., Zuo, Y. J., Hilliou, L., Ashokkumar, M., and Hemar, Y. (2016). Viscosity and hydrodynamic radius relationship of high-power ultrasound depolymerised starch pastes with different amylose content. *Food Hydrocolloids*, 52, 183–191.

Karaca, K., Sharma, J. M., and Nordgren, R. (1995). Nitric oxide production by chicken macrophages activated by acemannan, a complex carbohydrate extracted from Aloe Vera. *International Journal of Immunopharmacology*, 17, 183–188.

Kardos, N. and Luche, J.-L. (2001). Sonochemistry of carbohydrate compounds. *Carbohydrate Research*, 332, 115–131.

Khandpur, P. and Gogate, P. R. (2015). Effect of novel ultrasound based processing on the nutrition quality of different fruit and vegetable juices. *Ultrasonics Sonochemistry*, 27, 125–136.

Kim, Y. S. (2006). Carbohydrates. In *New Perspectives on Aloe* (eds. Y. I. Park and S. K. Lee). Springer, Boston, MA.

Kiran, P. and Rao, P. S. (2014). Rheological and structural characterization of prepared aqueous *Aloe vera* dispersions. *Food Research International*, 62, 1029–1037.

Kumar, S. and Tiku, A. B. (2016). Immunomodulatory potential of acemannan (polysaccharide from *Aloe vera*) against radiation induced mortality in Swiss albino mice. *Food and Agricultural Immunology*, 27, 72–86.

Lad, V. N. and Murthy, Z. V. P. (2013). Rheology of *Aloe barbadensis* Miller: A naturally available material of high therapeutic and nutrient value for food applications. *Journal of Food Engineering*, 115, 279–284.

Lee, K. Y., Weintraub, S. T., and Yu, B. P. (2000). Isolation and identification of a phenolic antioxidant from *Aloe barbadensis*. *Free Radical Biology and Medicine*, 28, 261–265.

Lee, S., Do, S.-G., Kim, S. Y., Kim, J., Jin, Y., and Lee, C. H. (2012). Mass spectrometry-based metabolite profiling and antioxidant activity of *Aloe vera* (*Aloe barbadensis* Miller) in different growth stages. *Journal of Agricultural and Food Chemistry*, 60, 11222–11228.

Lemmens, L., Colle, I., Knockaert, G., Van Buggenhout, S., Van Loey, A., and Hendrickx, M. (2013). Influence of pilot scale in pack pasteurization and sterilization treatments on nutritional and textural characteristics of carrot pieces. *Food Research International*, 50, 526–533.

León-Martínez, F. M., Rodríguez-Ramírez, J., Medina-Torres, L. L., Méndez Lagunas, L. L., and Bernad-Bernad, M. J. (2011). Effects of drying conditions on the rheological properties of reconstituted mucilage solutions (*Opuntia ficus-indica*). *Carbohydrate Polymers*, 84, 439–445.

Li, S.-W., Yang, T.-C., Lai, C.-C., Huang, S.-H., Liao, J.-M., Wan, L., *et al.* (2014). Antiviral activity of aloe-emodin against influenza A virus via galectin-3 up-regulation. *European Journal of Pharmacology*, 738, 125–132.

Li, W., Wang, Z., Sun, Y.-S., Chen, L., Han, L.-K., and Zheng, Y.-N. (2011). Application of response surface methodology to optimise ultrasonic-assisted extraction of four chromones in Radix Saposhnikoviae. *Phytochemical Analysis*, 22, 313–321.

Lim, Z. X. and Cheong, K. Y. (2015). Effects of drying temperature and ethanol concentration on bipolar switching characteristics of natural *Aloe vera*-based memory devices. *Physical Chemistry Chemical Physics*, 17, 26833–26853.

Lin, C. C., Kao, S. T., Chen, G. W., and Chung, J. G. (2005). Berberine decreased *N*-acetylation of 2-aminofluorene through inhibition of *N*-acetyltransferase gene expression in human leukemia HL-60 cells. *Anticancer Research*, 25, 4149–4155.

Lin, J.-G., Chen, G.-W., Li, T.-M., Chouh, S.-T., Tan, T.-W., and Chung, J.-G. (2006). Aloe-emodin induces apoptosis in T24 human bladder cancer cells through the p53 dependent apoptotic pathway. *Journal of Urology*, 175, 343–347.

Lin, M.-L., Lu, Y.-C., Su, H.-L., Lin, H.-T., Lee, C.-C., Kang, S.-E., *et al.* (2011). Destabilization of CARP mRNAs by aloe-emodin contributes to caspase-8-mediated p53-independent apoptosis of human carcinoma cells. *Journal of Cellular Biochemistry*, 112, 1176–1191.

Liu, J., Willför, S., and Xu, C. (2015). A review of bioactive plant polysaccharides: Biological activities, functionalization, and biomedical applications. *Bioactive Carbohydrates and Dietary Fibre*, 5, 31–61.

Lucini, L., Pellizzoni, M., Pellegrino, R., Molinari, G. P., and Colla, G. (2015). Phytochemical constituents and in vitro radical scavenging activity of different Aloe species. *Food Chemistry*, 170, 501–507.

Machado, N. F. L. and Marques, M. P. M. (2010). Bioactive chromone derivatives – structural diversity. *Current Bioactive Compounds*, 6, 76–89.

Mandal, G. and Das, A. (1980a). Structure of the d-galactan isolated from aloe barbadensis miller. *Carbohydrate Research*, 86, 247–257.

Mandal, G. and Das, A. (1980b). Structure of the glucomannan isolated from the leaves of *Aloe barbadensis* Miller. *Carbohydrate Research*, 87, 249–256.

Manna, S. and Mcanalley, B. H. (1993). Determination of the position of the *O*-acetyl group in a β-(1 → 4)-mannan (acemannan) from *Aloe barbardensis* Miller. *Carbohydrate Research*, 241, 317–319.

Masaldan, S. and Iyer, V. V. (2014). Exploration of effects of emodin in selected cancer cell lines: enhanced growth inhibition by ascorbic acid and regulation of LRP1 and AR under hypoxia-like conditions. *Journal of Applied Toxicology*, 34, 95–104.

McAnalley, B. H. (1993). Process for preparation of Aloe products. *United States of America patent application* 89902414.5.

McConaughy, S. D., Kirkland, S. E., Treat, N. J., Stroud, P. A., and McCormick, C. L. (2008a). Tailoring the network properties of Ca^{2+} crosslinked *Aloe vera* polysaccharide hydrogels for in situ release of therapeutic agents. *Biomacromolecules*, 9, 3277–3287.

McConaughy, S. D., Stroud, P. A., Boudreaux, B., Hester, R. D., and McCormick, C. L. (2008b). Structural characterization and solution properties of a galacturonate polysaccharide derived from *Aloe vera* capable of in situ gelation. *Biomacromolecules*, 9, 472–480.

Medina-Torres, L., Calderas, F., Minjares, R., Femenia, A., Sánchez-Olivares, G., Gónzalez-Laredo, F. R., *et al.* (2016). Structure preservation of *Aloe vera* (*barbadensis* Miller) mucilage in a spray drying process. *LWT – Food Science and Technology*, 66, 93–100.

Nejatzadeh-Barandozi, F. and Enferadi, S. (2012). FT-IR study of the polysaccharides isolated from the skin juice, gel juice, and flower of *Aloe vera* tissues affected by fertilizer treatment. *Organic and Medicinal Chemistry Letters*, 2, 33.

Ni, Y., Turner, D., Yates, K. M., and Tizard, I. (2004a). Isolation and characterization of structural components of *Aloe vera* L. leaf pulp. *International Immunopharmacology*, 4, 1745–1755.

Ni, Y., Yates, K. M., and Tizard, I. R. (2004b). Aloe polysaccharides. In *Aloes: The genus Aloe* (ed. T. Reynolds). CRC Press, Boca Raton, FL.

Nindo, C. I., Powers, J. R., and Tang, J. (2007). Glass transition and rheological properties of *Aloe vera* (*Aloe barbadensis*, L.) dried by different methods. ASABE Annual International Meeting Sponsored by ASABE, Minneapolis, Minnesota. *Transactions of the American Society of Agricultural and Biological Engineers.*

Nindo, C. I., Powers, J. R., and Tang, J. (2010). Thermal properties of *Aloe vera* powder and rheology of reconstituted gels. *Transactions of the American Society of Agricultural and Biological Engineers*, 53, 1193–1200.

Olennikov, D. N., Zilfikarov, I. N., and Penzina, T. A. (2013). Use of microcolumn HPLC for analysis of aloenin in *Aloe arborescens* raw material and related drugs. *Pharmaceutical Chemistry Journal*, 47, 494–497.

Ovodova, R. G., Lapchik, V. F., and Ovodov, Y. S. (1975). Polysaccharides of *Aloe arborescens. Chemistry of Natural Compounds*, 11, 1–2.

Pan, Q., Pan, H., Lou, H., Xu, Y., and Tian, L. (2013). Inhibition of the angiogenesis and growth of aloin in human colorectal cancer in vitro and in vivo. *Cancer Cell International*, 13, 1–9.

Park, J. H. and Kwon, S. W. (2006). An epitome of chemical components and low molecular compounds. In *New Perspectives on Aloe* (eds. Y. I. Park and S. K. Lee). Springer, Boston, MA.

Park, M. Y., Kwon, H. J., and Sung, M. K. (2011). Dietary aloin, aloesin, or aloe-gel exerts anti-inflammatory activity in a rat colitis model. *Life Sciences*, 88, 486–492.

Patist, A. and Bates, D. (2008). Ultrasonic innovations in the food industry: From the laboratory to commercial production. *Innovative Food Science and Emerging Technologies*, 9, 147–154.

Pérez, S., Rodríguez-Carvajal, M. A., and Doco, T. (2003). A complex plant cell wall polysaccharide: rhamnogalacturonan II. *A structure in quest of a function. Biochimie*, 85, 109–121.

Piao, L. Z., Park, H. R., Park, Y. K., Lee, S. K., Park, J. H., and Park, M. K. (2002). Mushroom tyrosinase inhibition activity of some chromones. *Chemical and Pharmaceutical Bulletin*, 50, 309–311.

Popov, S. V. and Ovodov, Y. S. (2013). Polypotency of the immunomodulatory effect of pectins. *Biochemistry Moscow*, 78, 823–835.

Pothuraju, R., Sharma, R. K., Onteru, S. K., Singh, S., and Hussain, S. A. (2016). Hypoglycemic and hypolipidemic effects of *Aloe vera* extract preparations: A review. *Phytotherapy Research*, 30, 200–207.

Povey, M. J. W. and Mason, T. J. (1998). *Ultrasound in Food Processing*, Blackie Academic and Professional, London.

Radha, M. H. and Laxmipriya, N. P. (2015). Evaluation of biological properties and clinical effectiveness of *Aloe vera*: A systematic review. *Journal of Traditional and Complementary Medicine*, 5, 21–26.

Ramachandra, C. T. and Rao, P. S. (2008). Processing of Aloe vera leaf gel: a review. *American Journal of Agricultural and Biological Sciences*, 3, 502–510.

Ray, A. and Aswatha, S. M. (2013). An analysis of the influence of growth periods on physical appearance, and acemannan and elemental distribution of *Aloe vera* L. gel. *Industrial Crops and Products*, 48, 36–42.

Ray, A., Dutta Gupta, S., Ghosh, S., Aswatha, S. M., and Kabi, B. (2013). Chemometric studies on mineral distribution and microstructure analysis of freeze-dried *Aloe vera* L. gel at different harvesting regimens. *Industrial Crops and Products*, 51, 194–201.

Ray, A., Ghosh, S., Ray, A., and Aswatha, S. M. (2015). An analysis of the influence of growth periods on potential functional and biochemical properties and thermal analysis of freeze-dried *Aloe vera* L. gel. *Industrial Crops and Products*, 76, 298–305.

Reynolds, T. (1985). The compounds in Aloë leaf exudates: a review. *Botanical Journal of the Linnean Society*, 90, 157–177.

Reynolds, T. (2004). Aloe chemistry. In *Aloes: The Genus Aloe* (ed. T. Reynolds). CRC Press, Boca Raton, FL.

Reynolds, T. and Dweck, A. C. (1999). *Aloe vera* leaf gel: a review update. *Journal of Ethnopharmacology*, 68, 3–37.

Rodríguez, E. R., Martín, J. D., and Romero, C. D. (2010). *Aloe vera* as a functional ingredient in foods. *Critical Reviews in Food Science and Nutrition*, 50, 305–326.

Rodríguez-González, V. M., Femenia, A., González-Laredo, R. F., Rocha-Guzmán, N. E., Gallegos-Infante, J. A., Candelas-Cadillo, M. G., *et al.* (2011). Effects of pasteurization on bioactive polysaccharide acemannan and cell wall polymers from *Aloe barbadensis* Miller. *Carbohydrate Polymers*, 86, 1675–1683.

Rodríguez-González, V. M., Femenia, A., Minjares-Fuentes, R., and González-Laredo, R. F. (2012). Functional properties of pasteurized samples of *Aloe barbadensis* Miller: Optimization using response surface methodology. *LWT – Food Science and Technology*, 47, 225–232.

Shahidi, F. and Naczk, M. (2003). *Phenolics in Food and Nutraceuticals*, Taylor and Francis, London.

Shahidi, F., Janitha, P. K., and Wanasundara, P. D. (1992). Phenolic antioxidants. *Critical Reviews in Food Science and Nutrition*, 32, 67–103.

Sharma, K., Mittal, A., and Chauhan, N. (2015). *Aloe vera* as penetration enhancer. *International Journal of Drug Development and Research*, 7, 31–43.

Sila, D., Yue, X., Vanbuggenhout, S., Smout, C., Loey, A., and Hendrickx, M. (2007). The relation between (bio-)chemical, morphological, and mechanical properties of thermally processed carrots as influenced by high-pressure pretreatment condition. *European Food Research and Technology*, 226, 127–135.

Sila, D. N., Van Buggenhout, S., Duvetter, T., Fraeye, I., De Roeck, A., Van Loey, A. *et al.* (2009). Pectins in processed fruits and vegetables: Part II – Structure–function relationships. *Comprehensive Reviews in Food Science and Food Safety*, 8, 86–104.

Simões, J., Nunes, F. M., Domingues, P., Coimbra, M. A., and Domingues, M. R. (2012). Mass spectrometry characterization of an *Aloe vera* mannan presenting immunostimulatory activity. *Carbohydrate Polymers*, 90, 229–236.

Sood, N., Baker, W. L., and Coleman, C. I. (2008). Effect of glucomannan on plasma lipid and glucose concentrations, body weight, and blood pressure: systematic review and meta-analysis. *American Journal of Clinical Nutrition*, 88, 1167–1175.

Soria, A. C. and Villamiel, M. (2010). Effect of ultrasound on the technological properties and bioactivity of food: a review. *Trends in Food Science and Technology*, 21, 323–331.

Sun, Y. N., Kim, J. H., Li, W., Jo, A. R., Yan, X. T., Yang, S. Y., and Kim, Y. H. (2015). Soluble epoxide hydrolase inhibitory activity of anthraquinone components from aloe. *Bioorganic and Medicinal Chemistry*, 23, 6659–6665.

Sun, Y. N., Li, W., Yang, S. Y., Kang, J. S., Ma, J. Y., and Kim, Y. H. (2016). Isolation and identification of chromone and pyrone constituents from Aloe and their anti-inflammatory activities. *Journal of Functional Foods*, 21, 232–239.

Swami Hulle, N. R., Patruni, K., and Rao, P. S. (2014). Rheological properties of *Aloe vera* (*Aloe barbadensis* Miller) juice concentrates. *Journal of Food Process Engineering*, 37, 375–386.

Talmadge, J., Chavez, J., Jacobs, L., Munger, C., Chinnah, T., Chow, J. T., *et al.* (2004). Fractionation of *Aloe vera* L. inner gel, purification and molecular profiling of activity. *International Immunopharmacology*, 4, 1757–1773.

t'Hart, L. A., Van Den Berg, A. J., Kuis, L., Van Dijk, H., and Labadie, R. P. (1989). An anti-complementary polysaccharide with immunological adjuvant activity from the leaf parenchyma gel of *Aloe vera*. *Planta Medica*, 55, 509–512.

Toma, M., Vinatoru, M., Paniwnyk, L., and Mason, T. J. (2001). Investigation of the effects of ultrasound on vegetal tissues during solvent extraction. *Ultrasonics Sonochemistry*, 8, 137–142.

Tseng-Crank, J., Do, S.-G., Corneliusen, B., Hertel, C., Homan, J., Yimam, M., *et al.* (2013). UP780, A chromone-enriched aloe composition, enhances adipose insulin receptor signaling and decreases liver lipid biosynthesis. *Open Journal of Genetics*, 3, 78.

Tummalapalli, M., Berthet, M., Verrier, B., Deopura, B. L., Alam, M. S., and Gupta, B. (2016). Composite wound dressings of pectin and gelatin with aloe vera and curcumin as bioactive agents. *International Journal of Biological Macromolecules*, 82, 104–113.

Turner, C. E., Williamson, D. A., Stroud, P. A., and Talley, D. J. (2004). Evaluation and comparison of commercially available *Aloe vera* L. products using size exclusion chromatography with refractive index and multi-angle laser light scattering detection. *International Immunopharmacology*, 4, 1727–1737.

Vega-Gálvez, A., Miranda, M., Aranda, M., Henriquez, K., Vergara, J., Tabilo-Munizaga, G., *et al.* (2011). Effect of high hydrostatic pressure on functional properties and quality characteristics of *Aloe vera* gel (*Aloe barbadensis* Miller). *Food Chemistry*, 129, 1060–1065.

Vogler, B. K. and Ernst, E. (1999). *Aloe vera*: a systematic review of its clinical effectiveness. *British Journal of General Practice*, 49, 823–828.

Wang, H., Wei, G., Liu, F., Banerjee, G., Joshi, M., Bligh, S., *et al.* (2014). Characterization of two homogalacturonan pectins with immunomodulatory activity from green tea. *International Journal of Molecular Sciences*, 15, 9963.

Wu, X., Ding, W., Zhong, J., Wan, J., and Xie, Z. (2013). Simultaneous qualitative and quantitative determination of phenolic compounds in *Aloe barbadensis* Mill by liquid chromatography–mass spectrometry-ion trap-time-of-flight and high performance liquid chromatography-diode array detector. *Journal of Pharmaceutical and Biomedical Analysis*, 80, 94–106.

Yagi, A. (2014). Possible efficacy of aloe vera gel metabolites in longterm ingestion to insulin sensitivity. *Journal of Gastroenterology and Hepatology Research*, 3, 996–1005.

Yagi, A., Hamano, S., Tanaka, T., Kaneo, Y., Fujioka, T., and Mihashi, K. (2001). Biodisposition of FITC-labeled aloemannan in mice. *Planta Medica*, 67, 297–300.

Yagi, A., Kabash, A., Okamura, N., Haraguchi, H., Moustafa, S. M., and Khalifa, T. I. (2002). Antioxidant, free radical scavenging and anti-inflammatory effects of aloesin derivatives in *Aloe vera*. *Planta Medica*, 68, 957–960.

Yagi, A., Hegazy, S., Kabbash, A., and Wahab, E. a.-E. (2009). Possible hypoglycemic effect of *Aloe vera* L. high molecular weight fractions on type 2 diabetic patients. *Saudi Pharmaceutical Journal*, 17, 209–215.

Yaron, A. (1993). Characterization of *Aloe vera* gel before and after autodegradation, and stabilization of the natural fresh gel. *Phytotherapy Research*, 7, S11–S13.

Yaron, A., Cohen, E., and Arad, S. M. (1992). Stabilization of aloe vera gel by interaction with sulfated polysaccharides from red microalgae and with xanthan gum. *Journal of Agricultural and Food Chemistry*, 40, 1316–1320.

Zhao, L.-C., Liang, J., Li, W., Cheng, K.-M., Xia, X., Deng, X., *et al.* (2011). The use of response surface methodology to optimize the ultrasound-assisted extraction of five anthraquinones from *Rheum palmatum* L. *Molecules*, 16, 5928.

Zhong, J., Huang, Y., Ding, W., Wu, X., Wan, J., and Luo, H. (2013). Chemical constituents of *Aloe barbadensis* Miller and their inhibitory effects on phosphodiesterase-4D. *Fitoterapia*, 91, 159–165.

Zhong, J. S., Wan, J. Z., Liu, Y. P., Ding, W. J., Wu, X. F., and Xie, Z. Y. (2014). Simultaneous HPLC quantification of seven chromones in *Aloe barbadensis* Miller using a single reference standard. *Analytical Methods*, 6, 4388–4395.

Zhu, F. (2015). Impact of ultrasound on structure, physicochemical properties, modifications, and applications of starch. *Trends in Food Science and Technology*, 43, 1–17.

Index

Page numbers in *italics* refer to figures.
Page numbers in **bold** refer to tables.

black beans, phenolic compounds   97

blackcurrant, on α-amylases   31

black tea, phenolic compounds and starch   32

blood–brain barrier, aging   230

blood pressure

   acemannan on   267

   ginsenosides on   215

blueberry

   on α-amylases   31

   polyphenols   212–213

bone marrow, SCFA on   145

brain *see* central nervous system

branched volatile fatty acids, molecular weights of fibers on   3

bread

   addition of fiber   83, 84, **85**

   antioxidants   86

   barley kernel-based, on glucose metabolism   149

   guar gum, molecular weights   2–3

   melanoidins   209–210

breakfast cereals   84–86

breast cancer, Mediterranean diet   237

breast feeding, *see also* human milk oligosaccharides

   on microbiota   216–217

   prebiotics   140

bulking, feces   8

butyric acid

   anticancer activity   105, 151

   arabinoxylans on   130

   causing apoptosis   183–184

   on colon   124

   colorectal cancer   137, 183

     resistance   180

   on detoxifying enzymes   102

   exopolysaccharides on   140

   G protein-coupled receptors for   187

   on 4-hydroxy-2-nonenal (HNE)   185

   on inflammation   135, 184

   molecular weights of fibers on production   3

   protecting DNA   184–185

   on reactive oxygen species   185

   sources   126, 181

   sugar types producing   11

C

cacao beans, beverage from   65

Caesalphinia pulcherrima   59

caffeic acid, gastrointestinal absorption   35

calcium

   absorption   127

   obesity and   65

Canada, microbiota   220

cancer   231–236, 237, *see also* anticancer activity; chemoprevention; colorectal cancer

   Aloe vera   271

   pectins on   268

carcinogens   137

   glucuronide metabolites   108

cardiovascular disorders, *see also* cholesterol; lipids (serum); triglycerides

   dietary fiber types on   **161**

   microbiota and   149–150

care (long-term), on microbiota   219

Caribbean, sugar-sweetened beverages   45–46

carnitine, anticancer activity of SCFAs and   151

Caromax (Nutrinova; carob fiber)   60–65

carrot peel   82

case-control studies   191–192

caspase-dependent pathways, phenolic compounds on   25

cassava bagasse   148

catalase   102

catechins

   molecules   *25*

   from polyphenols   213

   on starch viscosity   30

cation-exchange capacity   7

cavitation, ultrasound   275

Ccne2 gene, *CDKN1&2A* genes, common bean fiber on expression   112

celiac disease   224

cell cultures, anticancer activity measurement in   108–110